AN ORAL HISTORY OF NEUROPSYCHOPHARMACOLOGY

THE FIRST FIFTY YEARS

Peer Interviews

Volume One: Starting Up

Thomas A. Ban (series editor)
AN ORAL HISTORY OF NEUROPSYCHOPHARMACOLOGY

Edward Shorter (volume editor)
VOLUME 1: STARTING UP

Library of Congress Cataloging-in-Publication Data
Thomas A. Ban, Edward Shorter (eds):
An Oral History of Neuropsychopharmacology: The First Fifty Years, Peer Interviews
Includes bibliographical references and index
ISBN: 1461009642
ISBN-13: 978-1461009641

1. Neuropsychopharmacology - history 2. Psychotropic drugs
3. Behavioral pharmacology
4. American College of Neuropsychopharmacology

Publisher: ACNP
ACNP Executive Office
5034A Thoroughbred Lane
Brentwood, Tennessee 37027
U.S.A.
Email: acnp@acnp.org
Website: www.acnp.org

Cover design by Jessica Blackwell; JBlacwell Design www. Jblackwelldesign.com

AMERICAN COLLEGE OF NEUROPSYCHOPHARMACOLOGY

AN ORAL HISTORY OF NEUROPSYCHOPHARMACOLOGY
THE FIRST FIFTY YEARS
Peer Interviews

Edited by
Thomas A. Ban

Co-editors

Volume 1: Starting Up - Edward Shorter

Volume 2: Neurophysiology - Max Fink

Volume 3: Neuropharmacology - Fridolin Sulser

Volume 4: Psychopharmacology - Jerome Levine

Volume 5: Neuropsychopharmacology - Samuel Gershon

Volume 6: Addiction - Herbert D. Kleber

Volume 7: Special Areas - Barry Blackwell

Volume 8: Diverse Topics - Carl Salzman

Volume 9: Update - Barry Blackwell

Volume 10: History of the ACNP - Martin M. Katz

VOLUME 1

STARTING UP
&
OVERVIEW OF THE SERIES

ACNP
2011

PROLOGUE

Hollister: I think these kinds of interviews are very good, historically, but I'm still a print man. This project with all the visuals is important but I still would like to see something in print.

Ban: We seem to have the necessary information in these interviews to present in print a coherent account on the history of the field. Do you think it would be a worthwhile undertaking?

Hollister: I think it's a worthwhile undertaking, yes. Many organizations start off with no concept that they are going to want someday to know what their history was, and so they ignore it for the first decade or two. And then, all of a sudden, someone says, "Gee whiz, we've got a history!"

Ban: We are ready to do it. That's all I can say.

(Leo E. Hollister, Interview with Thomas A. Ban, December 9, 1996.)

Thomas A. Ban

OVERVIEW OF THE SERIES
&
Interviewees & Interviewers

OVERVIEW OF THE SERIES

The field of neuropsychopharmacology is now more than a half-century old. In the 1990s the American College of Neuropsychopharmacology began an interviewing program to draw on the memories of the American pioneers. The collection of 238 interviews, presented in this ten volume series, is a resource for historians of neuropsychopharmacology of the future, and also a source of enlightenment and inspiration for scientists and clinicians today.

It was the therapeutic and commercial success in the mid-1950s of chlorpromazine for the treatment of schizophrenia that generated interest within the pharmaceutical industry in developing drugs for other psychiatric conditions.[1] By the end of the 1950s there were several effective drugs in clinical use for the treatment of psychosis, depression and anxiety. The psychiatric establishment received the new drugs incredulously. Yet with the help of the pharmaceutical industry, by the end of the 1950s, pharmacotherapy with psychotropic drugs had become an accepted treatment modality, and psychopharmacology had become part of the teaching curriculum at medical schools.[2.]

The term "psychopharmacology" was introduced in 1920 by David Macht, an American pharmacologist at Johns Hopkins University, for describing the effects of the antipyretics, quinine and acetylsalicylic acid on neuromuscular coordination tests.[3] The term was used as a synonym for "pharmacopsychology," a term introduced in 1892 by Emil Kraepelin, for describing the "psychic effects" of morphine, alcohol, paraldehyde, chloral hydrate, ether and amyl-nitrate.[4] The scope of psychopharmacology was gradually extended to all experimental investigations of the psychometric and "psychic" effects of drugs. By the 1940s, with the availability of lysergic acid diethylamide, psychopharmacology embraced research with psychotomimetics (also referred to as hallucinogens, psychodysleptics, psychotopathics, etc.), and by the 1950s it included clinical investigations of the therapeutic effects of a rapidly growing number of new psychotherapeutic drugs used in the treatment of psychiatric disorders.[5] Simultaneously, with the availability of effective psychotropic drugs in mental illness, such as chlorpromazine, reserpine, imipramine, and iproniazid, there was a shift in the understanding of the nature of synaptic transmission from a purely electrical to a chemically mediated event; by the end of the 1950s seven neurotransmitters had been identified in the central nervous system: acetylcholine, epinephrine, dopamine, γ-amino butyric acid, norepinephrine, serotonin, i.e., 5-hydroxytryptamine, and substance P.[6] Recognition of chemical mediation at the site of the synapse, coupled with the introduction of the spectrophotofluorometer,[7] an instrument with a resolution power to detect drug-induced changes in the concentration of neurotransmitter monoamines and their metabolites, led to the development of neuropharmacology, a branch of pharmacology that deals with the detection and identification of structures responsible for the psychotropic effects of centrally acting drugs. Previously, research dealing with centrally acting drugs was restricted to behavioral pharmacology[8] and neurophysiological measures. Spectrophotofluorometry provided direct access to the detection of the biochemical changes that might be responsible for therapeutic effects. Spectrophotofluorometry has also opened the path for the development of neuropsychopharmacology, a new discipline that studies the relationship between neuronal and mental processing in the brain with the employment of centrally acting drugs.[5]

The first neuropharmacological studies with the aid of spectrophotofluorometry revealed: (1) that administration of reserpine, a Rauwolfia alkaloid, produced a decrease in brain serotonin and norepinephrine levels;[9,10] (2) that administration of iproniazid, an inhibitor of the enzyme responsible for the breakdown of monoamines,[11] increased brain serotonin levels;[12] (3) that pretreatment with iproniazid attenuated reserpine-induced depletion of serotonin and catecholamines;[13,14] and (4) that only those Rauwolfia alkaloids[15] and benzoquinolizines[16] (a group of synthetic substances) that depleted serotonin had tranquilizing, or sedating, action. A possible relationship between mood and cerebral monoamine levels was based on clinical reports which indicated that treatment with iproniazid induced euphoria, a feeling of well-being in some tubercular patients,[17,18] whereas treatment with reserpine induced depressed mood or dysphoria in about 15% of hypertensive patients.[19,20] The "birth" of neuropsychopharmacology in the mid-1950s was the result of combining these clinical observations with findings in neuropharmacological research.[21] The foundation of the new discipline was tenuous. There were reports that isoniazid, the parent substance of iproniazid, had similar effects on mood to those of iproniazid without virtually any effect on monoamine oxidase activity.[22, 23, 24] There was also a report on the favorable effects of reserpine in anxious and depressed patients.[25, 26]

One of the first to recognize that neuropsychopharmacology opened up a new perspective in the understanding of psychiatric illness was Abraham Wikler, an American psychiatrist.[27.] In his monograph on The Relation of Psychiatry to Pharmacology, he suggested that studying the mode of action of psychotropic drugs with known therapeutic effects might provide information on the biochemical basis of mental disorders.[28] By generating information on molecular changes in psychiatric illness, findings in neuropsychopharmacological research were to guide the development of rational drug treatments. The notion that drugs with known therapeutic effects might provide the key for bridging the gap between neuronal processing and mental pathology has remained the driving force for research in the new field.

By the end of the 1950s the "neurotransmitter era," the first epoch in the history of neuropsychopharmacology, had taken form. Research in the pathophysiology and treatment of mental illness had become guided by knowledge derived from the effect of psychotropic drugs on neurotransmitter dynamics and metabolism.[29] In the 1960s neuronal re-uptake and pre-synaptic mechanisms became the focus of interest. Yet as time passed, attention shifted to receptors and post-synaptic mechanisms. In the late 1970s the scope of research was extended from cerebral monoamines to neurotransmitter modulators, neuropeptides and prostaglandins.[30] With the recognition in the mid 1980s that communication in the brain is not restricted to "wiring transmission" (based on neurotransmitter dynamics) in which one neuron connects directly with another, but also involves "volume transmission" that takes place in the extra-cellular space,[31] the neurotransmitter era was approaching its end. Yet it was only after the introduction of molecular genetic technology in the 1990s that a genetic era in neuropsychopharmacology emerged.[2]

During its first 50 years neuropsychopharmacology had a major impact on the development of psychiatry. The site of psychiatric practice shifted from the psychiatric hospital to the community; the scope of psychiatry was extended from the psychoses and neuroses to dimensional anomalies of abnormal psychology; and pharmacological therapy has come to dominate treatment in most psychiatric disorders. By supplying drugs with demonstrated therapeutic efficacy, together with information on their mode of action in the brain, the pharmaceutical industry had played an important role in changing the thinking of psychiatrists from psychological to biological and reintegrating psychiatry with the other medical disciplines.[6]

Recognition of the need in research for continuous dialogue between clinicians and basic scientists resulted in the founding of associations that would provide a platform for interaction among the various disciplines of the new field. The first major organizations to provide such platforms were the Collegium Internationale Neuro-Psychopharmacologicum (CINP), founded in 1957,[32] and the American College of Neuropsychopharmacology (ACNP), founded in 1961.[33] Both the International and the American organizations have also offered a venue for communicating information about new psychotropic drugs. With the support of the US Public Health Service and the pharmaceutical companies, by the mid-1960s, research in neuropsychopharmacology flourished in the United States. The annual meetings of the American College of Neuropsychopharmacology were to become signposts in the development of the discipline.

By the mid-1990 the pioneer generation was fading away; to preserve their legacy, the late Oakley Ray, at the time ACNP's Secretary, generated funds from Solway Pharmaceuticals for the founding of the ACNP-Solway Archives in Neuropsychopharmacology. Ray also arranged for the videotaping of peer-interviews with the pioneers at annual meetings, to be stored at the archives. The endeavor that was to become known as the "oral history project" was gradually extended to include videotaped interviews with members of the College, and later also with non-members, who contributed to the development of the field. Most of these interviews were conducted by peers. Furthermore with ACNP's Fiftieth Anniversary approaching in 2011, a few special interviews were videotaped with a focus on the history of the college and on interviewees' contributions to the activities of ACNP.

In this series of ten volumes the edited transcripts of these biographical interviews collected over a period of 14 years (from December 1994 to December 2008) are presented. The material is based on 235 videotaped interviews conducted by 66 interviewers – most of them peers, knowledgeable in the same field of inquiry – with 213 interviewees who contributed to the development of neuropsychopharmacology. Of the 235 interviews, 212 were done at ACNP's annual meetings and 23 between meetings; 229 involved a single interviewer, five involved two interviewers and one was a group interview. Some interviewees were the subjects of several interviews.

The series covers the first 50 years in the history of neuropsychopharmacology. Volume 1 deals with the state of the art in psychiatry and pharmacology at the time of the emergence of neuropsychopharmacology; and Volumes 2 through 8 with various areas of research, clinical activities and education in the discipline. Volume 9 is focused on the changes over the years and Volume 10 on the history of ACNP. The transcripts of Volumes 1 through 8 are based on first interviews, and of Volume 9 on second (update) interviews. Volume 10 includes, in addition to interview transcripts, material relating to the history of ACNP excerpted from transcripts presented in prior volumes. Introductions by some of the volume editors provide an overview of developments in the particular area within neuropsychopharmacology covered in that volume, and a Preface by the series editor draws together the contributions presented in the various volumes into a history of the field as a whole. Volume 10 also includes a Postscript by the editor outlining the present status of neuropsychopharmacology; a Quotation selected from each interview followed by a Chronological List of Publcations in neuropsychopharmacology based on interviewees contributions and references in editor's Preface in the volumes; and Acknowledgements of the numerous contributors to this project, which has taken more than 16 years to reach fruition.

In the information overload created by the online accessibility of virtually all information that is not protected by patent or copyright, authentic primary sources are often indistinguishable from inaccurate or trivial information. By presenting the first-hand accounts of ACNP members about their contributions to the field, this series provides a guide to recover the historical record from the flood of non-replicable research reports and time-bound reviews contaminated by reviewers' biases. It complements David Healy's three-volume series (*The Psychopharmacologists*) which includes the edited transcripts of audiotaped interviews with 78 psychopharmacologists selected for their significant contributions to the development of the field.[34, 35, 36] It complements as well CINP's four-volume series (*The History of Psychopharmacology and the CINP, As Told in Autobiography*), which includes the autobiographical accounts of about 250 leaders of psychopharmacology from more than 50 countries.[37, 38, 39, 40] These three series of source books offer historians reliable material for reconstructing the early history of neuropsychopharmacology. The original videotapes will be available in ACNP's International Archives in Neuropsychopharmacology.

REFERENCES

1   Ban TA. Fifty years chlorpromazine. A historical perspective. Neuropsychiat Dis Treat 2007; 3: 483–8.
2   Ban TA, Ucha Udabe R. The neurotransmitter era in neuropsychopharmacology. In: Ban TA, Ucha Udabe R. editors. The Neurotransmitter Era in Neuropsychopharmacology. Buenos Aires: Polemos; 2006. p. 265–74.
3   Macht DL. Contributions to psychopharmacology. Bull Johns Hopkins Hosp 1920; 31: 167–73.
4   Kraepelin E. Über die Beeinflussung einfacher psychischer Vorgänge durch einige Arzneimittel. Jena: Fischer; 1892.
5   Ban TA. Neuropsychopharmacology and the history of pharmacotherapy in psychiatry.A review of developments in the 20th century. In: Ban TA, Healy D, Shorter E, editors. Reflections on Twentieth-Century Psychopharmacology. Budapest: Animula; 2004. p.697–720.
6   Ban TA. Academic psychiatry and the pharmaceutical industry. Prog Neuropsychopharmacol Biol Psychiatry 2006; 30: 429–41.
7   Bowman RL, Caulfield PA, Udenfriend S. Spectrophotometric assay in the visible and ultraviolet. Science 1955; 122: 32–3.
8   Simon P. Behavioural pharmacology. In: Ban TA, Healy D, Shorter E, editors. The Rise of Psychopharmacology and the Story of CINP. Budapest: Animula; 1998. p. 131–4.
9   Pletscher A, Shore PA, Brodie BB. Serotonin release as a possible mechanism of serotonin action. Science 1955; 122: 374–5.
10 Holzbauer M, Vogt M. Depression by reserpine of the noradrenaline concentration in the hypothalamus of the rat. J Neurochem 1996; 1: 8–11.
11 Zeller EA, Barsky JR, Fouts W, Kirchheimer WP, Van Orden LS. Influence of isonicotinic acid hydrazide (INH) and 1-isonicotinyl-2-isopropyl hydrazide (IIH) on bacterial and mammalian enzymes. Experientia 1952; 8: 349–50.
12 Pletscher A. Beeinflussung des 5-Hydroxytryptamin-stoffwechsels im Gehirn durch Isonikotinsäurehydrazide. Experientia 1956; 12: 479–80.
13 Besendorf H, Pletscher A. Beeinflussung zentraler Wirkungen von Reserpin und 5-Hydroxytryptamin durch Isonikotinsäurehydrazide. Helv Physiol Pharmacol Acta 1956; 14: 383–90.
14 Carlsson A, Rosengren E, Bertler A, Nilsson, J. Effects of reserpine on the metabolism of catecholamines. In: Garattini S, Ghetti V, editors. Psychotropic Drugs. Amsterdam: Elsevier; 1957. p. 363–72.

15   Brodie BB, Shore PA, Pletscher A. Limitation of serotonin releasing activity to those alkaloids possessing tranquilizing action. Science 1956; 123: 992–3.

16   Pletscher A. Release of 5-hydroxytryptamine by benzoquinolizine derivatives with sedative action.
Science 1957; 126: 507–8.

17   Flaherty JA. The psychiatric use of isonicotinic acid hydrazide: a case report. Del Med J 1952; 24:
298–300.

18   Selikoff IJ, Robitzek FH, Orenstein GG. Treatment of pulmonary tuberculosis with hydrazine derivatives
of isonicotinic acid. JAMA 1957; 150: 973–80.

19   Freis ED. Mental depression in hypertensive patients treated for long periods with large doses of reserpine. N Engl J Med 1954; 251: 1006–8.

20   Mueller JC, Pryor WW, Gibbons JJ, Orgain ES. Depression and anxiety occurring during Rauwolfia
therapy. JAMA 1955; 159: 836–9.

21   Ban, T.A. The birth of neuropsychopharmacology. Neuropsychopharmacol Hung 2008; 3(Suppl 2):
S12–3.

22   Delay J, Laine B, Buisson JF. Note concernant l'action de l'isonicotinyl dans le traitement des états
dépressives. Ann Med Psychol (Paris) 1952; 110; 689–92.

23   Salzer HM, Lurie ML. Anxiety and depressive states treated with isonicotinyl hydrazide (isoniazid). Arch
Neurol Psychiatry 1953; 70: 317–24.

24   Salzer HM, Lurie ML. Depressive states treated with isonicotinyl hydrazide (isoniazid). Ohio State Med
J 1955;51:437–41.

25   Davies DL, Shepherd M. Reserpine in the treatment of anxious and depressed patients. Lancet 1955;
2: 117–20.

26   Healy D. The Antidepressant Era. Cambridge: Harvard University Press; 1997. p. 72–4.

27   Hollister LE. Review of Wikler's The Relation of Psychiatry to Pharmacology. In: Ban TA, Ray OS, editors. A History of the CINP. Nashville: JM Productions; 1996. p. 339–43.

28   Wikler A. The Relation of Psychiatry to Pharmacology. Baltimore: Williams and Wilkins; 1957.

29   Pletscher A. The dawn of the neurotransmitter era in neuropsychopharmacology. In: Ban TA, Ucha
Udabe R, editors. The Neurotransmitter Era in Neuropsychopharmacology. Buenos Aires: Polhemos;
2006. p. 27–37.

30   Carlsson A. The 12th CINP Congress. In: Ban TA, Hippius H, editors. Thirty Years CINP. Berlin: Springer;
1986, p. 42–3.

31   Agnati LF, Fuxe K, Zoli M, Zini I, Toffano G, Ferraguti F. A correlation analysis of regional distribution
of central enkephalin and ß-endorphin immunoreactive terminals and of opiate receptor in adult and
old male rats. Evidence of the existence of two main types of communications in the central nervous
system: The volume transmission and the wiring transmission. Acta Physiol Scand 1986; 128: 201–7.

32   Ban TA. A history of the Collegium Internationale Neuro-Psychopharmacologicum (1957–2004). Prog
Neuro-Psychopharmacol Biol Psychiatry 2006; 30: 599–616.

33   Ray OS. The history of the American College of Neuropsychopharmacology. In: Ban TA, Healy D,
Shorter E, editors. Reflections on Twentieth-Century Psychopharmacology. Budapest: Animula; 2004.
p. 616–20.

34   Healy D. The Psychopharmacologists. Interviews by David Healy. London: Altman; 1996.

35   Healy D. The Psychopharmacologists II. Interviews by David Healy. London: Altman; 1998.

36   Healy D. The Psychopharmacologists III. Interviews by David Healy. London: Arnold; 2000.

37   Ban TA, Healy D, Shorter E, editors. The Rise of Psychopharmacology and the Story of CINP. Budapest:
Animula; 1998.

38   Ban TA, Healy D, Shorter E, editors. The Triumph of Psychopharmacology and the Story of CINP.
Budapest: Animula; 2000.

39   Ban TA, Healy D, Shorter E, editors. From Psychopharmacology to Neuropsychopharmacology in the
1980s and the Story of CINP.Budapest: Animula; 2002.

40   Ban TA, Healy D, Shorter E, editors. Reflections on Twentieth-Century Psychopharmacology. Budapest:
Animula; 2004.

List of Interviewees & Interviewers

Legend

(1)	interviewer is historian or mental health professional
(2)	interviewee is not affiliated with ACNP
(3)	interview focused on interviewee's contribution to ACNP
(4)	group interview
(5)	interview conducted between annual meetings
(6)	two interviewees interviewing each other in one interview
(7)	interviewee interviewed only in group interview
(8)	interview focused on the history of ACNP
(/)	two interviewers
(+)	more than one interview

	INTERVIEWEES	INTERVIEWERS
1.	Manfred Ackenheil	Andrea Tone (1)
2.	Martin W. Adler	Larry Stein
3.	George K. Aghajanian	Hollister / Ban
4.	Bernard W. Agranoff	Leonard Cook
5.	Huda Akil	James Meador-Woodruff
6.	Hagop S. Akiskal	Paula J. Clayton
7.	George S. Alexopoulos	Andrea Tone (1)
8.	Nancy C. Andreasen	Andrea Tone (1)
9.	Burton Angrist	David S. Janowsky
10.	Victoria Arango	Andrea Tone (1)
11.	Joseph Autry (2)	Leo E. Hollister
12.	Julius Axelrod	Leo E. Hollister
13.	Frank J. Ayd, Jr.	Hollister +Healy + Ban (5)
14.	Ross J. Baldessarini	Leo E. Hollister
15.	Thomas A. Ban	Hollister + W. Bunney, Jr
16.	Jack D. Barchas	Stanley Watson
17.	Samuel Barondes	Tone (1) / Ban
18.	Herbert Barry III	Thomas A. Ban
19.	Charles M. Beasley	William Z. Potter
20.	Robert H. Belmaker	Calabrese + Frazer (3, 4)
21.	Frank M. Berger	Leo E. Hollister
22.	Barry Blackwell	Donald S. Robinson
23.	Jack Blaine	Leo E. Hollister
24.	Dan G. Blazer II	Andrea Tone (1)

25.	Floyd E. Bloom	David J. Kupfer
26.	Charles L. Bowden	Andrea Tone (1)
27.	Philip B. Bradley (2)	Thomas A. Ban (5)
28.	Joseph V. Brady	Leo E. Hollister
29.	Walter A. Brown	John F. Greden
30.	William E. Bunney, Jr.	Thomas A. Ban
31.	Enoch Callaway III	Thomas A. Ban
32.	Arvid Carlsson	W.Bunney, Jr. + Frazer (3,4)
33.	William T. Carpenter, Jr.	Thomas A. Ban
34.	Charles Jelleff Carr	Thomas A. Ban (5)
35.	Bernard J. Carroll	Hollister / Ban
36.	Kanelios Charalampous	Thomas A. Ban
37.	Dennis S. Charney	William Z. Potter
38.	Thomas N. Chase	Thomas A. Ban
39.	Eva Ceskova (2)	Andrea Tone (1)
40.	Guy Chouinard	Andrea Tone (1)
41.	Paula J. Clayton	Thomas A. Ban
42.	Robert Cohen (2)	Thomas A. Ban (5)
43.	Jonathan O. Cole	Hollister + Ban (5) + Salzman (5)
44.	Keith C. Conners	Burton Angrist
45.	Leonard Cook	Larry Stein
46.	Thomas B. Cooper	Thomas A. Ban
47.	Erminio Costa	Stephen H. Koslow
48.	Joseph T. Coyle	William E. Bunney Jr
49.	Svein G. Dahl	Andrea Tone (1)
50.	Annica Dahlström (2)	Andrea Tone (1)
51.	John M. Davis	David Healy
52.	Kenneth L. Davis	Stanley J. Watson
53.	José M. Delgado	Joel Braslow (1)
54.	Claude de Montigny	Andrea Tone (1)
55.	Thomas Detre	B.S. Bunney + Kupfer (3,5)
56.	Peter B. Dews	John A. Harvey
57.	James Dingell	Leo E. Hollister
58.	Edward F. Domino	Christian J. Gillin
59.	David L. Dunner	Thomas A. Ban
60.	Michael H. Ebert	Benjamin S. Bunney
61.	Burr S. Eichelman	Thomas A. Ban
62.	Joel Elkes	Sulser + Sulser (3,5)
63.	Jean Endicott	Darrel Regier
64.	Salvatore Enna	Elizabeth Bromley (1)
65.	Jan A. Fawcett	Frederick K. Goodwin

66.	Irwin Feinberg	Leo E. Hollister
67.	Hans Christian Fibiger	Thomas A. Ban
68.	Max Fink	Cole + Healy
69.	Barbara Fish	Meldrum (1,5) / Bromley (1,5)
70.	Ellen Frank	William E. Bunney, Jr.
71.	Alan Frazer	Stephen H. Koslow
72.	Alfred M. Freedman	Thomas A. Ban (5)
73.	Arnold J. Friedhoff	Benjamin S. Bunney
74.	Kjell Fuxe	Thomas A. Ban
75.	Donald M. Gallant	Thomas A. Ban (5)
76.	Silvio Garattini	Leo E. Hollister
77.	George Gardos	Thomas A. Ban
78.	Peter Gaszner (2)	Andrea Tone (1)
79.	Mark S. George	Robert M. Post
80.	Samuel Gershon	Thomas A. Ban
81.	Christian A. Gillin	William E. Bunney, Jr.
82.	Alexander H. Glassman	Thomas A. Ban
83.	Ira D. Glick	Donald F. Klein
84.	Burton J. Goldstein	Thomas A. Ban
85.	Frederick K. Goodwin	Thomas Detre
86.	Louis A. Gottschalk	W. Bunney, Jr. + Ban (5)
87.	John F. Greden	Thomas A. Ban
88.	Paul Greengard	Eric J. Nestler
89.	Angelos Halaris	Thomas A. Ban
90.	Uriel M. Halbreich	Daniel P. van Kammen
91.	Katherine A. Halmi	Thomas A. Ban
92.	Ernest Hartmann	Thomas A. Ban
93.	George E. Heninger	Thomas A. Ban
94.	Fritz A. Henn	Andrea Tone (1)
95.	Hanns F. Hippius	Andrea Tone (1, 5)
96.	Gerard Hogarty	Andrea Tone (1)
97.	Leo E. Hollister	Ayd + Ban
98.	Philip S. Holzman	Thomas A. Ban
99.	Turan M. Itil	Ban + Tone (1)
100.	Leslie L. Iversen	Thomas A. Ban
101.	Jerome H. Jaffe	Leo E. Hollister
102.	David J. Janowsky	Hollister + Angrist
103.	Murray Jarvik	Thomas A. Ban
104.	Donald R. Jasinski	Leo E. Hollister
105.	Dilip V. Jeste	Thomas A. Ban
106.	Lewis L. Judd	Andrea Tone (1)

107.	Samuel C. Kaim	Leo E. Hollister
108.	Eric R. Kandel	Huda Akil
109.	John M. Kane	Thomas A. Ban
110.	Shitij Kapur	Elizabeth Bromley (1)
111.	Alexander G. Karczmar	Erminio Costa
112.	Martin M. Katz	Endicott + Koslow +Ban (3)
113.	Seymour Kaufman	Thomas A. Ban
114.	Robert M. Kessler	Andrea Tone (1)
115.	Seymour Kety	Irwin J. Kopin
116.	Eva K. Killiam	Keith F. Killiam (6)
117.	Keith F. Killiam	Eva K. Killiam (6)
118.	Herbert D. Kleber	Andrea Tone (1)
119.	Gerald D. Klee	William T. Carpenter, Jr. (5)
120.	Donald F. Klein	Hollister + Davis
121.	Rachel G. Klein	Healy + Leckman
122.	Joel E. Kleinman	Elizabeth Bromley (1)
123.	James C. Klett	Leo E. Hollister
124.	Joseph Knoll (2)	Thomas A. Ban (5)
125.	James H. Kocsis	Joel Braslow (1)
126.	Irwin J. Kopin	Thomas A. Ban
127.	Conan Kornetsky	Koob + Ban
128.	Stephen H. Koslow	Thomas A. Ban
129.	Mary Jean Kreek	Lisa H. Gold
130.	David J. Kupfer	Alan F. Schatzberg
131.	Albert A. Kurland	Leo E. Hollister (5)
132.	Harbans Lal	Elizabeth Bromley (1)
133.	Salomon Z. Langer	W. Bunney, Jr. + Frazer (3,4)
134.	Louis C. Lasagna	Donald F. Klein
135.	Paul Leber	Thomas A. Ban
136.	Yves Lecrubier (2)	Andrea Tone (1)
137.	Heinz E. Lehmann	William E. Bunney, Jr.
138.	Jerome Levine	Gershon + Carpenter
139.	Alfred J. Lewy	Thomas A. Ban
140.	Jeffrey A. Lieberman	Shitij Kapur
141.	Sarah H. Lisanby	Andrea Tone (1)
142,	Vincenzo G. Longo (2)	Leonard Cook
143.	Roger Maickel	Leo E. Hollister
144.	Arnold J. Mandell	David Healy
145.	Aleksander A. Mathé	Leo E. Hollister
146.	William T. McKinney	Thomas A. Ban
147.	Douglas McNair	Leo E. Hollister

148.	Herbert Y. Meltzer	Koslow + Tamminga
149.	Roger E. Meyer	Thomas R. Kosten
150.	Charles R. Nemeroff	Thomas A. Ban
151.	Ernest P. Noble	Edythe D. London
152.	Charles O'Brien	Hollister / Ban
153.	John E. Overall	Thomas A. Ban (5)
154.	Gregory F. Oxenkrug	Thomas A. Ban
155.	Steven M. Paul	Thomas A. Ban
156.	Eugene S. Paykel	Thomas A. Ban
157.	Candace B. Pert	Leo E. Hollister
158.	Roy Pickens	Leo E. Hollister
159.	Alfred Pletscher	Ban (5) + Tone (1,5)
160.	Robert M. Post	Thomas A. Ban
161.	William Z. Potter	Thomas A. Ban
162.	Arthur J. Prange	Robert H. Belmaker
163.	Benny J. Primm (2)	Nancy Campbell (1,5)
164.	Frederic Quitkin	Thomas A. Ban
165.	Judith L. Rapoport	David Healy
166.	Allen Raskin	Leo E. Hollister
167.	Barry Reisberg	Elizabeth Bromley (1)
168.	Elliott Richelson	Thomas A. Ban
169.	Karl Rickels	David Healy
170.	Trevor Robbins	Alan Frazer (4,8)
171.	Donald S. Robinson	Joel Braslow (1)
172.	Carl Salzman	Roger F. Mayer
173.	Paul R. Sanberg	Matthew J. Wayner
174.	Elaine Sanders-Bush	Joel Braslow (1)
175.	Merton Sandler	David Healy
176.	Gerald J. Sarwer-Foner	Awad + Braslow (1)
177.	Alan F. Schatzberg	Thomas A. Ban
178.	Joseph Schildkraut	David Healy
179.	Joseph C. Schooler	David Healy
180.	Nina R. Schooler	Thomas A. Ban
181.	Richard L. Shader	Carl Salzman
182.	Eric M. Shooter	Thomas A. Ban
183.	Marc A. Schuckit	Andrea Tone (1)
184.	Charles R. Schuster	Thomas A. Ban
185.	Baron Shopsin	Andrea Tone (1)
186.	George M. Simpson	L. Hollister + T. Ban (5)
187.	Solomon H. Snyder	Floyd E. Bloom
188.	Louis Sokoloff	Thomas A. Ban

189.	Sydney Spector	Fridolin Sulser
190.	Stephen M. Stahl	Andrea Tone (1)
191.	Larry Stein	Arvid Carlsson
192.	Arthur A. Sugerman	Thomas A. Ban
193.	Fridolin Sulser	Leo E. Hollister
194.	Stephen Szára	Leo E. Hollister (5)
195.	Gary D. Tollefsen	Joel Braslow (1)
196.	William J. Turner	Jo Ann Engelhardt (1)
197.	Eberhard H. Uhlenhuth	Jerome Levine
198.	Daniel P. van Kammen	Thomas A. Ban
199.	Herman van Praag	Healy + Belmaker
200.	Oldrich Vinar	Leo E. Hollister
201.	Nora D. Volkow	Charles O'Brien
202.	E. Leong Way	Lynn E. DeLisi
203.	Matthew J. Wayner	Paul R. Sanberg
204.	Daniel Weinberger	Steven Potkin
205.	Myrna M. Weissman	Thomas A. Ban
206.	Paul H. Wender	Thomas A. Ban
207.	David Wheatley (2)	Leo E. Hollister
208.	Peter C. Whybrow	Andrea Tone (1)
209.	Andrew Winokur	Andrea Tone (1)
210.	James H. Woods	David Healy
211.	Joseph Wortis	Leo E. Hollister
212.	Richard J. Wurtman	Thomas A. Ban
213.	Joseph Zohar	Alan Frazer (4,8)

VOLUME 1

Edward Shorter

STARTING UP

Preface
Thomas A. Ban

Dedicated to the Memory of Heinz E. Lehmann, President ACNP, 1965

PREFACE
Thomas A. Ban

Naturally occurring substances have been used to heal the mind and induce ecstasy throughout history. Yet the story that leads to the development of neuropsychopharmacology begins only in the early nineteenth century with the emergence of organic chemistry, pharmacology.[1] and the pharmaceutical industry.[2] The rapidly growing drug companies during the second half of the nineteenth century were instrumental to the introduction of several centrally acting drugs. By the end of the 1890s morphine,[3,4]a substance isolated from opium[5] along with apomorphine, and hyoscine (scopolamine) were extensively used in the control of excitement and agitation; chloral hydrate[6,7] and paraldehyde[8] for calming and inducing sleep; and potassium bromide[9] for relieving restlessness, anxiety and tension. The use of these drugs provided day- and night time sedation in the asylums, and reduced the need for physical restraint.[1] It was during this period – between 1850 and 1900 – that academic psychiatry was born with more than 20 academic departments established in German-speaking universities alone.[4]

By the end of the 19th century, pharmacological control of behavior made it possible to study the symptoms and signs of psychiatric patients during the entire course of their illness.[1] The information collected opened the path for the further development of psychopathology, the discipline that deals with the symptoms and signs of psychiatric disease[10, 11]and psychiatric nosology, the discipline that deals with the methodology of synthesizing and classifying diseases.[12,13] During the first half of the 20th century, psychopathology provided a common language for the description of the mental state of patients, and nosology the necessary orientation points to classify them into groups with some predictability of behavior and response to treatment. In the new classification, the psychoses – which originally included all mental pathologies[14] – are split into "organic" and "endogenous,"[15, 16] the "endogenous psychoses" are divided into manic-depressive insanity (illness) and dementia praecox (schizophrenia),[17, 18] the "exogenous (toxic) psychoses"[19] are distinguished from the "reactive (psychogenic) psychoses,"[20] and the "psychoses" (manifestations of disease),[21] are separated from the "personality disorders" (manifestations of anomalous development).[10]

Simultaneously with the development of modern psychiatry, the armamentarium of drugs used in psychiatric disorders had grown. In 1903, the barbiturates,[22] a group of sedative drugs appeared; they found their place in clinical practice in a variety of disorders, including insomnia, epilepsy,[23] and inhibited catatonia.[24] They were also used in general anesthesia and in the facilitation of psychotherapy.[23] In 1936, after the recognition of their central nervous system stimulating effect (initially described in 1927[25]), the amphetamines entered the psychiatric scene; Benzedrine (amphetamine sulfate) was shown to have therapeutic effect in narcolepsy[26] and in calming hyper-excitable and hyperactive children.[27] In the 1940s, with the introduction of nicotinic acid[28] and penicillin,[29] cerebral pellagra[30] and cerebral syphilis[31] were wiped out in psychiatry; and with the introduction of thiamine[32] and diphenylhydantoin[33] the psychiatric population with amnestic syndrome[34, 35] and epilepsy[33] was drastically decreased.[1] The use of drugs in the study of mental pathology – advocated in the mid-nineteenth century by Moreau de Tours[36] – was re-vitalized with the introduction of phenomenological psychopathology, the branch of psychopathology that deals with the subjective experiences of psychic life.[10] Initially, phenomenological studies with mescaline, the active ingredient of peyote (a cactus plant),[37] were in vogue.[38, 39, 40] Interest shifted to lysergic acid diethylamide (LSD), an ergot alkaloid, after its accidental discovery in 1943 by Hofmann[41] while working with synthetic ergot alkaloids in order to develop a nikethamide-like analeptic[42] in the laboratories of Sandoz, a Swiss pharmaceutical company. LSD was more than 1,000 times more potent than mescaline; it was active in 0.5 to 1 microgram per kilogram.[43] The possibility that a chemical in such minute amounts could induce hallucinations had fuelled the contemporary hypothesis that undetectable traces of psychoactive substances produced by the body might be responsible for the pathogenesis of some mental illness.

The idea that autointoxication plays a role in the pathogenesis of some psychoses entered psychiatry in the 1930s with Rolv Gjessing's finding of nitrogen retention in certain phases of periodic catatonia[44]. His postulation that the alteration of metabolism by the production of mescaline-like substances in the body is responsible for periodic catatonia profoundly affected psychiatric thinking in the 1940s and '50s. John Cade,[45] stimulated by the work of Gjessing[44] and Hofmann,[41] hypothesized that mania, as thyrotoxicosis, was a state of intoxication by a product of the body in excess, and melancholia, as myxedema, was a state of deficiency of the same substance.[46] The hypothesis was wrong, but it led to the serendipitous discovery of the therapeutic effect of lithium in mania in the late 1940s.[46]

Autointoxication, combined with Walter Cannon's findings about the role of the adrenals in the adaptation to stress, is at the core of Osmond and Smythies'[47] postulation that schizophrenia is the result of stress-induced anxiety and a failure in the metabolism of norepinephrine. Harley-Mason[47] suggested that a trans-methylation product of norepinephrine, DMPEA (3, 4- dimethoxyphenylalanine) – a toxic substance that could induce experimental catatonia[48] – was responsible for the pathogenesis of schizophrenia; Hoffer,

Osmond and Smythies[49] proposed that adrenochrome, an oxidation product of epinephrine,[50] was the culprit. Both hypotheses were wrong. Yet they
stimulated research in the biochemistry of mental illness in a period (1950s)
when psychodynamic schools dominated psychiatry in North America, and
schizophrenia ("schizophrenic reactions") was perceived as the outcome of
poor mothering manifesting as narcissistic withdrawal with regression to early
autoerotic stages of ego development.[51]

It was against this background that within a period of five years five effective pharmacological treatments appeared on the psychiatric scene.

The *first, chlorpromazine* (CPZ), was synthesized on December 11, 1950
in the Laboratories of Rhône-Poulenc, a French pharmaceutical company, in a
program that aimed to develop drugs for use in general anesthesia.[52] Its potential use in psychiatry was recognized by Laborit in the course of using artificial
hibernation for the prevention of surgical shock,[53] and its therapeutic effect in
psychoses and especially in schizophrenia was demonstrated by Delay and
Deniker [54, 55, 56, 57, 58, 59, 60] at Ste. Anne's Hospital in Paris. CPZ was released for
clinical use in France in November 1952.

The *second, reserpine*, was isolated from the Rauwolfia root in 1952 by
Mueller, Schlittler and Bein[61] in the laboratories of CIBA, a Swiss pharmaceutical company. The substance was responsible for about 50% of the antihypertensive and tranquilizing action of the snakeroot plant (Rauwolfia serpentina)
that had been in use for hundreds of years in various preparations by Ayurvedic
practitioners in India.[62] In 1954, Delay et al.,[63] Kline,[64] and Noce, William and
Rapoport[65] independently demonstrated the therapeutic effect of the substance in schizophrenia. In the same year, Steck reported on the similarities
in therapeutic and adverse effects of reserpine and CPZ.[66] Yet another line of
research indicated that reserpine may induce depression and depletes monoamines (serotonin and norepinephrine) in the brain (*see* Overview).

The *third, meprobamate* (2-methyl-2-n-propyl-prapanediol), was synthesized in 1950 by Ludwig at Wallace Laboratories in New Jersey (U.S.) in order
to prolong the duration of mephenesin's "tranquilizing and muscle relaxant" action. Mephenesen had been discovered during the mid-1940s in the laboratories of British Drug Houses in London by Frank Berger[67] while trying to develop
non-toxic antibacterial agents that would inhibit the growth of Gram-negative
micro-organisms that caused enzymatic destruction of penicillin[68] (*see* Berger,
Volumes 3 and 9). In 1956, Lowell Selling reported on the therapeutic effect of
meprobamate in anxiety and tension states, and a few months later the substance was introduced for clinical use in the United States.[69]

The *fourth, imipramine,* a dibenzazepine, was selected from the chemical library of Geigy, a Swiss pharmaceutical company, by psychiatrist Roland Kuhn.
Because of its structural similarity to CPZ he hoped that it would have similar

therapeutic effects in schizophrenia.[70] His expectations were not fulfilled, but he found the drug effective in endogenous depression in which "vital distur-bance" was in the background. Kuhn presented and published his findings in 1957.[71]

The *fifth, iproniazid*, was synthesized in 1951 by Herbert Fox at Roche Laboratories in Nutley, New Jersey for the chemotherapy of tuberculosis.[72] The following year, Zeller et al.[73] at Northwestern University in Chicago, dem-onstrated the monoamine oxidase inhibiting properties of the substance. In 1952 there were also reports that iproniazid induced euphoria and overactive behavior in some tubercular patients.[74, 75] In 1956, Alfred Pletscher, working as a visiting scientist in Bernard Brodie's laboratory at the (U.S.) National Heart Institute – on leave from his position as research director of Roche – showed that iproniazid increased brain serotonin levels[76] and attenuated reserpine-in-duced depletion of serotonin.[77] (*See* Pletscher, Volumes 3 and 9). Finally in 1957, Crane,[78] and Loomers, Saunders and Kline[79] independently published their findings on the "psychic energizing"/"antidepressant" effect of the drug. Iproniazid was the first psychotropic drug introduced with a proposed rational for its possible mode of action.

By 1957 the pharmaceutical industry, recognizing the potential market for psychopharmaceuticals, was moving ahead industriously synthesizing and developing new drugs for psychiatric disorders. Pharmacology was ready to meet the challenge of identifying new drugs that might have similar clinical effects to the ones already in use by adopting a behavioral methodology, and developing a suitable methodology (neuropharmacology) for the detection of the mode of action of psychotropic drugs. The onus was on psychiatry to pro-vide the necessary feedback by identifying the populations (e.g., diagnoses) and/or mental activities (e.g., forms of experience) affected by the new drugs, in order for neuropsychopharmacology to progress. (*See* Overview). Yet there were only a few psychiatrists, like the late Fritz Freyhan, an American pioneer of neuropsychopharmacology, who recognized the need for the development of an empirically derived, pharmacologically valid psychiatric nosology[1] in or-der to translate the mode of action of drugs into pathomechanisms of illness. Mainstream psychiatry was split into a small group that flatly rejected the new drugs as chemical strait-jackets that interfered with psychotherapy and a large group that accepted the new drugs as more effective treatments than any other pharmacological treatment in the past but attributed their effectiveness to fa-cilitation of the natural healing process. In the case of CPZ, for example, the idea was that the drug freed the psyche from the disruptive interference of excessive affect without grossly interfering with cognitive processes, allowing the "patient's psyche to reorganize" itself.[40]

Interviewees & Interviewers

Volume 1 covers the state of the art in psychiatry and pharmacology at the time of the emergence of neuropsychopharmacology. It includes transcripts of 22 videotaped biographical interviews with clinicians and basic scientists of whom all but one (Robert Cohen) are affiliated with ACNP. It is a distinguished group; fourteen (Ayd, Brady, Carr, Cook, Dews, Domino, Elkes, Freedman, Gottschalk, Hollister, Kurland, Lehmann, Sarwer-Foner and Turner) are founders, and seven (Cook, Detre, Elkes, Freedman, Hollister, Lasagna, and Lehmann) past-presidents of the College. Three (Hippius, Hollister and Lehmann) are past presidents of CINP.

The interviews were conducted from 1994 to 2004 and with the exception of six (Carr, Cohen, Freedman, Hippius, Kurland and Szara) they were done at ACNP's annual meetings. One of the interviews (Hippius') was conducted at CINP's biennial congress, another (Carr's) in Nashville, and four at the home of the interviewees.

The 22 interviewees were interviewed by 13 interviewers. Eleven of the interviewers are peers of the interviewees, knowledgeable in the same field; one (Tone) is a medical historian; and one (Engelhardt) a mental health professional and former associate of the interviewee. Ten of the interviewers conducted one interview, and three conducted multiple interviews, i.e., 2 (Bunney), 3 (Ban), or 4 (Hollister.)

By the time the editing of Volume 1 began, four of the interviewees (Carr, Hollister, Turner and Wortis) and one of the interviewers (Hollister) had passed away; for reasons of health, three were unable to complete the editing of their transcripts.

Contributions of Intervewees

In the following section some of the contributions made by interviewees to the development of psychopharmacology are reviewed.

Four of the interviewees (Wortis, Cohen, Gottschalk and Sarwer-Foner), all psychiatrists, had some **background in psychoanalysis**. *Joseph Wortis* was psychoanalyzed by Sigmund Freud himself. He did not become a psychoanalyst but introduced insulin coma and convulsive treatment with pentylenetetrazol (Cardiazol, Metrazol) in the United States.[80] In the early 1960s, Wortis studied the effects of chlorpromazine on brain tissue preparations.[81]

Robert Cohen was analyzed by Frieda Fromm-Reichman. In 1952 he moved from Chestnut Lodge, one of the fortresses of psychoanalysis, to the National Institutes of Health, and during the 1960s and '70s, he was the moving force in developing the intramural research program of the National Institute of Mental Health (NIMH). (*See* Kety, Volume 2).

Louis Gottschalk (*see* also Volume 9) was trained under Franz Alexander and Thomas French at the prestigious Chicago Institute for Psychoanalysis. He became interested in objective measurements and developed an instrument with the capability of monitoring drug-induced changes by content analysis of speech.[82]

Gerald Sarwer-Foner (*see also* Volume 9) in parallel with his psychoanalytic training became involved in the clinical evaluation of the new psychotropic drugs, e.g., reserpine, imipramine, phenelzine, perphenazine, trifluoperazine, and haloperidol.[83] His postulation that psychotropic drugs exert their effect by shifting "psychic defenses" was lauded by the psychoanalytic establishment. The idea was that in contrast to some of the old drugs, such as the barbiturates, which enforce defenses like regression, denial, and projection, some of the new drugs facilitate the operation of more constructive defense mechanisms, such as isolation, rationalization, and sublimation, allowing the patient's ego to work through to a better adaptation to the reality principle.[40] Alternative psychodynamic formulations were proposed by Azima[84] and Ostow.[85]

Two of the interviewees (Szára and Domino) made their mark in the arena of research that deals with **model psychoses.** *Steven Szára* was first to describe the psychomimetic properties of dimethyltryptamine (DMT), a psychotoxic end product of tryptophan metabolism.[86] His negative findings about the presence of adrenochrome in the plasma of normal subjects and schizophrenic patients[87] was the *coup de gr ce* of the adrenochrome hypothesis of schizophrenia.[49]

Edward Domino was instrumental to the research that led from phencyclidine (Sernyl)[88] to psychomimetic arylcyclohexylamines, e.g., ketamine, a group of drugs which selectively reduce the excitation of mammalian neurons induced by aspartate–like amino acids.[89]

Eight of the interviewees (Hippius, Lehmann, Hollister, Ayd, Kurland, Turner, Freedman and Detre) all psychiatrists, contributed to the **introduction of new psychotropic drugs**; seven in the United States, and one, Hippius, in Germany. *Hanns Hippius* was also instrumental in training a cadre of psychiatrists involved in research in the new field.[90, 91]

Heinz Lehmann, a Canadian psychiatrist, was the first to report in 1954 on the therapeutic effect of CPZ in psychotic patients in North America.[92] The impact of his paper was so profound that in 1957 he was presented with the prestigious Lasker Award of the American Public Health Association for "bringing the full practical significance of CPZ to the attention of the medical community." Lehmann was also first in North America to report on the effects of imipramine in the treatment of depression.[93]

Leo Hollister (*see also* Volume 9) was one of the leading figures in the introduction of new psychotropic drugs, e.g., reserpine, in the United States.[94] A sharp observer, Hollister noted that CPZ and reserpine not only controlled productive (positive) psychopathology, e.g., hallucinations and delusions, but made patients talk and interact with their environment. He was the first to report withdrawal reactions after prolonged high-dose use of several drugs, including CPZ, meprobamate, and chlordiazepoxide.[95]

Frank Ayd (*see also* Volumes 9 and 10) was among the first to report on the therapeutic and adverse effects of numerous psychotropic drugs, including chlorpromazine[96] and amitriptyline[97] in the 1950s and '60s. A prolific writer, he was quick to disseminate in his *Newsletter* newly emerging finding with psychotropic drugs in an era when findings in clinical research still traveled slowly. His *Lexicon of Psychiatry, Neurology and the Neurosciences* was to become a standard reference.[98]

Albert Kurland was Principal Investigator of one of the first Early Clinical Drug Evaluation Units (ECDEU), a program of the Psychopharmacology Service Center, sponsored by the NIMH. He was one of the first, in the mid-1950s, to compare the effects of chlorpromazine and reserpine in the treatment of schizophrenia.[99] Kurland was to become a proponent of LSD treatment of alcoholism[100] introduced by Hoffer and Osmond.[101]

William Turner was one of the investigators in the ECDEU program. He collaborated in the 1950s and '60s with Sydney Merlis in the clinical evaluation of trifluoperazine and numerous. other new psychotropic drugs.[102] To pursue their investigations in an inpatient setting in a large mental hospital, Turner adopted the Malamud-Sands Rating Scale for use by the ward personnel in the assessment of change in patients.[103] Turner was to become a proponent of the use of diphenylhydantoin in the control of aggression.

Alfred Freedman was instrumental in extending pharmacological treatment with psychotropic drugs from adult to child psychiatry. He was the first in the 1950s to study the effects of diphenhydramine, iproniazid, imipramine, iproniazid, and promethazine in children.[104] In the 1970s and '80s he contributed to the evaluation of the effects of cyclazocine, naloxone, etc., in narcotic addiction.[105]

Thomas Detre (*see also* Volume 10) was involved in clinical investigations with reserpine and some of the other new drugs in the 1950s.[106] As clinical director of Yale's New Haven Hospital during the 1960s, he was in the forefront in breaking the resistance of the psychoanalytic establishment to using psychotropic drugs.[107]

The steadily growing number of new psychotropics in the late 1950s created a need for the adoption of a **clinical methodology** for the demonstration of therapeutic efficacy. *Louis Lasagna* played an important role in the introduction of the placebo-controlled randomized clinical trial in psychopharmacological research.[108] He was also instrumental in developing clinical pharmacology into a distinct medical discipline in the United States.[109]

Registration of the new drugs called for adequate **toxicity requirements** to secure their safe use. Requirements were tightened after the thalidomide disaster in Europe in which the substance, taken as a hypnotic by pregnant mothers, caused phocomelia in the newborn. In the development of "regulatory toxicology," *Jelleff Carr* played an important in role in the United States.[110]

Four of the interviewees (Brady, Cook, Dews and Stein) were instrumental in introducing **behavioral pharmacology**[111] in the study of the new psychotropic drugs. The roots of behavioral pharmacology lie in the research of Ivan Petrovich Pavlov, a Russian physiologist, who studied the effects of bromides and caffeine,[112, 113] and of Horsley Gantt, his American disciple, who studied first the effects of alcohol,[114] acetylcholine, and adrenaline,[115] and then CPZ and reserpine,[116] on conditioned reflex (CR) behavior. Gantt was referred to as the first American psychopharmacologist by Wagner Bridger, an American psychiatrist who himself studied the effects of mescaline on the CR.[117] Pavlov and Gantt recognized that non-specific properties of a drug, e.g., color of the capsule, and events that regularly occur prior to its administration, could become signals for eliciting the specific effects of a substance.[117] This recognition was further elaborated by the American behaviorist school.[118] *Joseph Brady* demonstrated that drugs not only have signal function as do all other signals in the environment (classical paradigm of conditioning), but also function as "reinforcers" of activities that control behavior (instrumental-operant paradigm of conditioning).[119] In the 1940s, Brady developed a conditioned emotional response (CER) in animals and during the 1950s he studied the effects of the new psychotropic drugs on the CER.[120]

Peter Dews was the first to recognize the role of the operating schedule of reinforcement[121] on the behavioral effects of drugs. He also showed that if two different events maintain response on a fixed interval schedule, then a given drug will affect each behavior pattern in the same way.[122]

Leonard Cook was first to show that CPZ and drugs with similar clinical effects differ from barbiturates and old-time sedatives by selectively blocking the conditioned avoidance reflex, while leaving the unconditional escape response unaffected.[123, 124, 125]

Larry Stein was instrumental in bridging behavioral pharmacology with neurochemistry. He was the first to demonstrate the reward augmenting effect of dopamine agonists, such as apomorphine[126] and high dose amphetamine.[127]

The remaining two interviewees (Elkes and Gershon) contributed to **bridging basic and clinical research** in neuropsychopharmacology. *Joel Elkes* (*see also* Volume 10) conducted the first blind, controlled, crossover clinical trial with CPZ in chronic psychotic patients.[128] He also explored the effects of amobarbital, amphetamine, and mephenesine on catatonic stupor.[129] In collaboration with Philip Bradley, Elkes was first to study the effects of centrally acting drugs on the electrical activity of the brain in conscious animals.[130, 131.] (See also Bradley, Volume 2). The concept of signal transduction in the brain was shifting during the 1950s from a purely electrical to a chemically mediated event; Elkes mapped the cholinesterases, responsible for the formation and breakdown of acetylcholine, in various areas of the central nervous system.[132] He recognized that inhibition of the enzyme has an effect on the emergence of various inborn reflexes.[133] Acetylcholine was the first neurotransmitter identified in the brain. The role of acetylcholine in mental integration, as reflected in consciousness and memory, was to become one of the major areas of neuropsychopharmacological research.

While looking for pharmacological antagonists of morphine in the early 1950s, *Samuel Gershon* discovered that tetrahydroaminoacridane (THA), a cholinesterase inhibitor, antagonized both morphine-induced sedation and coma, and the aberrant behavior induced by atropinergic (anticholinergic) drugs, e.g., Ditran. His discovery yielded, many years later, the introduction of THA in the treatment of dementias. Gershon spearheaded research using drugs in the elucidation of the underlying molecular changes in psychopathology.[134, 135] He was first with his collaborators to show that the administration of amphetamine, a dopamine agonist, could induce not only "paranoid excited hyperactive states" but also symptoms like "anergia."[136] (See also Angrist, Volume 5). He and his collaborators were also the first to show that pharmacological interference with the formation of serotonin by the administration of p-chlorophenylalanine blocked the therapeutic effect of antidepressants, whereas interference with the formation of norepinephrine by the administration of α-methylparatyrosine left the therapeutic effect of antidepressants unaffected.[137] (See also Shopsin, Volume 5). Gershon was a member. of Trautner's team that defined the therapeutic window for lithium treatment. He provided further substantiation for the specificity of lithium treatment in manic-depressive disease; and was first to report on the effectiveness of lithium in the prophylactic treatment of bipolar affective disorder.[138] Gershon's research was instrumental in introducing lithium treatment in psychiatry in the United States.[139]

In Volume 1, the personal stories of the interviewees begin in a period in which the brain is perceived an unpenetrable "black box," and mental disease is conceptualized as the result of interaction between psychological and social factors.

The background of the interviewees varies widely. Their only common feature is that they all participated in starting up the new field.

Edward Shorter the editor of Volume 1 is a social historian with a background in the history of psychiatry and psychopharmacology. [4, 140, 141, 142, 143, 144]

In his Introduction, Dramatis Personae and biographic footnotes Shorter brings alive a period in history during which neuropsychopharmacology was born.

REFERENCES

1   Ban TA. Academic psychiatry and the pharmaceutical industry. Prog Neuro-Psychopharmacol Biol Psychiatry 2006; 30: 429–41.
2   Healy D. The Antidepressant Era. Cambridge: Harvard University Press; 1997. p.17–21.
3   Wood A. A new method of treating neuralgia by the direct application of opiates to the painful points. Edinb Med and Surg J 1855; 82: 265–81.
4   Shorter E. A History of Psychiatry from the Era of the Asylum to the Age of Prozac. New York: John Wiley & Sons; 2005.
5   Sertürner FW. Darstellung der reinen Mohnsäure (Opiumsäure) nebst einer Chemischen Utersuchurgen des Opiums mit vorzüglicher Hinsicht auf einen darin neu entdecten stoff und dahin gehörigen Bemerkungen. Journal der Pharmacie für Ärzten und Apotheken (Leipzig) 1806; 14: 47–93.
6   Liebig J. Über die Verbindungen welche durch die Einwirkung des Chlors auf Alcohol, Aether, Olbildendes Gas und Effiggeist Entstehen. Liebigs Annalen der Pharmazie 1832; 1: 182–230.
7   Liebreich MEP. Das Chloralhydrate, ein neues Hypnoticum und Anaestheticum, und dessen Anwendung in die Medizin. Eine Arzneimeittel-Untersuchung. Berlin: Müller; 1869.
8   Cervello V. Über die Physiologische Wirkung des Paraldehyds und Beiträge zu den Studien über das Chloralhydrate. Arch Exp Path Pharmacol 1882; 16: 265–90.
9   Joynt RJ. The use of bromides in epilepsy. Am J Diseases of Children 1974; 128: 362–3.
10   Jaspers K. Eifersuchtswahn: Entwicklung einer Persönlichkeit oder Prozess. Z Ges Neurol Psychiatr 1910; 1: 567–637.
11   Jaspers K. Allgemeine Psychopathologie. Berlin: Springer; 1913.
12   Boissier de Sauvages F. Nosologia Methodica. Amsterdam: Frat de Tournes; 1768.
13   Kahlbaum K. Die Gruppierung der psychischen Krankheiten und die Enteilung der Seelenstoerungen. Danzig: AW Kaufman; 1863.
14   Feuchtersleben E. Lehrbuch der Ärztlichen Seelenkunde. Vienna: Carl Gerold; 1845.
15   Bayle ALJ. Traité des Maladies du Cerveau et de ses Membranes. Paris: Gabon; 1826.
16   Möbius JP. Abriss der Lehre von den Nervenkrankheiten. Leipzig: Abel; 1893.
17   Kraepelin E. Psychiatrie. Ein Lehrbuch für Studierende und Ärzte. 5 Auflage. Leipzig: Barth; 1896.
18   Kraepelin E. Psychiatrie. Ein Lehrbuch der Studierende und Ärzte. 6 Auflage. Leipzig: Barth; 1899.
19   Bonhoeffer K. Zur Frage der exogenen Psychosen. Neur Zbl 1909; 32: 499–505.
20   Wimmer A. Psykogene Syndssygdomsformer. Copenhagen: Lunds; 1916.
21   Schneider K. Klinische Psychopathologie. 3 Auflage. Stuttgart: Thieme; 1950.
22   Fischer E, Mering von J. Über eine neue Klasse von Schlafmittels. Ther Ggw 1903; 44: 97–101.
23   Lehmann HE, Ban TA. Pharmacotherapy of Tension and Anxiety. Springfield: Charles C. Thomas; 1970. p.14–5.
24   Thorner NW. Psychopharmacology of Sodium. amytal. I. Catatonia. J Nerv Ment Dis 1935; 82: 299–303.
25   Alles GA. The comparative physiological action of phenylethanolamine. J Pharmacol 1927; 32: 121–33.
26   Prinzmetal M, Blumberg W. The use of Benzedrine in the treatment of narcolepsy. JAMA 935; 105: 2051–3.
27   Bradley CB. The behavior of children receiving Benzedrine. Am J Psychiatry 1937; 94; 577-80.
28   Elvehjem CA, Madden RJ, Strong FM, Wooley DW. The isolation and the identification of the anti-blacktongue factor. J Biol Chem 1937; 123: 137–49.
29   Fleming A. On the antibacterial action of cultures of penicillium with special reference to their use in the isolation of B influensae. Br J Exp Pathol 1929; 10: 226–36.
30   Fouts PJ, Helmer OM, Lepkovsky YS, Jukes TH. Treatment of human pellagra with nicotinic acid. Proc Soc Exp Biol Med 1937; 37: 405–7.
31   Stokes JH, Sternberg TH, Schwartz WH, Mahoney JF, Moore JE, Wood WB. The action of penicillin in late syphilis including neurosyphilis. JAMA 1944; 126: 73–9.
32   Jansen BCP, Donath WF. On the isolation of antiberiberi vitamin. Proc K Ned Akad Wet 1926; 29: 1390–400.

33   Putnam TJ. The demonstration of the specific anticonvulsant action of diphenylhydantoin and re-lated compounds. In: Ayd FJ, Blackwell B, editors. Discoveries in Biological Psychiatry. Philadelphia: Lippincott; 1970. p. 85–90.

34   De Wardener HE, Lennox B. Cerebral beri-beri (Wernicke's encephalopathy): review of 52 cases in Singapore prisoner-of-war hospital. Lancet 1947; 1: 11–7.

35   Wernicke C. Lehrbuch der Gehirnkrankheiten. Breslau: Schlettersche Buchhandlung; 1881.

36   Moreau de Tours J. Du Hachich et de L'Aliénation Mentale. Etudes Psychologiques. Paris: Fortin & Masson; 1845.

37   Lewin L. Phantastica: Narcotic and Stimulating Drugs. Their Use and Abuse. London: Routledge; 1931.

38   Beringer K. Mescaline Intoxication. Berlin: Springer; 1927.

39   Knauer A, Maloney WM. Psychic action of mescaline. J Nerv Ment Dis 1913; 40: 425–40.

40   Lehmann HE. Before they called it psychiatry. Neuropsychopharmacology 1993; 8: 291–303.

41   Stoll A, Hofmann A. Partial synthese von Alkaloiden Typus des Ergobasins. Helv Chim Acta 1943; 26: 944–7.

42   Hofmann A. The discovery of LSD and subsequent investigations with naturally occurring hallucino-gens. In: Ayd FJ, Jr, Blackwell B, editors. Discoveries in Biological Psychiatry. Philadelphia: Lippincott; 1970. p. 91–106.

43   Brown FC. Hallcinogenic Drugs. Springfield: Charles C. Thomas; 1972.

44   Gjessing R. Disturbances of somatic functions in catatonia with periodic course, and their compensa-tion. J Ment Sci 1938; 84: 608—21.

45   Cade JF. The story of lithium. In: Ayd FJ, Jr, Blackwell B, editors. Discoveries in Biological Psychiatry. Philadelphia: Lippincott; 1970. p. 218–29.

46   Cade JF. Lithium salts in the treatment of psychotic excitement. Med J Aust 1948; 2: 349–52.

47   Osmond H, Smythies J. Schizophrenia: a new approach. J Ment Sci 1952; 98: 309–15.

48   Noteboom L. Experimental catatonia by means of derivatives of mescaline and adrenaline. Proc Natl Acad Sci USA 1934; 37: 562–3.

49   Hoffer A, Osmond H, Smythies J. Schizophrenia: a new approach II. J Ment Sci 1954; 100: 39–45.

50   Green D, Richter D. Adrenalin and adrenochrome. Biochem J 1937; 31: 596–616.

51   Noyes AP, Kolb LC. Modern Clinical Psychiatry. Philadelphia: W. Saunders; 1958.

52   Caldwell AE. Origins of Psychopharmacology. From CPZ to LSD. Springfield: Charles C. Thomas; 1970. p. 23–35.

53   Laborit H, Huguenard P, Alluaume R. Un nouveau stabilisateur végétatif (le 4560 RP). Presse Méd 1952; 60: 206–8.

54   Ban TA. Fifty years chlorpromazine. A historical perspective. Neuropsychiat Dis Treat 2007; 3: 483–8.

55   Delay J, Deniker P. Le traitment des psychoses par une méthode neurolytique dérivée de l'hibernothérapie; le 4560 RP utilisée seul en cure prolongée et continué. CR Congr Méd Alién Neurol (France) 1952; 50: 497–502.

56   Delay J, Deniker P. 38 cas de psychoses traitèes par la cure prolongée et continué de 4560 RP. CR Congr Méd Alién Neurol (France) 1952; 50: 503–13.

57   Delay J, Deniker P. Réactions biologiques observées au cours du traitement par l'chlorhydrate de deméthylaminopropyl-N-chlorophénothiazine. CR Congr Méd Alién Neurol (France) 1952; 50: 514–8.

58   Delay J, Deniker P, Harl JM. Utilisation en thérapeutique d'une phénothiazine d'action centrale selec-tive. Ann Med Psychol (Paris) 1952; 110: 112–7.

59   Delay J, Deniker P, Harl JM. Traitement des états d'excitation et d'agitation par une méthode médica-menteuse dérivé de l'hibernothérapie. Ann Med Psychol (Paris) 1952; 110: 267–73.

60   Delay J, Deniker P, Harl JM, Grasset A. Traitements d'états confusionnels par l'chlorhydrate de dimé-thylaminopropyl-N-chlorophénothiazine (4560 RP). Ann Med Psychol (Paris) 1952; 110: 112–7.

61   Müller JM, Schlittler E, Bein HJ. Reserpin der sedative wirkstoff aus Rauwolfia serpentine benth. Experientia 1952; 8: 338–9.

62   Bein H. Biological research in the pharmaceutical industry with reserpine. In: Ayd FJ Jr, Blackwell B, editors. Discoveries in Biological Psychiatry. Philadelphia: Lippincott; 1970. p. 142–54.

63   Delay J, Deniker P, Tardieu Y, Lemperière Th. Premiers essais en thérapeutique psychiatrique de la réserpine, alcaloïde nouveau de la Rauwolfia Serpentina. CR Congr Méd Alién Neurol (France) 1954; 52: 836–41.

64   Kline NS. Use of Rauwolfia serpentina benth in neuropsychiatric conditions. Ann NY Acad Sci 1954; 59: 107–32.

65   Noce RN, Williams DB, Rapaport W. Reserpine (Serpasil) in the management of the mentally ill and the mentally retarded. JAMA 1954; 156: 821–4.

66   Steck H. Le syndrome extrapyramidal et diencéphalique au cours des traitements au Largactil et au Serpasil. Ann Med Psychol 1954; 112: 737–43.

67   Berger FM. Anxiety and the discovery of the tranquilizers. In: Ayd FJ Jr, Blackwell B, editors. Discoveries in Biological Psychiatry. Philadelphia: Lippincott; 1970. p. 115–29.

68   Berger FM. As I remember. In: Ban TA, Healy D, Shorter E, editors. The Rise of Psychopharmacology and the Story of CINP. Budapest: Animula; 1998. p. 59–62.

69   Burger A. History. In: Usdin E, Forrest IS, editors. Psychotherapeutic Drugs. Part I Principles. New York: Marcel Dekker; 1976. p. 11–57.

70   Kuhn R. The discovery of the tricyclic antidepressants and the history of their use in early years. In: Ban TA, Ray OS, editors. The History of the CINP. Brentwood: JM Productions; 1996. p. 425–35.

71   Kuhn R. Über die Behandlung depressives Zustande mit einem iminodibenzyl-derivat (G22355). Schweiz Med Wochenschr 1957; 87: 1135–40.

72   Fox HH, Gibbs JT Synthetic tuberculostats. VII. Monoalkyl derivatives of isonicotinylhydrazine. J Organic Chem 1942; 18: 994–1002.

73   Zeller EA, Barsky JR, Fouts W, Kirscheimer WF, Van Oden LS. Influence of isonicotinic acid hydrazide (INH) and 1-isonicotinyl-2-isopropl hydrazide (IIH) on bacterial and mammalian enzymes. Experientia 1952; 8: 349–50.

74   Flaherty JA. The psychiatric use of isonicotinic acid hydrazide: a case report. Del Med J 1952; 24: 298–300.

75   Selikoff IJ, Robitzek E.H, Orenstein GG. Treatment of pulmonary tuberculosis with hydrazide derivatives of isonicotinic acid. JAMA 1952; 150: 973–87.

76   Pletscher A. Beeinflussung des 5-Hydroxytryptamin–stoffwechsels im Gehirn durch Isonikotinsäuere hydrazide. Experientia 1956; 12: 479–80.

77   Besendorf H, Pletscher A. Beeinflussung zentraler Wirkungen von Reserpin und 5-hydroxytryptamin durch Isonicotinic–säuerhydrazine. Helv Physiol Acta 1956; 14: 383–90.

78   Crane GE. Iproniazid (Marsilid) phosphate a therapeutic agent for mental disorders. Psychiatr Res Reports 1957; 8: 142-54.

79   Loomer HP, Sanders JC, Kline NS. A clinical and pharmacodynamic evaluation of iproniazid as a psychic energizer. Psychiatr Res Rep Am Psychiatr Assoc 1957; 8: 129–41.

80   Wortis J, Lambert RH. Irreversible or hypoglycemic insulin coma. Am J Psychatry 1939; 96: 335–45.

81   Wortis J, Jackim E. Effects of chlorpromazine on brain tissue preparations. Am J Psychiatry 1962; 119: 363–6.

82   Gottschalk LA. Content Analysis of Verbal Behaviour: New Findings and Clinical Applications. Hillsdale, NJ: Lauwrence Erlbaum; 1995.

83   Sarwer-Foner GJ. Psychoanalytic theories of activity-passivity conflicts and of the continuum of ego defences: experimental verification using reserpine and chlorpromazine. Arch Neurol Psychiatry 1957; 78: 413–8.

84   Azima H. Psychodynamic alterations concomitant with Tofranil administration. Can Psychiatr Assoc J 1959; 4: 172–81.

85   Ostow M. Drugs in Psychoanalysis and Psychotherapy. New York: Basic Books; 1962.

86   Szára S. Dimethyltryptamine: its metabolism in man; the relation of its psychotic effect to serotonin metabolism. Experientia 1956; 12: 441–2.

87   Szára S, Axelrod J, Perlin S. Is adrenochrome present in the blood? Am J Psychiatry 1958; 115: 162–4.

88   Domino EF. Neurobiology of phencyclidine (Sernyl), a drug with unusual spectrum of activity. Int Rev Neurobiol 1964; 6: 303–47.

89   Domino EF, Chodoff P, Corssen G. Pharmacological effects of CI-581 (ketamine,) a new dissociative anesthetic in man. Clin Pharmacol Ther 1966; 6: 279–91.

90   Kalinowsky L, Hippius H. Pharmacological, Convulsive and Other Somatic Treatments in Psychiatry. New York: Grune & Stratton; 1969.

91   Benkert O, Hippius H. Psychiatrische Pharmakotherapie. Berlin: Springer; 1974.

92   Lehmann HE, Hanrahan GE. Chlorpromazine, new inhibiting agent for psychomotor excitement and manic states. Arch Neurol Psychiatry 1954; 71: 227–37.

93   Lehmann HE, Cahn CH, deVerteuil R. Treatment of depressive conditions with imipramine (G-22355) Can Psychiatr Assoc J 1958; 3: 155–64.

94   Hollister LE, Krieger GE, Kringel A, Roberts RH. Treatment of schizophrenic reactions with reserpine. NY Acad Sci 1955; 61: 92–100.

95   Hollister LE. Clinical Psychopharmacology of Psychotherapeutic Drugs. New York: Churchill Livingstone; 1978.

96   Ayd FJ. Treatment of psychiatric patients with Thorazine. South Med J 1955; 48: 177–86.

97   Ayd FJ. Amitriptyline (Elavil) therapy of depressive reactions. Psychsomatics 1960; 1: 320–5.

98   Ayd FJ. Lexicon of Psychiatry, Neurology and the Neurosciences. Second Ed. Philadelphia: Lippincott Williams & Wilkins; 2000.

99   Kurland AA. Comparison of chlorpromazine and reserpine in the treatment of schizophrenia. Arch Neurol Psychiatry 1956; 75: 510–3.

100   Kurland AA, Unger SM, Shaffer JW, Savage C. Psychedelic therapy utilizing LSD in the treatment of the alcoholic patient: a preliminary report. Am J Psychiatry; 123: 1202–9.

101   Hoffer A, Osmond H. New Hope for Alcoholics. New Hyde Park, NY: University Books; 1968.

102   Merlis S, Turner WJ. Drug evaluation and practice of psychiatric therapies. JAMA 1961; 177: 39–42

103   Turner WJ, Krumholz W, Merlis S. A modified Malamud-Sands Rating Scale for use by ward personnel. Psychopharmacol Serv Cent Bull 1962; 2: 11–4.

104   Freedman AM, Efron AS, Bender L. Pharmacotherapy in children with psychiatric illness. J Nerv Ment Dis 1955; 122: 479–85.

105   Freedman AM, Zaks A, Resnick R, Fink M. Blockade with methadone, cyclazocine and naloxone. Int J Addict 1970; 5: 507–15.

106   Detre T, Jarecki HG. Modern Psychiatric Treatment. Philadelphia: Lippincott; 1971.

107   Detre T. The way we were and the way we are. In: Ban TA, Healy D, Shorter E, editors. Reflections on Twentieth-Century Psychopharmacology. Budapest: Animula; 2004. p. 217–22.

108   Lasagan L. The controlled clinical trial. Theory and Practice 1955; 1: 353–67.

109   Lasagna L. Back to the future: evaluation and drug development. 1949–1998. In: Healy D. The Psychopharmacologists II: Interviews. London: Arnold; 1998. p. 135–65.

110   Carr CJ. Science on Trial. Regul Toxicol Pharmacol 1996; 24: 102–3.

111   Iversen SD, Iversen LL. Behavioral Pharmacology. Oxford Univesity Press; 1981.

112   Pavlov IP. Conditioned Reflexes. Translated by GV Anrep. Oxford: Oxford University Press; 1927.

113   Pavlov IP. Conditioned Reflexes and Psychiatry. Translated by WH Gantt. Chicago: International University Press; 1941.

114   Gantt WH. Effect of alcohol on cortical and subcortical activity measured by the conditional reflex method. Bull. Johns Hopkins Hosp 1935; 56: 61–83.

115   Freile M, Gantt WH. Effect of adrenalin and acetylcholine on excitation and inhibition and neuroses. Trans Am Neurol Assoc 1944; 70: 180–1.

116   Gliedman L, Gantt WH. The effect of reserpine, chlorpromazine and morphine on the orienting response. In: Gantt WH, editor. Physiological Basis of Psychiatry. Springfield: Charles C. Thomas; 1958. p. 196–206.

117   Stoff DM, Bridger W. Horsley W. Gantt: The first Amerian psychopharmacologist. In: McGuigan FJ, Ban TA, editors. Critical Issues in Psychology, Psychiatry and Physiology. New York: Gordon and Breach Science Publishers; 1987. p. 177–87.

118   Skinner BF. The Behavior of the Organisms: An Experimental Analysis. New York: Appleton-Century; 1938.

119   Brady JV. Comparative psychopharmacology: animal experimental studies on the effects of drugs on behavior. In: Cole JO, Gerard RW, editors. Psychopharmacology Problems in Evaluation. Washington: National Academy of Sciences – National Research Council; 1959. p. 46–63.

120   Brady JV. Assessment of drug effects on emotional behavior. Science 1956; 123: 1033–4.

121   Dews PB. The measurement of the influence of drugs on voluntary activity in mice. Br J Pharmacol 1953; 8: 46–8.

122   Dews PP. Studies on behaviour. I. Differential sensitivity to pentobarbital or pecking performance in pigeons depending on the schedule of reward. J Pharmacol Exp Ther 1955; 113: 393–401.

123   Cook L, Wesley E. Behavioral effects of some psychopharmacological agents. Ann NY Acad` Sci 1957; 66:740–52.

124   Cook L, Catania AC. Effect of drugs on avoidance and escape behavior in neuropsychopharmacology. Fed Proc 1964; 23: 818–35.

125   Cook L. Memoirs of psychopharmacology. From the Beginning. In Ban TA, Healy D, Shorter E, editors. The Triumph of Psychopharmacology and the Story of CINP. Budapest: Animula; 2000. p. 38–42.

126   Baxter BL, Gluckman MI, Stein L, Scerni RA. Self-injection of apomorphine in the rat: Positive rein-
       forcement by a dopamine receptor stimulant. Pharmacol, Biochem Behav 1974; 2: 387–91.
127   Stein L, Belluzzi JD, Ritter S, Wise D. Self-stimulation, reward pathways, norepinephrine vs dopamine.J
       Psychiatr Res 1974; 11: 115–24.
128   Elkes J, Elkes C. Effects of chlorpromazine on the behavior of chronically overactive psychotic pa-
       tients. Br Med J 1954; 2: 560–76.
129   Ban TA. Foreword. In: Ban TA, editor. Selected Writings of Joel Elkes. Budapest: Animula; 2001. p.
       11–21.
130   Elkes J, Elkes C, Bradley P. The effects of some drugs on the electrical activity of the brain and behav-
       iour. J Ment Sci 1954; 100: 125–8.
131   Bradley PB, Elkes J. The effects of some drugs on the electrical activity of the brain. Brain 1957; 80:
       77–117.
132   Elkes J, Todrick A. On the development of the cholinesterases in the rat brain. In: Waelsch H, editor.
       Biochemistry of the Developing Nervous System. New York: Academic Press; 1955.
133   Elkes J, Eyars JT, Todrick A. On the effect and the lack of effect of some drugs on postnatal develop-
       ment in the rat. In: Waelsch H, editor. Biochemistry of the Developing Nervous System. New York:
       Academic Press; 1955.
134   Soares JC, Gershon S. THA – historical aspects, review of pharmacological properties and theapeutic
       effects. Dementia 1995; 6: 225–34.
135   Gershon S, Olaria J. JB-329, a new psychotomimetic, its antagonism by tetrahydro-aminoacridane
       and its comparison with LSD, mescaline, and Sernyl. J Neuropsychiatry 1960; 1: 283–9.
136   Angrist, B, Gershon S. The phenomenology of experimentally induced amphetamine psychosis : pre-
       liminary observations. Biol Psychiatry 1970; 2: 95–107.
137   Shopsin B, Gershon S, Goldstein M, Friedman E, Wilk S. Use of synthesis inhibitors in defining the role
       for biogenic amines during imipramine treatment in depressed patients. Psychopharmacol Commun
       1975; 1: 239–49.
138   Gershon S, Trautner EM. Treatment of shock dependency by pharmacological agents. Med J Aust
       1956; 43: 783–7.
139   Gershon S, Yuwiler A. Lithium ion: A specific psychopharmacological approach to the treatment of
       mania. J Neuropsychiat 1960; 1: 229–41.
140   Shorter E. A Historical Dictionary of Psychiatry. Oxford: Oxford University Press; 2005.
141   Shorter E, Healy D. Shock Therapy: A History of Electroconvulsive Treatment of Mental Illness. New
       Brunswick, NJ: Rutgers University Press; 2007.
142   Swartz CM, Shorter E, Psychotic Depression. Cambridge: Cambridge University Press; 2007.
143   Shorter E. Before Prozac: The Troubled History of Mood Disorders in Psychiatry. Oxford: Oxford
       University Press; 2009.
144   Shorter E, Fink M. Endocrine Psychiatry: Solving the Riddle of Melancholia. Oxford: Oxford University
       Press; 2010.

CONTENTS

Overview of the Series, Thomas A. Ban ix
Interviewees & Interviewers xv

Volume 1 Starting Up

Preface, Thomas A. Ban xxv
Abbreviations xli
Introduction & Dramatis Personae, Edward Shorter xlv

Interviewees and Interviewers

Trialists 3

Frank J. Ayd, Jr. 5
 interviewed by Leo E. Hollister
Samuel Gershon 19
 interviewed by Thomas A. Ban
Hanns F. Hippius 35
 interviewed by Andrea Tone
Leo E. Hollister 39
 interviewed by Frank J. Ayd, Jr.
Albert A. Kurland 63
 interviewed by Leo E. Hollister
Heinz E. Lehmann 81
 interviewed by William E. Bunney, Jr.
William J. Turner 91
 interviewed by Jo Ann Engelhardt

Pharmacologists 102

Joseph V. Brady 105
 interviewed by Leo E. Hollister
Charles Jelleff Carr 115
 interviewed by Thomas A. Ban
Leonard Cook 121
 interviewed by Larry Stein

Peter B. Dews   145
      interviewed by John A. Harvey
Edward F. Domino   157
      interviewed by Christian J. Gillin
Louis C. Lasagna   169
      interviewed by Donald F. Klein
Larry Stein   177
      interviewed by Arvid Carlsson

Clinical Scientists   188

Robert A. Cohen   191
      interviewed by Thomas A. Ban
Thomas Detre   205
      interviewed by Benjamin S. Bunney
Joel Elkes   211
      interviewed by Fridolin Sulser
Alfred M. Freedman   225
      interviewed by Thomas A. Ban
Louis A. Gottschalk   265
      interviewed by William E. Bunney, Jr.
Gerald J. Sarwer-Foner   277
      interviewed by A. George Awad
Stephen Szára   289
      interviewed by Leo E. Hollister
Joseph Wortis   311
      interviewed by Leo E. Hollister

Index   327

ABBREVIATIONS

A1 allele	allele of the D2 receptor gene
ACNP	American College of Neuropsychopharmacology
AIDS	acquired immunodeficiency syndrome
AMA	American Medical Association
AMPT	α-methylparatyrosine
APA	American Psychiatric Association
BPRS	Brief Psychiatric Rating Scale
CA1	cornu ammonis area 1
CA3	cornu ammonis area 3
CCK	cholecystokinin
CER	conditioned emotional response
CINP	Collegium Internationale Neuro- Psychopharmacologicum
CNS	central nervous system
Col	colonel
CPDD	College on Problems of Drug Dependence
CPZ	chlorpromazine
CR	conditioned reflex
CRC	Clinical Research Center
CV	curriculum vitae
D	dopamine receptor
DC	District of Columbia
DET	diethyltryptamine
DFP	di-isopropylphosphorofluoridate
DMPEA	3, 4-dimethoxyphenylalanine
DMT	dimethyltryptamine
DNA	deoxyribonucleic acid
DSc	Doctor of Science
DSM-I	Diagnostic and Statistical Manual (of the American Psychiatric Association) [first edition]
DSM-II	Diagnostic and Statistical Manual, second edition
DSM-III	Diagnostic and Statistical Manual, third edition
DSM-IV	Diagnostic and Statistical Manual, fourth edition
ECT	electroconvulsive therapy
EEG	electroencephalography
EKG	electrocardiography
FDA	Food and Drug Administration
fMRI	functional magnetic resonance imaging

GC	gas chromatography
GI	Government Issue
GNP	gross natural product
GS	General Staff
HIV	human immunodeficiency virus
HLA	human leukocyte antigens
HMO	Health Maintenance Organization
IBM	International Business Machines Corporation
ICU	intensive care unit
IRB	Institutional Review Board
IMPS	Inpatient Multidimensional Psychiatric Scale
IQ	intelligence quotient
ISPP	International Society of Political Psychology
IUPHAR	International Union of Basic and Clinical Pharmacology
JAMA	Journal of the American Medical Association
LAAM	Levo-α-acetylmethadol
LISP	LISf Processing (programming language)
LOD	logarithm of the odds
LSD	lysergic acid diethylamide
M	mescaline
MAO	monoamine oxidase
MAOI	monoamine oxidase inhibitor
Mass	Massachusetts
MD	medical doctor
MEql	milliequivalent
MHRI	Mental Health Institute (Ann Arbor, Michigan)
MIT	Massachusetts Institute of Technology
MMPI	Minnesota Multiphasic Personality Inventory
MPTP	1-methyl-4-phenyl-1, 2, 3, 6-tetrahydropyridine
MRI	magnetic resonance imaging
MS	mass spectrometry
MS	Mississippi
NAMI	National Alliance on Mental Illness (originally known as National Alliance for the Mentally Ill)
NARSAD	National Alliance for Research on Schizophrenia and Depression
NASA	National Aeronautics and Space Administration
NIAA	National Institute of Alcohol and Alcoholism
NIDA	National Institute on Drug Abuse
NIH	National Institutes of Health
NIMH	National Institute of Mental Health

NMR	nuclear magnetic resonance
NY	New York
NYA	National Youth Administration
NYAS	New York Academy of Sciences
NYU	New York University
OB/GYN	obstetrics and gynecology
OSS	Office of Strategic Services
PCP	phencyclidine
PCPA	p-chlorophenylalanine
Penn	Pennsylvania
PET	positron emission tomography
PhD	doctor of philosophy
PI	principal investigator
Pitts	University of Pittsburgh
PSA	prostate specific antigen
PSC	Psychopharmacology Service Center
PSP	prostate specific antigen
PTD	Prevention and Treatment of Depression
Reed	Walter Reed Army Hospital/Medical Center
REM	rapid eye movement
RFP	request for proposals
RNA	ribonucleic acid
ROTC	Reserve Officers' Training Corps
SK&F	Smith, Kline & French
SKF-525-A	ß-dimethylaminoethyl diphenylpropylacetate hydrochloride
SSRI	Selective serotonin reuptake inhibitor
STP	2, 5-dimethoxy-4-methyl-amphetamine
TB	tuberculosis
THA	tetrahydroaminoacridane
THC	tetrahydrocannabinol
TV	television
UCI	University of California Irvine
UCLA	University of California Los Angeles
UCSF	University of California San Francisco
UOEH	University of Occupational and Environmental Health
USPHS	United States Public Health Service
VA	Veterans' Administration
Washington U	Washington University (St. Louis, Missouri)
WHO	World Health Organization
WPA	World Psychiatric Association
Vs	versus

INTRODUCTION & DRAMATIS PERSONAE
Edward Shorter

The individuals in this volume had ringside seats at one of the great dramas in the history of modern medicine – and modern society – the triumph of biological thinking in psychiatry. They are in this volume because they were all pioneers, and they advanced knowledge in a subject that was considered at the time to be a non-subject: drugs that meliorate the symptoms of psychiatric illness. How could there be such a subject! In the 1950s and '60s the Freudian psychoanalysts who dominated psychiatry widely believed that the cause of psychiatric symptoms was psychogenic, that illness arose from psychic conflict within the mind. The brain was considered to have nothing to do with this. Hence a subject such as neuropsychopharmacology was almost by definition a non-subject – like an Orwellian non-person – irrelevant to clinicians because the brain was thought not to matter.

Yet outside the offices of the psychoanalysts, especially in the state hospitals where patients were unreachable with psychoanalysis, psychoactive drugs were indeed used. What was the status of psychopharmacology at the time? Psychoactive drugs had been used in medicine since time out of mind – black hellebore goes back to the Middle Ages. Thanks to the scientists of the German organic chemical industry, synthetic sedatives began appearing in the last third of the nineteenth century, capped by the barbiturates in 1901. 1930 is considered by some the beginning date of psychopharmacology as William Bleckwenn at the University of Wisconsin successfully employed amobarbital (sodium amytal) in the treatment of catatonia. The amphetamines began to be used in psychiatry with the advent of Smith, Kline & French's Benzedrine (amphetamine) sulfate in 1935. These were all important advances in the relief of anxiety, insomnia, and other behavioral conditions. Psychosis and melancholic depression remained, however, unreachable.

It was in the early 1950s that the revolution in psychopharmacology occurred. At the beginning, it was literally outside the compass of the medical imagination. Jelleff Carr, interviewed in this volume, was at the time a pharmacologist at the Psychopharmacology Service Center (PSC) of the National Institute of Mental Health (NIMH). He said of the late 1950s: "The whole subject of psychopharmacology was foreign to the thinking of physicians and people in general. It was a very unique moment in history. . . . It was believed for hundreds of years that when people got crazy that was the end of it. Now, we were saying that one can give them a pill and they will get better."

Even within the pharmaceutical industry, the notion that psychoactive drugs could modify behavior was met with disbelief. It was Smith, Kline & French (SK&F) that in the 1930s developed the amphetamines, and certainly by the early 1950s SK&F was indicating dextroamphetamine for minor depression. Yet the big illnesses, such as schizophrenia, seemed out of reach. Len Cook started working for SK&F as their head of pharmacology in the early 1950s, just as they were developing chlorpromazine, the first antipsychotic agent. Cook recalls in his interview with Larry Stein, "Even people in our research commit- tee felt that it was not possible that a drug could affect your thoughts and your mind, as a drug could affect the pumping action of the heart or be a diuretic. . . . For decades people felt that behavior was a free will thing and that drugs, really, didn't affect the mind as they did, for example, the heart."

Psychiatry, with its Freudian history of insisting on the mind's independence from the brain, was even more resistant than pharmacology. Psychoanalyst Jules Masserman, a leading light in psychiatric circles, is said to have scorned chlorpromazine, the first of the antipsychotic agents, as a "glorified seda- tive."[1] Yet with the advent of new medications, psychiatric practice began to steer away from depth psychotherapy and back towards biological perspec- tives. This occurred with the so-called "tranquilizers": reserpine (Serpasil), chlorpromazine (Thorazine, Largactil), and meprobamate (Miltown, Equanil), all launched in a brief window between 1953 and 1955. It was in 1955 that Thomas Detre, later chair of psychiatry at the University of Pittsburgh, began his residency at Yale, still very much under the influence of psychoanalysis. He said in his interview with Benjamin ("Steve") Bunney in this volume that at the first teaching conference he attended at Yale, the resident presented a female patient with agitated schizophrenia: "I proposed that instead of treating this young woman just with psychotherapy, we might want to give her some chlor- promazine. Jules Coleman (an analyst who was a big figure at Yale) just stared, but one of my fellow residents . . . said, 'This guy is for the birds.' That was the attitude. Things got even worse when I became . . . chief resident of the Yale Psychiatric Institute, where to the consternation of everyone, I suggested that the era of neuropsychopharmacology had arrived."

The era of neuropsychopharmacology had arrived. Who knew? It was like the fat pashas of the late Ottoman Empire who glimpsed in the distance the horsemen of the Young Turks. Could change be coming? Why did this revolu- tion not occur earlier with the barbiturates or amphetamines? Both drug classes had been highly effective in various psychiatric disorders. Why did the revolu- tion not begin with them? In the early 1950s two new circumstances appeared: (1) The awakening of scientific interest in the neurotransmitters, which offered a theoretical mechanism for getting from drug action to behavioral illness;[2] (2) the advent of a technique for measuring the concentration of biogenic amines in neural tissue. The spectrophotofluorometer originated in 1955 and made it possible to link specific pharmacologic agents and neurochemicals to given behavioral changes.

What difference did these scientific events make in the lives of patients? In his interview William J. Turner, on staff at Central Islip State Hospital on Long Island, one of the largest and most desolate psychiatric hospitals in the United States, recalls Henry Brill, chief of the New York State Hospital system, mandating that patients be treated with chlorpromazine: "It was a hoard of miracles to see people who came in (to Central Islip), in a terrible state, accompanied by a husband who is tormented and distraught and to see that same patient leave the hospital a couple of weeks later, radiant, buoyant with life, with her husband cheerful, running with the daughter, running up to see the mother. Thorazine, in just a couple of weeks, transformed this woman from the drab terrified person to a happy mother."

Thus, the epochal changes that began in neuroscience and in clinical science resulted in great improvements in public health. The interviews in this volume offer a cross-section across these changes, from trialists, to pharmacologists, to clinical scientists. For example, a key contribution came in 1956 from psychologist Joseph Brady at Walter Reed Hospital on the mental effects of reserpine[3] (See Brady, in this volume). It was Brady who championed "behavioral pharmacology," which means roughly the same as psychopharmacology. A host of researchers attributed their formation in the new science to Brady at "the Reed."

Many pioneers of psychopharmacology are not featured in this volume. Some, such as Daniel Freedman, chair of psychiatry at the University of Chicago, passed on before they could be interviewed. Others, such as German trialist Arno Voelkel, were never members of the American College of Neuropsychopharmacology (ACNP). Numerous pioneers are distributed throughout other volumes in this series. Thus, the pioneers of psychopharmacology in this volume do not by any means represent a comprehensive list.

Yet there are key figures here. Almost all, with a few exceptions such as Robert Cohen (born 1909), William Turner (born 1907), Joseph Wortis (born 1906) or Larry Stein (born 1932) were born in the 1910s and 1920s, and accordingly were in their thirties and forties – and in strategic positions – as the psychopharmacological revolution started to break across the psychiatric landscape. There is a heavy representation of Americans, appropriately so because the new drugs tended to be *developed* in the US, although many – such as chlorpromazine – were *discovered* in Europe. This is because in the 1950s the American pharmaceutical industry was just starting to flex its muscles, disposing of material resources of which their European colleagues could only dream. And the individuals featured here are – alas – all men, because in the 1950s and early '60s female scientists, though present, were not numerous. For various reasons, therefore, it takes a bit of cheek to call this volume "The Pioneers of Psychopharmacology." Yet pioneers they were.

Dramatis Personae

The following pages introduce the dramatis personae of this volume in enough detail to give a framework for understanding their achievements.

The interviewees are grouped into trialists, who demonstrated the efficacy and the pitfalls of the new drugs; pharmacologists, who attempted to discover their mechanism of action; and clinical scientists, who tried to put the changes into the context of clinical care.

Trialists

Frank J. Ayd, Jr. is remembered as one of the classic trialists, conducting large numbers of early and important drug trials from his clinical base at Taylor Manor Hospital near Baltimore. He became attracted to biological approaches to psychiatry when he saw the dramatic effect of electroconvulsive treatment on his own father. He became intrigued with psychopharmacology in the early 1950s when Squibb asked him to conduct a clinical trial on mephenesin, a muscle relaxant that Frank Berger had introduced to American psychiatry. The short duration of action of mephenesin made it unsuitable for psychiatric use. But in 1953 SK&F prevailed upon him to undertake trials for Thorazine, the drug that launched psychopharmacology. Ayd was closely identified with trials for the tricyclic antidepressant amitriptyline (Merck's Elavil), and it was at the company's urging that Ayd wrote what was probably the first psychopharmacology bestseller, *Recognizing the Depressed Patient*; the company distributed 50,000 copies.[4]

Ayd was a key figure in founding ACNP, among the people, including Leo Hollister, whom Ted Rothman talked to about getting a group together for a weekend at the Barbizon-Plaza Hotel in New York in November 1960.[5] Six years later, in 1966, he began editing the influential *International Drug Therapy Newsletter*.

Ayd, an intensely observant Catholic, will also be remembered for a series of broadcasts over Vatican Radio that he conducted from 1962 to 1965 on the subject of medicine. The most enduring monument that he leaves behind is the massive *Lexicon of Psychiatry, Neurology and the Neurosciences*, the first edition of which was published by Williams & Wilkins in 1995. Of the second edition (2000), reviewer Ronald Pies, at the Tufts University School of Medicine in Boston, said, "Dr. Ayd has created an invaluable – indeed a monumental –

contribution to the professional reference library."[66] Ayd did not have a regular academic appointment, and was said to have been looked down on for his drug trial work by some of the snooty academics at Johns Hopkins University, in those days still mired in psychoanalysis.[7] Yet he clearly figures as one of the founders of psychopharmacology.

It was *Samuel Gershon* who brought lithium to the US.[8] Yet Gershon himself had much wider interests. The story begins with Gershon's residency in psychiatry in Melbourne in the early 1950s and his fellowship in pharmacology. In the department of pharmacology he worked with expatriated German physiologist Edward Trautner in early clinical studies of lithium, discovering for example that in manic-depressive illness maintenance lithium therapy could replace maintenance electroconvulsive therapy (ECT). In 1959/60 Gershon briefly joined Ralph Gerard's "Schizophrenia and Psychopharmacology" project at the University of Michigan before returning to Melbourne. Gershon's definitive migration to the US occurred in 1963, when Max Fink asked him to beef up the pharmacology side of their research at the Missouri Institute of Psychiatry. Although the focus of Gershon's research in those years was more on psychotogens such as phencyclidine rather than lithium, Gershon's 1960 article, co-written with Arthur Yuwiler, is nonetheless considered the formal introduction of lithium to the US scientific community.[9] In 1965, Arnold Friedhoff recruited Gershon to the department of psychiatry of New York University (NYU). Interest in lithium was now blossoming in US psychiatry, although lithium was not admitted by the Food and Drug Administration (FDA) until 1970.

At NYU Gershon organized a lithium clinic, where the doctrine of lithium's specificity in mania was further fortified. In his interview with Thomas Ban, Gershon said of those years, "Studies were done in a schizophrenia group and a schizoaffective group and it appeared fairly clearly that in that group, lithium was dramatically less effective than the neuroleptic. . . . It appeared to increase pathology."

In 1965 Gershon founded the Neuropsychopharmacology Research Unit at NYU, which he directed until his departure in 1980 for Detroit. As well, at NYU he and colleagues developed one of the early centers for the study of Alzheimer's disease. Thomas Ban spoke teasingly of the NYU years: "So these were the activities in the famous Sam Gershon unit at NYU?"

Gershon: "Right. The psychopharmacology group was not only a vehicle for research. It was also a production line for very talented people to become successful."

Gershon moved from Detroit to Pittsburgh at Tom Detre's behest, as Associate Vice-Chancellor for Research at the University of Pittsburgh from 1988 to 1995 and director of the Alzheimer's Disease Research Center. Under the influence of Detre and Gershon, Pittsburgh became a world power in psychopharmacology research.

After his retirement from the University of Pittsburgh, Gershon moved to Miami to become vice-chair of academic affairs in the department of psychiatry at the University of Miami. He continued to do research, studying for example inositol in treatment-resistant depression.

Ban: "So, this was your last publication?"

Gershon: "Don't say the last. That's a horrible thing to say. Most recent. . . . "

It was *Hanns Hippius* who led German psychiatry away from its National Socialist past and back into the international scientific community. He reached twenty just as the Second World War ended, graduating in medicine five years later; he studied immunology for two years at the Institute for Experimental Therapy in Marburg, then began training in psychiatry at the Free University of Berlin in 1953. Hippius came on staff in the department of psychiatry and organized a psychopharmacology group, searching for an antipsychotic with fewer extrapyramidal effects than those of chlorpromazine. In 1957 they settled on the phenothiazine perazine (Taxilan), an antipsychotic agent few outside of Germany have ever heard of. In 1971 Hippius became professor of psychiatry and head of the university psychiatric clinic in Munich, a city that once had been the epicenter of German psychiatry, where Emil Kraepelin fifty years earlier not only was professor of psychiatry but established the German Psychiatric Research Institute (Deutsche Forschunsanstalt für Psychiatrie). Hippius re-established an international profile for the department.

Meanwhile, the Wander pharmaceutical company in Berne, Switzerland, had produced a series of five tricyclic agents with a chemical similarity to dibenzepine. Wander offered them to the Berlin group for testing. One of these was clozapine, the first of the "atypical" antipsychotics. A Zurich group under Jules Angst conducted the first randomly controlled trials on clozapine, and both the Berlin and Zurich researchers were glad about the positive results in psychosis. Wander was then acquired by Sandoz; shortly thereafter agranulocytosis was noted as a clozapine side effect, and the development of the drug was put on hold for twenty years. It was really the agitation by Hippius, Angst, and several others that motivated Sandoz to revive clozapine.[10] It was licensed for the American market in 1990.

Hippius had a strong interest in the history of psychiatry, and in 2004 headed a team that wrote the richly illustrated volume, *The University Department of Psychiatry in Munich: From Kraepelin and His Predecessors to Molecular Psychiatry*.[11]

It is a measure of *Leo Hollister s* distinction that he became the dean of American psychopharmacology without having ever studied either psychiatry or pharmacology. (He became interested in drugs while working in a drug store as an undergraduate at the University of Cincinnati.) Hollister qualified as an internist in 1951, then spent the rest of his career – with the exception of a few final years at the University of Texas Medical School in Houston –- at the Veterans' Administration (VA) Hospital in Palo Alto, California, which was then basically a psychiatric facility.

Hollister arrived at Palo Alto in 1953 as chief of the medical service, later becoming associate chief of staff and senior medical investigator. He became drawn into psychopharmacology after he introduced reserpine at the VA as an antihypertensive, and saw that it had antipsychotic effects. At Palo Alto he pioneered randomly controlled trials using a parallel design on the entire first drug set of the 1950s and early '60s; his interests ranged from the psychotomimetics[12] to the benzodiazepines.[13] (It was at Palo Alto, incidentally, that Ken Kesey worked as an orderly, before going on to write *One Flew Over the Cuckoos Nest* in 1962.) Hollister was also a force in the VA Cooperative Studies Program, which ran the first large multi-center trials confirming the effectiveness of the new agents, an achievement for which the VA has never been sufficiently recognized. In addition to several decades of wise advice about the conduct of clinical trials, Hollister stoked interest in psychiatry in lysergic acid diethylamide (LSD) and the psychotogens; later he fought against the unfair stigmatization of the benzodiazepines as being somehow terribly addictive. He also wrote in 1978 a widely consulted psychopharmacology manual.[14] He was president of the ACNP in 1974. His tall gaunt figure was a familiar sight at psychopharmacology meetings, and an entire generation of clinicians and scientists looks back fondly on his memory.

Albert Kurland is among the most engaging yet controversial figures in the often colorful history of psychopharmacology. He grew up in Pennsylvania and earned his MD at the University of Maryland in 1940. After training at military facilities during the Second World War (and seeing extensive combat), he had a fellowship in neuropsychiatry at the Sinai Hospital in Baltimore. Kurland came on staff at the state hospital in Spring Grove, Maryland, in 1949, becoming director of medical research in 1953. He stayed at Spring Grove in various capacities for the rest of his career, deploying his energy to build the Maryland Psychiatric Research Center. But that was evidently not where his heart lay.

In 1953 Charles Savage at NIMH induced Kurland to undertake research on LSD; in 1960 Kurland conducted an open trial of the agent as an adjuvant in psychotherapy; this was followed by a controlled trial. He also used LSD to treat patients with illnesses such as cancer[15] and other highly experimental indications, publishing relatively little of this work[16] and in marginal journals.[17] In 1979 he was disqualified as an investigator by the FDA. Kurland saw himself as a scientist, not a hippie, though he often took LSD and other psychotomimetic substances (but so did numerous other investigators in the 1960s). The op-probrium that later struck his work was as much a matter of political disfavor as of any shortcomings on his part, save perhaps a tin-ear to growing societal conservatism about "psychedelics."

Heinz Lehmann, director of the Verdun Protestant Hospital in a suburb of Montreal, Canada, and professor of psychiatry at McGill University, organized the first North American trials of chlorpromazine,[18] imipramine,[19] and the first trial in which the monoamine oxidase (MAO) inhibitor iproniazid (Marsilid) was shown to be effective.[20] (Lehmann's report on iproniazid appeared in January 1958, Nate Kline's in June, though Kline gets credit for mentioning the effectiveness of iproniazid at a psychiatric meeting the previous year.) Lehmann was a trialists' trialist.

Heinz Edgar Lehmann was born in Berlin in 1911, the son of a Jewish father and a non-Jewish mother, and gained his medical degree at the University of Berlin in 1935, two years after Hitler's seizure of power. (For a thumbnail biography see Shorter 2005, pp. 160–161[21]) He interned at the Jewish General Hospital and the Martin Luther Hospital in Berlin then fled the country. Without any postgraduate training, he took a post in 1937 at the Verdun Protestant Hospital (now the Douglas Hospital), where initially he had, according to one biographer, "a caseload of 600 patients." He said, "That was my postgraduate training in psychiatry."[22] From 1947 to 1966 Lehmann was clinical director of the hospital, thereafter director of medical education and consultant. He was emerited as professor of psychiatry at McGill in 1981.

In 1958 Lehmann was joined by Thomas Ban, from Budapest, Hungary. Ban became the spark plug that drove forward many of the Verdun Hospital's trials. "There's hardly any drug, between 1952 and 1970, that we didn't do clinical trials with," Lehmann said in the interview. In the late 1950s Lehmann and Ban figured among the chief trialists of NIMH's Psychopharmacology Service Center, established in 1956. Lehmann was actually not a great believer in biological psychiatry, though he was grateful that the drugs were effective. As he remarked in the interview, he thought there was a "physical substrate" to the psychoses but not to the neuroses. He remained his life long a proponent of the virtues of psychotherapy and even psychoanalysis. (He had read Freud's works while in high school and never lost his enthusiasm for depth psychiatry.) He was skeptical of rating scales and large trials with undifferentiated diagnoses, preferring like many clinicians of his generation, such as Swiss psychiatrist Roland Kuhn (who initially discovered the effectiveness of imipramine), the close observation of individual patients. Yet in an institution such as Verdun, the patients were often very sick, and the effectiveness of the new agents lay at hand, regardless of whatever one thought of psychotherapy for what were then called "the walking wounded."

Lehmann was also a shrewd nosologist, and came out early against the large American overdiagnosis of "schizophrenia."[23] He coined in 1961 the term "antipsychotic," a more exact description of the action of the phenothiazines and butyrophenones than "neuroleptic."[24] Somewhat against his will, he said wryly, he became one of the founders of ACNP.

When *William Turner* attended the founding meeting of ACNP at the Barbizon-Plaza Hotel in New York on November 12, 1960, he was one of the older members. At the time a research psychiatrist at the Central Islip State Hospital on Long Island under Sidney Merlis, Turner was already 53. He had begun his scientific career in the VA Hospital system in 1937 at the North Little Rock hospital in Arkansas, where he was simply told that he was "a psychiatrist." In 1941 he migrated to the Northport, New York, VA hospital, where he opened the first research division of a VA facility. Turner took credit for the first use of electroencephalography in the VA. After the Second World War he served on the staff of the Huntington Hospital in New York State, where he stayed for the rest of his career, simultaneously beginning a private practice in Huntington. Supported by financier Jack Dreyfus, Turner set up a Dilantin (phenytoin) clinic at Huntington for people with lesser psychiatric symptoms. In 1954 Turner volunteered to help out as research psychiatrist at Central Islip, where he participated in drug evaluations for the Early Clinical Drug Evaluation program of NIMH. He recalled on one occasion, "We were the first or the second (and often the only ones) to test some 30 different compounds on patients." He and his colleagues, led by Wilhelm Krumholz, prided themselves on "a most enviable record of never approving for further study a drug which later had to be withdrawn, and only once failing to approve a drug which later became widely used." He was simultaneously professor of psychiatry at the State University of New York at Stony Brook.

In 1994 Turner moved from New York to Albuquerque, where, on staff in the department of psychiatry of the New Mexico State University, he published his discovery of greatest resonance: that there was a likely gene for homosexuality on the X chromosome.[25]

Turner was involved in efforts to integrate discharged psychiatric patients in the community, and served on the board of several halfway houses. Of the "Clubhouse," which he helped found, he wrote, "It is amazingly effective in bringing men and women, formerly hospitalized for years, into the community of employed, self-directed citizens." He added modestly, "I must emphasize that, *not I*, but the workers and the members of the Clubhouse are responsible for this."[26]

Pharmacologists

Joseph Brady pioneered the realm of behavioral pharmacology, beginning with his graduate work in psychology at the University of Chicago in the late 1940s and progressing through his appointment at Walter Reed Hospital as deputy director of the division of neuropsychiatry in 1963. At Walter Reed in the 1950s, Brady amplified the research of James Olds and Peter Milner[27] on pleasure centers in the brain that responded to electrical stimulation, and coined the term "self-stimulation."[28]

It was the program of research on the conditional reflex leading from this discovery that interested Brady: Not only did drugs function as biochemical agents in the central nervous system, Brady said, "They functioned as signals, and this is where the whole drug discrimination area has come from." Using the conditional emotional response, or CER, Brady investigated behavioral sequelae of a number of members of the "first drug set," as the pharmacologic agents of the 1950s are sometimes called. As Brady's biographer puts it, "Brady clearly saw the potential for widespread application of schedule-controlled operant behavior to the pharmaceutical industry and became a very early advocate for applying these procedures to preclinical drug discovery efforts."[29]

In 1967 Brady became professor of behavioral biology at Johns Hopkins, where his interests migrated to drug abuse and addiction. Brady, in a scientific career spanning more than 50 years, implemented the "mobile methadone maintenance treatment approach" in Baltimore.

In 1949 *Charles Jelleff Carr*, a pharmacologist at the University of Maryland, co-authored one of the early textbooks, *The Pharmacological Principles of Medical Practice*, published by Williams & Wilkins; it was said by a biographer to be "the standard in the education of generations of physicians, in North and South America, India, Australia, South Africa and the Philippines. His scientific influence touched uncounted millions of people in four continents."[30] Yet Carr grew tired of the continuing ardor required to keep a textbook in ever new editions: "I had to spend my whole time to keep the stuff going," he said in the interview. Carr turned a page when Jonathan Cole, director of the Psychopharmacology Service Center (PSC) at NIMH, asked him in 1957 to become senior pharmacologist there. Jelleff thus found himself at the very eye of the storm, as the PSC commissioned the important early drug trials in psychopharmacology. After leaving NIMH, in 1963 Carr founded a journal, *Regulatory Toxicology and Pharmacology,* directed at consultants who advised pharmaceutical companies about product safety before submitting New Drug Applications for regulatory approval. Interviewer Thomas Ban concluded the session by noting, "Your work has had a major impact on toxicology."

Carr: "I like to think that."

Carr died in 2005.

The interview with pharmacologist *Leonard (Len) Cook* will be a brisk wake-me-up for those who think "Prince of Darkness" whenever they hear "pharmaceutical industry." Beginning with SK&F in 1951, Cook spent 45 years directing neuropharmacological research in industry laboratories, and coming up with fundamental insights about differential drug effects. Yet even when he was a graduate student at Yale in the late 1940s, academics held the pharmaceutical industry in bad odor. Cook told his professor that his starting salary at Smith Kline would be a thousand dollars more than the professor was currently making. The professor stood "speechless," and then washed his hands of Cook as a "prostitute."

In devising preclinical behavioral tests for chlorpromazine, it was Cook who determined that conditioned avoidance would single out the antipsychotics, while "the conflict and fixed interval test" would select the anxiolytics. This was a fundamental insight, the more so given that among the antipsychotics the correlation between clinical efficacy and conditioned avoidance was an astonishingly high 0.9.

All perfect with industry? Not really, says Cook. Between 1954 and 1994, he argues, management has increasingly intruded upon the independence of industry's scientific process of drug discovery with "concerns about resources, specific goals and 'bang for the buck.'" There has been much agonizing about "empty pipelines" in the discovery of new drugs, but Cook puts his finger on one of the root causes: "What you have lost in this program of research discovery is the ingenuity of the individual scientists to follow their nose, and how long they should continue on something, because it's pretty hard to put a timetable on discovery. . . . Today planning committees tell the scientists in industry exactly what they're going to do, when they're going to do it and even though there's a little latitude for individual contribution, it's not what it really should be or was at the time."

Among the leaders of behavioral pharmacology – studying behavioral not just physiological results of drug action – was *Peter Dews*, born in Ossett, England, in 1922. Dews graduated in medicine at the University of Leeds, England, in 1944. He lectured in pharmacology there then crossed the ocean to work in the Wellcome Research Laboratories in Tuckahoe, New York, in 1948–49. In 1951 he earned a PhD in physiology at the University of Minnesota.

Dews ended up working on the pharmacology of behavior as a result of a chance encounter in 1953 with the Harvard behaviorist B. F. Skinner. Dews pioneered the use of such behavioral techniques as "schedules of reinforcement" and "fixed interval schedules" in pharmacology. A key early paper appeared in the *Journal of Pharmacology and Experimental Therapeutics* in 1955.[31] Dews went on to elaborate a "molecular" hypothesis of "schedule controlling methods." His assumption was that the schedules of daily life might have a bio-chemical platform, and that illnesses such as depression or psychosis might have a "scheduling" component as well. According to one of his biographers, "The experimental findings generated by Dews's [sic] research, blending the sophisticated use of behavior and pharmacological principles together with the elegant manner of their presentation and far-reaching implications, provided the force and momentum to establish and direct behavioral pharmacology for several decades."[32]

In the founding years of ACNP, an important contingent came from the University of Michigan, whose Department of Pharmacology and Mental Health Research Institute were world-class centers. Pharmacologist *Edward Domino* figured among these, born in Chicago and trained in medicine and pharmacology at the University of Illinois Medical School. Just as a number of other Chicagoans, such as neurophysiologist Ralph Gerard, drifted north to Michigan – Gerard going to a new research institute in Ypsilanti – Domino joined the pharmacologists in Ann Arbor. The legendary Maurice H. Seevers was head of that department and told Domino, "Ed, if you're good and you can make it here I'll promote you to assistant professor. If you're no damn good, then in six or nine months I'll let you know and you're out of here on the street at the end of the year." Domino remained at Michigan for the rest of his career. In this interview with Chris Gillin, Domino was quite frank about what drove his research: the need for grants. Somewhat tongue in cheek, he says that as intellectual fashions changed, so did his work, cycling through anti-Parkinsonian agents, drugs of addiction, and other issues that had caught the attention of the grant-givers. Domino's modesty and self-deprecation are charming, yet his interview is a reality check for beginning researchers who want to keep their heads above water.

Louis Lasagna, sometimes called "the father of clinical pharmacology," founded the first program in the United States at Johns Hopkins University in 1954. "The very discipline of clinical pharmacology . . . owes its beginnings to Lou Lasagna," stated one of his obituarists.[33]

Lasagna was born to Italian immigrant parents in New York City in 1923, and, after serving in the Navy, graduated MD from Columbia University in 1947; he trained in internal medicine at Maimonides Hospital. Taken on staff in the department of pharmacology at Johns Hopkins University in 1950, he went up to Boston two years later to work on an anesthesia project at Massachusetts General Hospital – his first involvement in pharmacology – then returned to Hopkins in 1954. At Massachusetts General Hospital he conducted the first random placebo-controlled trial in psychopharmacology in the US (he used parallel groups), publishing "a comparison of hypnotic agents" (chloral hydrate, pentobarbital, methylparafynol and placebo) in 1954.[34] In 1956 he brought out the results of a placebo-controlled trial of hypnotics using a "Latin squares" design (starting the 44 patients randomly at a given position in the Latin square and then rotating them about the squares on the different medications in the study). The drugs were methyprylon (Noludar), meprobamate (Miltown, Equanil), and three barbiturates. He discovered that the two new drugs in the study – meprobamate and methyprylon – did have hypnotic properties but that the barbiturates were superior in inducing sleep.[35] In 1970 he became professor of pharmacology at the University of Rochester, founding the Center for the Study of Drug Development in 1976. The center migrated with him in 1985 to Tufts University in Boston, as he became dean of the Sackler School of Graduate Biomedical Sciences. The heart of Lasagna's academic interests remained psychopharmacology, although he also campaigned against over-regulation by the Food and Drug Administration, and in general strode upon the public stage in testifying before Congress or serving on blue-ribbon commissions.[36] Among his other accomplishments were to follow in Harry Gold's footsteps, reminding people of the importance of the placebo. He scorned puffed-up controlled trials as a gateway to knowledge about the body: "We know that most of our knowledge about disease, drug treatment, and drug toxicity has, in fact, come, not from controlled trials, but from naturalistic observations by smart physicians using their past knowledge and experience as control."[37]

In the heady days of the 1950s, as behavioral psychopharmacology was just being opened up, *Larry Stein* at the Walter Reed Army Institute for Research sat at the very center of the action. He had Joseph Brady as a mentor. A few miles away Bernard Brodie at the Heart Institute of the National Institutes of Health (NIH) was just teasing apart the behavioral effects of the neurotransmitters. And the NIMH was at the halfway point in its decade-long transition from research on psychoanalysis to neurobiology. With his work on amphetamine and chlorpromazine at the Reed and the VA Hospital in Pittsburgh later in the 1950s -- and at Wyeth Laboratories in the 1960s-- Stein helped open up the "catecholamine theory of brain stimulation reinforcement."[38] In his interview he shares with Arvid Carlsson a kind of eureka moment: "By God, I can still remember vividly Bruce Baxter (a co-worker at Wyeth) coming up to me one day very excited with the tracings, showing me that the rats loved to self-administer apomorphine!" (The prevailing view had been that apomorphine would make the rats vomit.) So, that was a very big early hint that dopamine should get more prominence in reward theory. By 1971 Stein had moved on to the concept of schizophrenia representing "a reward system out of control."[39]

In 1979 Stein accepted the chair of pharmacology at the University of California, Irvine campus. He remained fully an adept of behaviorism. In the interview Carlsson asked rather puckishly if Stein believed that "a single cell could have a mind?"

Stein: "All this makes me a little bit uncomfortable because I was brought up in a very behavioristic tradition – to me, mind is almost a naughty word."

Clinical Scientists

Talk about being present at the formative years of biological psychiatry: Nobody had more of a ringside seat than *Robert A. Cohen*, who spent most of his career at NIMH as a senior administrator. Cohen had studied neurophysiology with Ralph Gerard at the University of Chicago, gaining in 1935 an MD at the same time as a PhD. He then drifted into the ambit of psychoanalysis, and after serving in the Navy during the war, was on staff at Chestnut Lodge Sanatorium, a psychoanalytically oriented private hospital in Rockville, Maryland, where he was analyzed by Frieda Fromm-Reichmann. In 1952 Robert Felix, another analyst and founding director of NIMH, asked Cohen to come over to Bethesda and help administer the research program. Cohen arrived the following year. There followed the most extraordinary decade in the history of biological psychiatry as federally-supported scientists and clinicians, figures such as Seymour Kety, David Hamburg, Louis Sokoloff, and Joel Elkes, achieved a trail of discoveries.

Interestingly, in 1981 Cohen left NIMH to return to Chestnut Lodge. What was the reason for summoning back this, by now very senior clinician and administrator? Because the Lodge leadership were unable to persuade their younger clinical staff to prescribe, and thought that Cohen's influence might steer the Lodge a bit more towards psychopharmacology!

Tom Detre, along with Steve Szára and Thomas Ban, belongs to a cohort of thoughtful Hungarian physicians who decided to exchange Communism for the brilliant scientific beacon that American medicine offered after the Second World War. With an MD from the University of Rome in hand, Detre sought training first at Mount Sinai Hospital in New York, then at Yale. He had the independence of mind to shun the psychoanalysis that both institutions had on offer and to enter the world of clinical trials and neuroscience. Fritz Redlich at Yale, who accepted Detre into the program, had the gift of being able to reconcile both worlds, that of biological psychiatry and of psychoanalysis, and presided over a very fruitful decade in his chairmanship of that department from 1950 to 1967. In 1973 Detre left Yale for Pittsburgh, taking with him a host of colleagues who had made themselves unpopular at Yale with their chatter about neuroscience. As head of psychiatry, and later as vice-president of the University of Pittsburgh Medical Center, Detre built Pitts into a scientific powerhouse. In his interview with Steve Bunney, he describes the first phase of this ascent.

Born in 1913 in Königsberg, Germany, the son of a distinguished physician, *Joel Elkes* grew up in nearby Kovno, Lithuania, filled with the spirit of science and the love of physics.[40] In 1930, at seventeen, he left Kovno to study medicine at St. Mary's Hospital Medical School in London, his course of study broken by intermittent financial difficulties – these were not easy times for Jews in Central Europe. He graduated in medicine in 1941 and, still animated by the desire to combine physics and biochemistry (though the term had not yet been invented), he accepted in 1942 a fellowship in pharmacology at the University of Birmingham. Elkes later insisted that his interest in psychiatry at the time was minimal, yet in 1937 he began training in psychoanalysis (completing a diploma in 1955 in Washington DC). At Birmingham, Elkes plunged into the study of lipoproteins and ended up working on myelin in the central nervous system. This was the beginning of his efforts to establish a physical, neurochemical basis for psychiatric phenomena.

After a year in the US as a Fulbright Fellow, in 1951 Elkes returned to Birmingham and became the founding director of the Department of Experimental Psychiatry, which had the mission of linking the University's basic science laboratories to the behavior of patients in the psychiatric wards of the University of Birmingham Hospitals. Supported by the Rockefeller Foundation and the Medical Research Council of England, they had at their disposition experimental animal laboratories plus a forty-patient ward in the former Cadbury mansion in Birmingham that they called the "Uffculme Clinic." This seems to have been the first experimental facility in the world dedicated to psychiatry and psychopharmacology. As Elkes said in the *University of Birmingham Gazette* in 1955, "The laboratory work of the Department rests on the assumption that the various manifestations of gross mental disorder and milder dysfunction have their counterpart in a disturbed physiology of the brain, and that the study of the chemistry, the cellular constitution, and the electrical activity of the brain may contribute to an understanding of its function as the highest integrating organ."[41]

In his interview in this volume, Elkes recalls the excitement as they began to discover the specificity of drug action. Although they were not the first to document the therapeutic effect of the barbiturates on catatonic stupor, they did note that, unexpectedly, amphetamine deepened it. At Winson Green Hospital in Birmingham, Elkes and his wife Charmian Elkes, who was the chief investigator, conducted one of the earliest controlled trials of chlorpromazine, publishing the results in the *British Medical Journal* in 1954.[42] "This is one of the milestones in psychopharmacology," said interviewer Fridolin Sulser.

In 1957 Elkes left Birmingham for the NIMH in Bethesda, Maryland. "The field was developing very fast in the United States, and I wanted to be part of it," he said in the interview. He established the Behavioral and Clinical Studies Center at St. Elizabeths Hospital in Washington DC; Elkes also directed its homologue at NIMH, the Clinical Neuropharmacology Research Center. At NIMH, Elkes' interest in regional neurochemistry intensified – he considered this kind of research among his most important life accomplishments – and in 1961 he and Seymour Kety published the proceedings of an agenda-setting conference on the subject.[43] In his subsequent tenure as chair of psychiatry at Johns Hopkins University, Elkes inspired an entire generation of American biological psychiatrists. "My job was to cultivate talent," he said. Eugene Paykel later referred to Elkes as "the father of neuropsychopharmacology."[44]

The name *Alfred Freedman* is indissolubly bound with the two-volume *Comprehensive Textbook of Psychiatry* that he, Harold Kaplan and Benjamin Sadock published with Williams & Wilkins in 1975. But it is not generally appreciated that Freedman pioneered the psychopharmacology of children in the United States.

Freedman grew up in Albany, New York, his parents Jewish emigrants from Eastern Europe who lived in the most straitened of circumstances. These were the 1930s, a time when Jews felt acutely the kiss of the lash of American anti-Semitism, and strict restrictions on Jewish admissions kept him from entering any of the East Coast medical schools to which he applied, despite a brilliant undergraduate record. He was finally accepted in medicine at the University of Minnesota (which also had a numerus clausus but applied it somewhat less restrictively), and warmed to the basic biological sciences. In the Army during the Second World War he began to drift towards psychiatry, with a view "to study the biochemistry of mental illness" (though, he like so many clinicians of his generation, also qualified in psychoanalysis). He trained as a resident on the children's ward of the psychiatric division of Bellevue Medical Center in New York City, and then stayed on staff. Were psychopharmaceuticals for children needed? Later in life, Freedman would tell groups skeptical of the use of drugs: "If they had seen Bellevue Hospital . . . they would have an appreciation of what the new drugs did. There was a pervasive smell of formaldehyde mixed with urine and feces that hit you when you entered the disturbed wards with patients wandering up and down babbling in camisoles. It was really bedlam." At Bellevue, Freedman discovered the effectiveness of diphenhydramine (Benadryl) in psychotic illness in children, and his chief, Lauretta Bender, became a big advocate of it. Freedman also conducted early chlorpromazine trials in children.

Freedman had always been politically active for progressive causes, and in the early 1970s permitted an alternative group within the American Psychiatric Association (APA) to advance his candidacy for president against the official slate. Freedman won, and undertook such steps as removing homosexuality from the disease classification as a diagnosis. As he said later, "I attribute my [winning] most of all to the general feeling in APA of electing someone not a member of the 'old boys' network' who would bring about change and a fresh wind in APA."[45]

In 1960 Freedman became chair of psychiatry at New York Medical College, a post he occupied for the next thirty years, turning the rather moribund psychiatric unit into a major force, its clinical base at Metropolitan Hospital. Because both the department and the hospital were in East Harlem, Freedman thought that a focus on drug abuse made sense. Over the years his group pioneered the study of such agents as cyclazocine and naloxone as narcotic antagonists. Freedman also tried to interest ACNP in the study of addiction and drug abuse. His judgment on the outcome of the war on drugs is rather sobering: "Now we recognize that the billions of dollars that have been spent on drug programs have been a waste."

For many of the founding figures of psychopharmacology, their sometime involvement with psychoanalysis turned into a story of apostasy: Many simply turned their backs on Freud and his teachings, either silently or publicly. For *Louis Gottschalk,* founding chair of psychiatry at the Irvine campus of the University of California, there was no apostasy. Yet he simultaneously harbored a deep interest in psychopharmacology; he was the first research scientist at NIMH as the Institute opened its doors in 1951. At the University of Cincinnati College of Medicine in the 1950s and '60s, Gottschalk developed means of inferring internal psychological states from a content analysis of the patients' language, a technique since adopted worldwide. In Cincinnati, Gottschalk was influenced by such researchers as analyst Arthur Mirsky (who displayed the same fascination with biology as Gottschalk) and analyst Maurice Levine. Gottschalk found, for example, that anxiety scores from content analysis correlated well with benzodiazepine blood levels. The main theme running through his more than fifty years of scientific research has been "the precision of measurement, whether it's a measurement of psychological states and traits . . . or the accuracy of measurement from blood levels."

Gottschalk's judgment of psychoanalysis in retrospect was that "it's pretty much an art form." Yet it had made him more sensitive to patients: "It probably has influenced my willingness to listen to people for a long time, as it has probably influenced you," he told interviewer William E. ("Biff") Bunney.

It is a testimonial to the openness of spirit of the federal scientific establishment that the NIH has been willing to take on scientists from the four corners of the globe, not just the United States, in the search for excellence. One of those scientists was the Hungarian *Stephen Szára,* who, like Thomas Ban, fled Hungary during the uprising of 1956 and ended up in the world of US research.

In Budapest, Szára earned a PhD in chemistry in 1950 and a medical degree in 1951. Until the uprising, he taught microbiology and biochemistry at the Medical University. This marked the onset of his interest in psychopharmacology, as he became interested in the psychotogens (but was unable to get Sandoz to send any samples of LSD behind the Iron Curtain), and in Abram

Hoffer's "adrenochrome" hypothesis of schizophrenia. Finally, Szára settled on studying the active principles of cohoba, a plant used as a hallucinogen by South American Indians, choosing first the plant's constituent dimethyltrypt-amine (DMT). Just as his DMT research began – all the colleagues flocking about begging to try some too – the uprising broke out.

After fleeing, Szára's first stops included Vienna and West Berlin, where he was a "visiting scientist," in fact just taken in and given shelter. But in Vienna Hans Hoff, the professor of psychiatry, gave him some LSD to let Szára com-pare the hallucinatory experiences with it and DMT. In 1958 Szára came on staff as a visiting scientist at NIMH, with the promise of an appointment at Joel Elkes' Clinical Neuropharmacology Research Center, situated at St. Elizabeths Hospital. But when Szára arrived in Washington, the labs weren't ready yet, so he spent the next two years working with Julius Axelrod in Building 10 of NIH on the metabolism of diethyltryptamine (DET).

In 1961 Szára became chief of the psychopharmacology section of NIMH; a decade later he was pushed out of the intramural side in an internal political struggle and had to give up lab research. He found himself, in 1971, as an ad-ministrator on the extramural side: chief of the clinical drug studies section of the Center for Studies of Narcotics and Drug Abuse in Rockville, Maryland. In 1974 the Center was enlarged to become the National Institute on Drug Abuse (NIDA), and Szára became chief of the biomedical research branch, organiz-ing controlled clinical research on marijuana. Szára's last move in the federal establishment was to become chief in 1980 of the biomedical branch in NIDA's division of preclinical research. He retired in 1990; Leo Hollister interviewed him for the ACNP in 1997.

In the years when psychoanalysis was all the rage, *Gerald Sarwer-Foner* was a medical student at the Université de Montréal. Of course his attention was captured by Freud's doctrines, as was everyone else's in the late 1940s and early '50s. Yet Sarwer-Foner's eye also fastened on several articles in the medical journal of the Paris hospitals by Henri Laborit advocating prometha-zine as part of a "lytic cocktail" for use in surgery. Sarwer-Foner went on to train in psychoanalytic psychiatry, encountering "such psychoanalytic greats as Gregory Zilboorg," as he said elsewhere.[46] He spent the early 1950s at several American centers, then returned in 1953 to the Queen Mary Veterans' Hospital in Montreal to complete his training.

Yet Sarwer-Foner never lost his curiosity about pharmacological approach-es to psychiatry and endeavored over the years to reconcile psychopharmacol-ogy and psychoanalysis. After joining the department of psychiatry at McGill University – then the preeminent training center in Canada and one of the larg-est in the world – Sarwer-Foner wrote extensively about psychotropics, usually considering their mechanism in an analytic context. He summed up his views in 1960 in the book *The Dynamics of Psychiatric Drug Therapy*.[47] Over the next several decades, Sarwer-Foner continued these efforts at reconciliation,[48] often to an increasingly disbelieving audience. Many of the pioneers of psychopharmacology had, as Sarwer-Foner, initially been trained as analysts and then put it behind them. But Sarwer-Foner never did. As he wrote in 1989, "Our work established a theory of how the neuroleptic drugs work in schizophrenic patients, in terms of the patients' overall mastery of his schizophrenic illness." Sarwer-Foner listed a number of conditions that had to be met for improvement to occur "in relationship to the drug action." One such precondition was: "This symptom complex must represent for the patient his/her inability to face and master himself and his most feared impulses . . . core or inner conflict he cannot solve for himself. In the face of this inability, shattered defenses and regression into schizophrenic illness."[49] In 1971, Sarwer-Foner left McGill to take a professorship at the University of Ottawa; it is a measure of the success he had in bridging the two worlds of psychoanalysis and psychopharmacology that in 1976/77 he served as "Sandoz Visiting Professor of Psychiatry to Canadian Medical Schools."

In the force field between psychoanalysis and biological psychiatry, *Joseph Wortis* occupies a distinctive position: right in the middle. He was analyzed by Sigmund Freud while he was a "Havelock Ellis" fellow in Vienna in 1934-35. (Wortis had been asked by the widow of a Harvard professor, a closet gay who had suicided, to study sexuality, and Ellis advised him.) At the same time in Vienna, Wortis knew Manfred Sakel and learned insulin coma therapy.

Wortis grew up in Brooklyn. As he said in an interview with social scientist Todd Dufresne (his interview in this volume is with Leo Hollister), "My mother was French, and my father was Russian born. They were both Jewish, but they were deeply imbedded in their respective ancestral cultures."[50] English was the only language the parents had in common and, unlike his playmates, he grew up with no Yiddish. Still, he felt sufficiently attracted to German culture to study medicine in Vienna, graduating MD in 1932. He returned to the States to train at Bellevue Hospital in New York, setting up an insulin coma clinic. His 1937 article in the *American Journal of Psychiatry* launched insulin coma treatment in the US.[51]

During the war, Wortis worked as a psychiatrist for the War Shipping Administration and for the US Public Health Service. Use of insulin coma was coming to an end at this time anyway, pushed aside by electroconvulsive therapy and then by chlorpromazine. After the war, Wortis's interests shifted toward developmental disorders. Immersed in a left-wing milieu (though apparently not himself a member of the Communist Party), in 1950 he wrote a sympathetic account of Soviet psychiatry.[52] He refused in 1953 to answer questions of the Senate Internal Security subcommittee, and it was perhaps of his political notoriety that he left Bellevue a year previously. Among psychiatrists, he is perhaps best known for his longtime editorship of the journal *Biological Psychiatry*. Among the public, however, his fame rests on his 1954 book *Fragments of an Analysis with Freud*.[53] Asked later who "his hero" was, he chose, however, the English sexologist Havelock Ellis; one of Wortis's sons bears Havelock as a middle name.[54]

REFERENCES

1. Shorter E. A History of Psychiatry from the Age of the Asylum to the Era of Prozac. New York: Wiley, 1997. p. 254.
2. Ban TA. Pharmacotherapy of depression: a historical analysis. J Neural Transmission 2001; 108: 707–16.
3. Brady JV. Assessment of drug effects on emotional behavior. Science 1956; 123:1033–4.
4. Healy D. The Antidepressant Era. Cambridge: Harvard University Press; 1997. p.75.
5. Ayd F. The discovery of antidepressants, In: Healy D, editor. The Psychopharmacologists. London: Altman; 1996. p. 81–110.
6. Pies RW. Review of Ayd, Lexicon of Psychiatry, Neurology, and the Neurosciences, 2nd edition. J Clin Psychopharm 2001; 21: 466.
7. Cole J. The evaluation of psychotropic drugs. In: Healy D, editor. The Psychopharmacologists. London: Altman; 1996, pp. 239–264.
8. Gershon S, Daversa C. The lithium story: a journey from obscurity to popular use in North America. In: Bauer M, Grof P, Müller-Oerlinghausen B, editors. Lithium in Psychiatry: The Comprehensive Guide. London: Informa; 2006. p.17–24.
9. Gershon S. Yuwiler A. Lithium ion: a specific psychopharmacological approach to the treatment of mania. J Neuropsychiatr 1960; 1: 229–41.
10. Hippius H. The founding of the CINP and the discovery of clozapine. In: Healy D, editor. The Psychopharmacologists. London: Altman; 1996, p.187–214.
11. Hippius H, Möller H-J, Müller N, Neundörfer-Kohl G. The University Department of Psychiatry in Munich: From Kraepelin and His Predecessors to Molecular Psychiatry. Heidelberg: Springer Medizin Verlag; 2008.
12. Hollister LE, Degan RO, Schultz SD. An experimental approach to facilitation of psychotherapy by psychotomimetics drugs. J Mental Sci 1962; 108: 99–100.
13. Hollister LE. Valium: a discussion of current issues. Psychosomatics 1977; 18: 44–58.
14. Hollister LE. Clinical Pharmacology of Psychotherapeutic Drugs. New York: Churchill Livingstone; 1978.
15. Kurland AA, Pahnke WN, Unger S. Psychedelic psychotherapy (LSD) in the treatment of the patient with a malignancy. In: The Present Status of Psychotropic Drugs. Pharmacological and Clinical Aspects. Proceedings VI (CINP) International Congress. Amsterdam: Excerpta Medica; 1969. p. 432–4.
16. Kurland AA, Unger S. Shaffer JW, Savage C. Psychedelic therapy utilizing LSD in the treatment of the alcoholic patient: a preliminary report. Am J Psychiatry 1967; 123: 1202–9.
17. Savage C, McCabe OL, Kurland AA, Hanlon T. LSD-assisted psychotherapy in the treatment of severe chronic neurosis. Journal of Altered States of Consciousness 1973; 1: 31–47.
18. Lehmann HE, Hanrahan GE. Chlorpromazine: New inhibiting agent for psychomotor excitement and manic states. Arch Neurol Psychiatry 1954; 71: 227–37.
19. Lehmann HE, Cahn CH, De Verteuil RL. The treatment of depressive conditions with imipramine (G 22355). Can Psychiatr Assoc J 1958; 3: 155–64.
20. De Verteuil RL, Lehmann HE. Therapeutic trial of iproniazid (Marsilid) in depressed and apathetic patients. Can Med Assoc J 1958; 78:131–3.
21. Shorter E. A Historical Dictionary of Psychiatry. New York: Oxford University Press; 2005, p.160–1.
22. Cahn CH, Heinz Edgar Lehmann, 1911–1999. Roy Soc Can Proc (6th series) 2001; 12: 211–4.
23. Lehmann H. Discussion: A renaissance of psychiatric diagnosis? Am J Psychiatry 1969; 125 (Suppl.): 43–6.
24. Lehmann HE. New drugs in psychiatric therapy. Can Med Assoc J 1961; 85: 1145–51.

25. Turner WJ. Homosexuality, type 1, an Xq28 phenomenon. Arch Sex Behav 1995; 24: 109–34.
26. Turner WJ. Curriculum vitae. ACNP Archives.
27. Olds J, Milner P. Positive reinforcement produced by electrical stimulation of the septal area and other regions of rat brain. J Compar Physiol Psychol 1954; 47: 419–27.
28. Brady JV, Boren J, Conrad D, Sidman M. The effect of food and water deprivation upon intracranial self-stimulation. J Compar Physiol Psychol 1957; 50: 134–7.
29. Barrett JE. Pioneer in behavioral pharmacology: A tribute to Joseph V. Brady. J Exp Anal Behav 2008; 90: 405–15.
30. Carr SW. Charles Jelleff Carr. Neuropsychopharmacology 2006; 31: 895.
31. Dews PB. Studies on behavior. I. Differential sensitivity to pentobarbital of pecking performance in pigeons depending on the schedule of reward. J Pharmacol Exp Therap 1955; 113: 393–401.
32. Barrett JE. Behavioral determinants of drug action: The contributions of Peter B. Dews. J Exp Anal Behav 2006; 86: 359–70.
33. Greenblatt DJ, Shader RI. In memoriam: Louis Lasagna, MD, 1923–2003. J Clin Psychopharm 2004; 24: 243–4.
34. Lasagna L. A comparison of hypnotic agents. J Pharmacol Exp Therap 1954; 111: 9–20.
35. Lasagna L. A study of hypnotic drugs in patients with chronic diseases. J Chron Dis 1956; 3: 122–33.
36. Lasagna L. Drug discovery and introduction: Regulation and overregulation. Clin Pharmacol Therap 1976; 20: 507–11.
37. Lasagna L. Clinical trials of drugs from the viewpoint of the academic investigator (a satire). Clin Pharmacol Therap 1975; 18: 629–33.
38. Stein L. Effects and interactions of imipramine, chlorpromazine, reserpine and amphetamine on self-stimulation: possible neurophysiological basis of depression. In: Wortis J, editor. Recent Advances in Biological Psychiatry. New York: Plenum; 1962, p. 288–308.
39. Stein L, Wise CD. Possible etiology of schizophrenia: Progressive damage to the noradrenergic reward system by 6-hydroxydopamine. Science 1971; 171: 1032–36.
40. Shorter E. A Historical Dictionary of Psychiatry. New York: Oxford University Press; 2005, p. 95–6.
41. Elkes J. The department of experimental psychiatry. University of Birmingham Gazette, March 11, 1955.
42. Elkes J, Elkes C. Effect of chlorpromazine on the behaviour of chronically overeactive psychotic patients. Br Med J 1954; 2: 560–5.
43. Kety S, Elkes J, editors. Regional Neurochemistry: Proceedings of the Fourth International Neurochemical Symposium, Varrena (Italy), 1961. London: Pergamon; 1961.
44. Paykel E. Q and A discussion. CINP Newsletter, March 9, 2003.
45. Freedman AM. Chronicles of a past president. Psychiatric News, March 15, 1996.
46. Sarwer-Foner GJ. Personal reminiscences of the early days of psychopharmacology. In: Ban TA, Healy D, Shorter E, editors. The Rise of Psychopharmacology and the Story of CINP. Budapest: Animula, Budapest, 1998. p. 32–5.
47. Sarwer-Foner GJ. The Dynamics of Psychiatric Drug Therapy. Charles C Thomas, Springfield, 1960.
48. Sarwer-Foner GJ. Psychiatric symptomatology. Its meaning and function in relationship to the psychodynamic actions of drugs. In: Denber HCB, editor. Psychopharmacological Treatment: Theory and Practice. New York: M. Dekker; 1979. p. 179–221.
49. Sarwer-Foner GJ. The psychodynamic action of psychopharmacologic drugs and the target symptom versus the anti-psychotic approach to psychopharmacologic therapy: Thirty years later. Psychiatr J Univ Ottawa. 1989; 14: 268–78.
50. Dufresne T. An interview with Joseph Wortis. Psychoanalytic Rev 1996; 83: 589–610.
51. Wortis J. Bowman KM. Further experiences at Bellevue Hospital with hypoglycemic insulin treatment of schizophrenia. Am J Psychiatry 1937; 94: 153–8.
52. Wortis J. Soviet Psychiatry. Williams & Wilkins, Baltimore, 1950.
53. Wortis J. Fragments of an Analysis with Freud. Simon and Schuster, New York, 1954.

INTERVIEWEES & INTERVIEWERS

Trialists

FRANK J. AYD, Jr.

Interviewed by Leo E. Hollister
San Juan, Puerto Rico, December 11, 1994

LH: Frank,* you are one of the older hands in the field of psychopharmacology. I think you were one of the faces on the historic photograph taken at the Woodner Hotel a number of years back where the founding fathers met together. How did you get into the field?

FA: Well, Leo, I got into psychopharmacology because I had some experience before I graduated from medical school with the impact of electroconvulsive therapy (ECT) on my father, who happened to be a manic-depressive. I saw the dramatic effect of ECT on my dad. He made a fairly prompt recovery and didn't require hospitalization again. At the time we didn't have succinyl chloride, intravenous barbiturates, the machinery that we have today. So it was a rather crude thing. Still, it worked. But it did produce a lot of memory impairment.

LH: That is what got you into the biological side of it.

FA: I had started a residency in pediatrics but got called to active duty by the Navy. In the incomprehensible way the Navy does things I was assigned to surgery at Bethesda Naval Hospital with no manual dexterity whatsoever and no interest in surgery.

LH: You actually went to surgery from pediatrics.

FA: That's right. Quite a change! At any rate, Admiral Hogan was commanding officer at the Naval Hospital at Bethesda, and I knew him. He happened to be Roman Catholic and we had been at a couple of retreats together at the Jesuit retreat house at the Naval Academy. So I had no hesitancy in saying to him: "hey, Ben, somebody's made a terrible mistake." He looked at my credentials and said: "well, we need psychiatrists. I'm going to send you to Bainbridge and they'll loan you to the VA hospital at Perry Point." So I went into that program. I thought it was a fate worse than death, because I had no real interest in psychiatry. But I was determined that I could take care of the physical aspects of things. It didn't take me very long, Leo, to realize that chronic schizophrenics are a different breed from the rest of us; they have altered temperature and pain sets. The only physical treatments at that time were insulin coma and ECT and since I had seen what ECT did for my father I volunteered to do the ECT. While at Perry Point, I was approached in my third year by Squibb. They had mephenesin, a muscle relaxant.

---

* Frank J. Ayd, Jr. was born in Baltimore, Maryland in 1920 and graduated in 1945 from the University of Maryland School of Medicine. From 1955 until his retirement in 2003 he was chief of psychiatry at Franklin Square Hospital in Baltimore. He was also director of education at Taylor Manor Hospital in Ellicott City, Maryland, and president of Ayd's Communications. Ayd died in 2008.

LH: That was sort of a meprobamate-like drug?

FA: That's correct. It preceded meprobamate. Anyhow, they were interested in somebody doing a study to see whether it had any value as a sedative drug. I did a small study in a number of chronic schizophrenics, and it did absolutely nothing. But it got me identified as an individual who might be interested in doing research with pharmaceuticals in psychiatric illnesses. As a consequence, when I left Perry Point and went into private practice, I received a phone call from a psychiatrist by the name of Bill Long. Bill was with Smith, Kline & French (SK&F). He knew me because his brother had taught me. And he said: "I hear you've got some interest in testing drugs." And I said: "I do." And he said: "Well, we've got one from Rhône-Poulenc, and we're looking for people who will take a look at it." I agreed that I would take a look at it. That was in December, 1952.

LH: Needless to say that the drug was chlorpromazine.

FA: It was chlorpromazine. I tested initially the 10–25 mg dose. Within a year, I had enough data to prepare a paper. I presented the paper at the Southern Medical Association meeting in St. Louis. Titus Harris and Doug Goldman were the discussants. The paper was well received and CIBA had somebody at the meeting. I don't remember his name.

LH: Dick Roberts?

FA: No, it was somebody that I didn't know. But somebody from CIBA approached me after I had given my paper and wanted to know if I would be interested in taking a look at reserpine. I said, "Well, I'll try it." So I did. And the following year I gave a paper on both chlorpromazine and reserpine at the American Psychiatric Association (APA) meeting in Atlantic City. And from there on it's just been plucking at one drug after another, trying to determine not only whether they work, but also how do they work, and at what price.

LH: I take it that your initial experiences with chlorpromazine and reserpine impressed you pretty much about their efficacy.

FA: That's correct; mainly the experience with chlorpromazine. Reserpine worked, but the price was too much in the way of side effects. I was never convinced that reserpine was a depressogenic agent. It certainly produced enough, not dangerous, but uncomfortable side effects. I considered it really wrong to persuade a patient to take this stuff for a long time because the benefits were not that apparent as they were with chlorpromazine.

LH: So you got launched in the field after working with those two drugs, and you say you've studied God knows how many. How many drugs did you study?

FA: Well, I really don't know the exact number, but practically speaking, every neuroleptic that ever got on the market in this country except for Clozaril (clozapine) and Risperdal (risperidone). I've looked at both after they were marketed. I don't do any more research prior to marketing. It's impossible to do that now.

LH: Why?

FA: Well, first of all, managed care is having its impact on your capacity to do research. I'm in private practice and if you are not approved with a particular insurance carrier, then you lose the patient unless they can pay out of their own pocket. The number of my new referrals decreased because I have not become a Health Maintenance Organization (HMO) or preferred provider doctor. And I don't want to be. I want to maintain my autonomy and independence. That's the first problem. The second problem is, you know as well as I Leo, the Food and Drug Administration (FDA) criteria for baseline data has increased tremendously. A lot of people just don't want to do electrocardiograms (EKGs), electroencephalograms (EEGs), and maybe even ophthalmological examinations, often at their own expense, to get a medication and a general physical free. So research with outpatients is declining. At any rate, I looked at not only the antipsychotics, but also the antidepressants. Nate Kline and I were good friends up until the day he died. But Nate got very angry with me because I published a paper on Marsilid (iproniazid) in the *American Journal of Psychiatry*. It was just a brief report, but he felt that I did it to steal his thunder, which was not the case.

LH: Oh.

FA: Nate was the man who got the credit for the discovery that monoamine oxidase inhibitors (MAOIs) were psychic energizers. As you know, it was disputed whether it was him who deserved the credit. In fact, I ended up with Henry Brill testifying along with Jack Howard in a court case.

LH: In Saunders' suit?

FA: Saunders' suit against Nate. Saunders didn't sue the first time when Nate got the Lasker Award for reserpine. But when he got the second one, he said I should have gotten that.

LH: Well, I don't think Lawrence Saunders was very active in Nate's work with reserpine, but he was probably intimately involved in the work with Marsilid.

FA: I'm sure he was. He left CIBA to join Nate at Rockland State. But, as you know it did end up in the courtroom. It was finally settled, and Nate got the credit.

LH: Well, that's not the first time that a major prize has been disputed.

FA: No.

LH: I think somebody disputed Waksman's Nobel Prize for streptomycin.

FA: Yes, I know that only too well.

LH: I can't tell you anything you don't know.

FA: He went to Israel when the Waksman Institute was dedicated. On his way back he stopped to have an audience with the Pope, and I interviewed him for the Vatican radio. At the luncheon after the interview, we got talking about different things, and he mentioned that he had been almost sued, so to speak.

LH: You indicated that early on you did a whole lot of clinical studies, but it is difficult to do these studies now in private practice.

FA: Oh, yes. Number one, it was easier to do clinical studies then. Number two, there was no competition. I was a pioneer. There weren't many people around doing clinical studies with drugs. It's no secret, Leo, in my hometown of Baltimore I was looked upon as an oddball, the guy who instead of thinking about the id and ego was interested in what's going on in the brain of people who have different psychiatric disabilities, and trying to treat them with chemical restraints, as they called it in those days.

LH: Oh, really?

FA: Oh, yes. I was different. There were very few psychiatrists at either the University of Maryland or at Hopkins working with drugs.

LH: I can't think of anybody from Baltimore in the early days. How about this fellow Winkelman in Philadelphia? How did he get on to work with chlorpromazine?

FA: Well, Bill worked in Philadelphia. He's an analyst working in private practice, but he always had some interest in physical methods of therapy.

LH: I thought he was a prominent neuropsychiatrist and neuropathologist.

FA: That's correct. Bill was serving as a consultant to SK&F, he and Bill Long. Long was an eclectic psychiatrist. That's how Winkelman got chlorpromazine.

LH: Were you aware of his work at that time?

FA: When I first went to meet Dr. Long he told me about Bill. In fact, it was just about that time that Bill's article appeared in JAMA (Journal of the American Medical Association). So he was really the first in the United States to do enough patients to get a paper together.

LH: Now, of course, you knew Heinz Lehmann as well.

FA: Oh, yes. I knew Heinz very early. He was the first in North America, not just in Canada. I also met, of course, John Kinross-Wright. In 1953, Bill Winkelman, Frank Jay and John Kinross-Wright were the three people who did the early work with chlorpromazine in the United States.

LH: I guess reserpine was only Nate.

FA: Nate Kline was the principal man with reserpine. I did some work with reserpine, but I didn't go on beyond the first 50 or so patients, I then stopped.

LH: I don't know whether that chap out in Augusta State Hospital who also got that Lasker Award for reserpine was working about the same time as Nate. I can't remember his name.

FA: I can't think of his name either. I guess that shows where we are.

LH: So much for glory. While we are talking about studies here, what was the drug that impressed you most?

FA: Well, obviously, chlorpromazine was tremendously impressive; mainly because of its immediate impact on agitation and anxiety. You could take a pretty disturbed individual and in a matter of hours you could see a change. They were still hallucinating and they were still deluded, but by God they were changed. In the antidepressant field it was impressive to see patients respond to imipramine almost as well as some responded to ECT. They were not the psychotically depressed patients, but what you would call in those days endogenous depressed patients; those patients, who come in with a history of recent weight loss, have early onset of their disease and late insomnia. You know, they're melancholic; they have a lot of vegetative symptoms and so forth. With an adequate dose of imipramine in a matter of four to six weeks you saw a lot of dramatic improvement in these patients.

LH: When you go from nothing to something that works, that's a huge jump. But then after that, the jumps become incremental.

FA: That's very true. But you see they opened a whole new field. I mean it was the first really good option in the treatment of depression beside ECT. The MAOIs had also a place in the treatment of depression. They still have a very valuable place. But you had the problems of the side effects of Marsilid (iproniazid) which were not necessarily dangerous, but troublesome. Then you had the problem of jaundice.

LH: I got that on the third patient I used Marsilid on.

FA: A couple of patients died, and that really hurt. For awhile it looked like the end of the MAOIs, and would have been the end if SK&F had not already started looking at tranylcypromine.

LH: Well, the peculiar thing is that Marsilid was first for tuberculosis. It was used in tubercular patients when the famous picture was published in which patients at the Public Health Service hospital in Staten Island were dancing.

FA: Dancing on the ward.

LH: Yes, but because of the problems with iproniazid, it was replaced by isoniazid.

FA: Right.

LH: And a number of studies done with isoniazid were negative.

FA: Right.

LH: The reason for this was that isoniazid was unlike iproniazid. It did not block MAO.

FA: Well, be that as it may, as you know, the MAOIs came close to death themselves.

LH: Well, I think Zeller was first to point out the fact that there was a difference between iproniazid and isoniazid. If they had gone on with isoniazid and found nothing going, this group of drugs would have dropped dead right there.

FA: Right. Well, it didn't take long to realize that MAOIs interacted with foods. We now know it was tyramine and sympathomimetics that created the trouble.

LH: That was a big deterrent for a long while, but lately people don't seem to be as much concerned about it as they used to be.

FA: Well, I think partly because they warn patients, and they give them a list of dietary substances that should be avoided. They warn them about taking over-the-counter preparations that contain sympathomimetics. And I think that in actual fact phenelzine is safer, and probably even tranylcypromine is probably a little bit safer than Marsilid, although I don't know of any direct comparison studies.

LH: I don't know any studies either.

FA: But the MAO inhibitors definitely have a place in treatment. We owe a lot to people like Fred Quitkin here, and Will Sargant and his group in England, because they stuck with them. And I've stuck with them even to this day. I prescribe more I'm sure, than most people in my geographic area because I'm convinced of their value in certain types of patients. When you think about it, you've got an alternative to MAO inhibitors and you have an alternative to ECT with imipramine. That really opened the gate for developments.

LH: Well, some of the earlier comparisons, I think one that Milton Greenblatt was part of, seem to indicate that the tricyclics were not a whole lot better than placebo; that ECT was better than tricyclics. Do you think that was because they were looking at very severely ill patients?

FA: Well, I think that may be part of the answer. I think the other part was dosage. Greenblatt's study also included phenelzine, if you recall, and the patients only got 30 mg of phenelzine a day when most patients with a moderate to severe depression require 90 mg. So it was a question of too low a dosage for too short a period of time. It was a methodologically flawed study.

LH: It almost did him in, too, didn't it?

FA: Yes, it almost did him in. Because Milton was a very fine man and very prestigious, and here he is at Harvard and working at the Mass Mental Health Center.

LH: Well, it's amazing how the drugs survive. You weren't at the Paris meeting in 1954 on chlorpromazine, were you?

FA: No. My wife was there, and she gave my paper for me.

LH: I had occasion to review the proceedings of that, and I didn't remember your name. What was the first big meeting you recall on these drugs in the US?

FA: Well, I guess the first really big one was the one on Thorazine (chlorpromazine) that SK&F sponsored, in Philadelphia.

LH: But that was a private session, wasn't it?

FA: Yes, it was private, but there were several hundred people there. And they published a little monograph of the papers that were presented, and they did the same thing later when they launched trifluoperazine, Stelazine. I guess the APA meeting in 1956 probably was the first big meeting where there were a number of papers not only on chlorpromazine but also on other drugs, such as my paper on reserpine. It was also the meeting where meprobamate was first mentioned. That gave cause for thinking about which way the wind was blowing. It certainly was blowing in the area of biological psychiatry.

LH: Yes, I think the pendulum still is on the side of biological psychiatry. Some people are arguing that perhaps it is too far over on the biological side. What do you think about that?

FA: Oh, I don't think so. I think that you can't lose sight of the fact that you are not just treating an illness but a human being who has the illness. You have to be aware of the physical status of that individual, and also of the fact that he is the one who has the illness and is going to react to the illness differently than somebody else who has the same illness. You can't treat just with drugs alone. There's got to be some psychoeducation, or whatever you want to call it, and some type of psychotherapy. I can't conceive of an internist treating a diabetic without at least giving the diabetic something besides diet and insulin in the way of counseling.

LH: Foot care, and other things.

FA: That's right. You have to do this. You are not just dispensing pills if you are practicing rational psychopharmacotherapy.

LH: You mentioned before a few people who were using chlorpromazine early. One of the people I think everybody often forgets is Mark Altschule.

FA: Mark was a very interesting person. He was a very intelligent man.

LH: A real scholar.

FA: No question about that. His wife had schizophrenia. She was in McLean Hospital. Mark really believed in the marriage contract. He stayed with her until she died, and he always looked for something that might help her. Yes, he definitely became very well informed about chlorpromazine at an early time.

LH: He was an internist, more interested, I think, in cardiology than in psychiatry, but he was one of the first people involved with the drug.

FA: Yes. One man we haven't mentioned so far is Fritz Freyhan. Fritz was involved very early with chlorpromazine. He was at Delaware State Hospital. Like everybody else working in a state institution or a Veterans' Administration (VA) hospital, he had hundreds of patients and no drugs. So he could really test drugs on a large number of patients very quickly. Fritz was a very astute clinician, I thought.

LH: Yes.

FA: Well trained in a German school. He was a very good observer. I learned a lot from him. I had more contact with him than I did with Heinz Lehmann in the beginning because Heinz was in Canada, and Fritz was in Wilmington, 60 miles away from where I was. He did a lot of studies for SK&F. We worked together on chlorpromazine. We looked also at prochlorperazine. He and I did two studies on prochlorperazine for SK&F, and we looked at trifluoperazine. Fritz also got interested in fluphenazine. Then we both looked at Temaril (trimeprazine), an antipyretic phenothiazine.

LH: Yes, but it has a different kind of pharmacology. It makes it more of an antihistamine.

FA: That's right. We tested it as a potential antipsychotic, and it just didn't work.

LH: Do you know Pacatal (mepazine)?

FA: Pacatal was the most anticholinergic antipsychotic, if it was an antipsychotic. It really was a very strong anticholinergic substance.

LH: Yes, it never went very far.

FA: No.

LH: And do you know Sparine (promazine)?

FA: Promazine, the Wyeth product. Again, there were some patients who improved, but only because it was sedative. As far as I'm concerned, it never had any true antipsychotic properties.

LH: Well, if you give patients enough promazine they get seizures.

FA: Oh, yes. But that's true for practically every psychoactive drug. If you give a high enough dose, you can produce a seizure.

LH: Well, not to the same extent as with promazine, I think.

FA: That's true.

LH: Fifty per cent seizures once you got up to about 1,200 mg.

FA: Yes, that's true.

LH: In a way it is interesting that truth won out. Some drugs fell by the way-side, like Pacatal and promazine, whereas others were more acceptable and efficacious and lasted. Well, I guess the early people in the field were pretty astute.

FA: Right. Anybody who has success with psychopharmaceuticals today owes a debt of gratitude to the people who pioneered these drugs.

LH: It is remarkable also that most of the people we have mentioned were outside of the academic community.

FA: That's true.

LH: Why do you think that was the case? Was it simply the fact that the academics were all psychoanalysts?

FA: Basically that's the truth. The medical schools in my area were dominated by psychoanalysts as they were practically everywhere else in the US, and there was no encouragement to think in terms of anything beyond the psyche, so to speak. I don't know of a medical school, in the beginning, that got into psychopharmacotherapy.

LH: Yes, it's hard to think of any. I guess you know that Kinross-Wright was at Baylor.

FA: Well, he actually was in Carolina first and then went to Baylor.

LH: Then, of course, Mark Altschule was in the department of medicine at Harvard.

FA: And Paul Hoch was at Columbia, at the New York State Psychiatric Institute.

LH: Did Paul do much with antipsychotics?

FA: He did a little, but not a great deal.

LH: He was more interested in hallucinogens.

FA: That's correct. But my point is that it was not easy to do what Henry Brill, Nate Kline and I were doing in those early days. Everybody was suspicious. But at the APA meeting in Atlantic City in 1956 that I mentioned before, the executive director of the National Mental Health Association was present. He got Henry, Nate and I to agree to go to Washington and testify before the senate and Mr. Hill's committee, and to tell them what was happening in our field with the hope of getting the federal government involved in funding research in psychopharmacology. And so Henry Brill, Nate and I went to Washington. We each gave a presentation, and suggested the formation within the National Institute of Mental Health (NIMH) of a division devoted solely to psychopharmacology. Senator Hill was very impressed and, as a matter of fact, he supported it. That accounted for another meeting in Washington. Lou Lasagna was there, so it was more than just psychiatry. We got pharmacologists involved.

Ralph Gerard from Michigan came. He was the man responsible for Jon Cole becoming the first director of the Psychopharmacology Service Center (PSC).

LH: Gerard was the author of that famous line: "Behind every twisted thought lies a twisted molecule," that I guess for a long while was kind of the moral of biological psychiatry.

FA: Yes, that's true. When you get to that point you begin to attract more attention. Before that, we were called medicine men. We were compared to the guys from the old wild-west going around selling snake oil. Reputable medical journals were not interested in publishing articles on the various psychopharmaceuticals. I gave a paper at the New York Academy of Sciences, Leo, one of the first papers I ever gave. The discussant was Nolan Lewis. You remember Nolan? He was president of the APA at one time. And the closing comment of his discussion of my paper was: "fellows, we ought to prescribe this stuff while it still works." Well, that's not a very good endorsement, is it?

LH: Well, I think that was the prevailing attitude in psychiatry in those days. Drugs couldn't work because they had been tried before and didn't. There had been over the years a lot of attempts to use drugs.

Well, what do you think was the biggest accomplishment that you've made? I know that's a tough question because you've made a lot of them.

FA: Well, I think aside from looking at the drugs and being persistent, I was sort of a St. John the Baptist in the wilderness preaching the gospel of the psychopharmaceuticals and their potential value for people. But as you know, some people called me for awhile Dr. Side Effect, because I was very interested in adverse effects. I felt that I should tell a balanced story that for every blessing there can be smite; you can help and you can smite people with these drugs. That was the first thing. The other one was that I started talking very early about the potential advantages and disadvantages for long-term therapy. I gave a paper at the Third World Congress of Psychiatry in Montreal on one-year continuous treatment with imipramine; then I published a paper in the *New England Journal of Medicine* on a year's clinical and toxicological experience with perphenazine. I've been interested in long-term therapy. In addition of testifying before Congress I was very much involved in getting the American College of Neuropsychopharmacology (ACNP) started. I also went to Milan for the initial meeting of what was to become the Collegium Internationale Neuro-Psychopharmacologicum (CINP). I played a role in the formation of the British College of Neuropsychopharmacology. I went over there at the request of David Wheatley, Tony Hordern and Max Hamilton and met with them for a couple days, told them how we started the ACNP. I've tried to extol the virtues as well as the liabilities of the drugs, because they are the only things that have really changed psychiatry. There is nothing new in the psychotherapy field. Well, you have cognitive therapy and so forth. But the concepts haven't changed.

LH: I think it's become a little less dogmatic.

FA: Yes, I would say that.

LH: Psychotherapeutics now embraces a whole variety of techniques.

FA: Right. Well, the challenge of the drugs, Leo, is that you give a pill and over a period of days or weeks, there is a change in the individual. Bernie Brodie and I became friends because my interest was in what happens. I would ask "what happens when you run a current from both temples through the midbrain, what did you do that suddenly changed a psychotic individual into a perfectly normal person?" And, in the early days, we didn't know how much of the drug was absorbed. We didn't know where it was going, how it got there. And so I was very interested from the beginning in what we call today pharmacokinetics and pharmacodynamics.

LH: Well, I think Bernie Brodie was probably the father of biochemical pharmacology, trying to explain drug action in biochemical terms.

FA: Right. I regretted that he wasn't around that I could have had him on the program of the symposium on Discoveries in Biological Psychiatry, because all we know today stems from his pioneering work. One of my benefits from starting the College was that I got to know him quite well. He, Jon Cole and I were on a committee, and we met frequently because Jon was still in Washington, he was in Washington and I was in Baltimore. I had ample opportunity to get to know him as a man.

LH: You mentioned earlier your testimony before Lister Hill's Committee. We were talking about political pressures in the early days. How about Mary Lasker's and Mike Gorman's work on the political front?

FA: Mike was the executive director of the National Mental Health Association. He was a very dynamic fellow. I don't know if you knew him personally?

LH: No.

FA: He really was a crusader for mental health. He believed in it, and used his contacts in Washington. He played a major role actually in putting pressure behind the scenes on the other members of the committee who may not have been as convinced as Senator Hill was. Right from the beginning, every one of us had a feeling that he listened attentively and seemed to believe that there was something to what we were saying. You know how a Congressional Committee is. They sit. They look.

LH: In those days it was easier to persuade a senator than your own colleagues.

FA: Oh, absolutely. That's very definitely the truth. Well, anyway, Mike played a major role in publicizing psychopharmaceuticals. He saw that it was the only concrete thing that really made a difference. And, of course, he had his connections everywhere. He had connections both in Washington and in New York with Mary Lasker. I strongly suspect that Mike played a role in Heinz Lehmann, Pierre Deniker and Nate Kline getting the Lasker Award.

LH: Do you think the reason that Hill became such an advocate of health was that his first name was Lister?

FA: I really don't know. But he definitely had an interest in this field. There's no question about that.

LH: You were almost a pediatrician and reluctantly, a surgeon.

FA: That was very short-lived. Three weeks.

LH: Sort of accidentally you became a psychiatrist. Do you have any regrets about the way things have turned out?

FA: No, none whatsoever. You know, when I was in medical school, psychiatry was not high on the list. Your exposure consisted of a few lectures, mostly on psychodynamics, and then a trip out to the state hospital. You were sort of taken on a guided tour: that's schizophrenia, this one's manic and that is mental retardation.

LH: Like a zoo, wasn't it?

FA: That's right. And, you know, there was nothing appealing about it whatsoever. But a few weeks after I got to Perry Point, I was assigned to what was euphemistically called continuous treatment service.

LH: That meant for people who were there for years.

FA: Well, there were 800 patients in the ward that I was assigned to, Leo. Most of those people were still under 60 years of age, but they had been in that hospital, most of them, 20–30 years.

LH: Many since World War I.

FA: That's it. Well, I even had one from the Spanish-American War, an old geriatric guy. But, actually, you learned one thing: schizophrenia was chronic and devastating. And it would be true if you put over the portal "abandon hope all ye who enter here," because your chances of leaving, outside of a pine box, were pretty slim.

LH: Well, it has been sort of gratifying, hasn't it, to see the changes that have occurred.

FA: Yes.

LH: Do you think we've gone too far in deinstitutionalizing people?

FA: Well, I think so.

LH: Is there still room for an asylum?

FA: Yes. And that's one of the things the New York Psychiatric Association and the ACNP ought to be taking a very strong stand on. Look, there are people who can be controlled with these medications in a structured environment, but they cannot be relied on to comply with a pharmaceutical program on their own out in the community, and they deteriorate. So, as you know, then tragic things happen. We had a woman in one of those so-called halfway houses in Baltimore some time back who was found dead in bed with a ruptured appendix when they did the autopsy. She was a deteriorated schizophrenic. She was put out of state hospital. She wasn't bothering anybody. She was too deteriorated to bother anybody.

LH: Schizophrenics seem to be so indifferent to pain.

FA: That's very true. When I got to Perry Point, the ward I had was approximately three-quarters of a mile to the dining hall, and three times a day the patients walked over to the dining hall. The attendants had to fight these guys in cold weather to put a coat on. And I remember one night, Leo, I was the officer of the day, and an attendant called and said a patient had gotten out from the shower and they couldn't find him. And, in my naivety, I said to him: "Oh, it's so cold now. He can't be gone long. He'll be back." This attendant was a farmer who worked part time at Perry Point. He said, "Doc, you don't know schizophrenics. If we don't find this man, he's going to be dead." And so he impressed me and we organized a search party. When we found this fellow he was hypothermic. We were lucky we saved his life. I didn't intend to become a psychiatrist when I went there, but made a resolution that I could take care of their physical needs. But I saw patients collapsing from ruptured ulcer who never complained. We had a couple of patients who developed nausea, vomiting, clearly meningitis, who must have had horrible headaches, but never complained. I remember one night a fellow stuffed himself with newspaper and ignited it. And when I got there he was pretty badly burned, but he was still sitting there, hallucinating and answering to voices. We never gave him any morphine. He didn't need it. You're right. Their pain and their temperature sense are quite different.

LH: It could be that Harry Beecher's old idea that pain is processed up here in our head, could explain this indifference to pain that psychotic people seem to have. Well, let me ask you before we quit: would you do it again?

FA: Yes, I would. In fact, when I look back, and I do that fairly often, I wish I had done more. But that's in retrospect. I couldn't have done it if I had wanted to if we didn't have what we have now. The excitement today is still as intense as it was back in 1953, '54, and in the 1960s, with the neuroimaging and all these other things that are happening.

LH: Yes, science is changing so rapidly, and even the vocabulary constantly changes.

FA: That's why I wrote my *Lexicon*.

LH: You have to know now what LOD scores are and all kinds of things that you have never thought of before.

Well, I think you can look back on a very interesting and illustrious career. You have already put some of your thoughts about this subject in writing and published them. I think this interview helped bring out a few more personal things than you would have put in your writings.

FA: That's true. I want to say one thing before we end, Leo. The credit for what I've accomplished should be given to my admiration of other people. You know, when I got involved with drugs, there weren't many people around I could turn to. ECT was not done at the medical schools, at either Maryland or at Hopkins. There was one fellow doing ECT, Lothar Kalinowsky, who was sort of looked upon as a renegade. So I wrote a letter to him and said "I would like to come and spend some time with you." He graciously agreed to have me. I went up for a week, stayed at a hotel, and spent one week with this man. He was one of my tutors. I did the same thing with Howard Fabing who was in Cincinnati. I called Doug Goldman, and I spent time with Doug Goldman. I went up to Canada and spent time with Heinz Lehmann. They were my mentors. These were the people who taught me. So did Titus Harris. He was not a biological psychiatrist. Still, he was a champion of physical methods of treatment, and developed one of the first departments of biological psychiatry in the US. There were a lot of people like that who played a major role. Well, even you. Look how much you've shared with me and taught me. That's been a lot.

LH: It's always mutual.

FA: No man accomplishes anything by himself.

LH: Well, thank you, Frank, for a rather interesting discussion, and anytime you want to say more. . . .

FA: Well, that's up to you.

LH: God, you're easy to interview.

FA: Thank you.

SAMUEL GERSHON

Interviewed by Thomas A. Ban

Acapulco, Mexico, December 15, 1999

TB: We are at the 38th annual meeting of the American College of Neuropsychopharmacology in Acapulco, Mexico. It is December 15, 1999, and I will be interviewing Dr. Sam Gershon* for the Archives of the American College of Neuropsychopharmacology. I'm Thomas Ban. So, Sam, let's start from the very beginning. Where were you born, brought up? If you could say something about your early interests, education, and how you got involved in neuropsychopharmacology.

SG: We'll start when I was born. It was in 1927, and that event was in Poland. Then, in 1929, we came to Australia and I had my education, including medical school, in Sydney, Australia. After that, I went for a psychiatric residency to Melbourne, and then towards the end of that residency, I had a fellowship in the physiology-pharmacology department at the University of Melbourne. Essentially, I continued in the various activities in that department till the end of my residency in '56. And then I went full time to the Department of Pharmacology at the University of Melbourne, and essentially stayed there till, pretty much, I left for the first time to the United States in 1959. Before I left, I was the acting chairman of the department of pharmacology. Then I went to the University of Michigan in Ann Arbor on a Pfizer Fellowship and I spent a year there.

TB: What did you do after that year?

SG: I went back to Australia, to the Department of Pharmacology in Melbourne. I stayed a year there, and then I returned to the United States to work in the Missouri Institute of Psychiatry in St. Louis for a couple of years. Then I went to New York University (NYU), and stayed there for seventeen years.

TB: You've jumped over several years of your activities in Australia. Could you talk about what you did in those years?

SG: During those years I was a resident in psychiatry. I had a mentor at the University of Melbourne, Dr. Trautner, who had started the first large study of lithium after the publication of Cade. Cade's publication was in 1949 and Trautner as soon as the beginning of 1950, started a large clinical trial

---

* Samuel Gershon was born in Lodz, Poland in 1927 and received a medical degree from the University of Sydney in 1950. He trained in psychiatry at the University of Melbourne then turned to pharmacology, becoming the acting head of the department at Melbourne in 1961. In 1963 he immigrated to the United States, taking a post at the Missouri Institute of Psychiatry. In 1965 he became director of the Neuropsychopharmacology Research Unit of New York University, spent the years from 1979 to 1988 as director of the Lafayette Clinic and chairman of psychiatry at Wayne State University, and from 1988 to 1995 as Associate Vice Chancellor for Research at the University of Pittsburgh. Currently he is Vice Chairman of Academic Affairs in the department of psychiatry at the University of Miami.

of lithium. He studied one hundred psychiatric subjects, more than any-body had before or for a long time after. He was also first to introduce the use of plasma lithium assays. It was possible for him to do that because about a year before, Dr. Victor Wynn at the University of Melbourne pub-lished on the use of flame photometry to assay electrolytes, including lithium. So, in all the patients he studied and published on in 1951, he had done plasma lithium assays. In his publication Trautner noted that one should monitor lithium levels to prevent potential toxicity. And that was an enormous advance for the clinical use of lithium. Cade had never used plasma lithium monitoring; he felt that adequate clinical observa-tions were sufficient. About the same time, two important events relevant to lithium treatment took place. First, in 1949, in the United States, many people died from lithium poisoning when lithium chloride was marketed as a substitute for sodium chloride for treating patients with hyperten-sion. Then, in 1951, Trautner pointed out that monitoring lithium levels indicated a therapeutic window of the drug. And, pretty much, he set the window the way it's always been for fifty years, from 0.6 mEql to 1.2 mEql. So, very early on after Cade's paper was published, Trautner's paper appeared and provided some essential information on how lithium should be used. Undoubtedly it was Cade who made the initial observa-tion on the therapeutic effects of lithium. But it was Trautner's work that made possible the broad clinical use of lithium. Trautner also highlighted that the action of lithium is pretty much restricted to its efficacy in typi-cal mania. He was supportive of the specificity of lithium for mania, an issue that has been debated during the past fifty years, and has remained pretty much unresolved. Following Trautner's first report, we conducted a series of other lithium studies. One of these studies, published in 1955, dealt with the teratology of lithium. It is interesting that at this annual meeting Dr. Manji referred to some of the teratological findings we had with lithium on tadpoles. In fact, all we found was a high rate of embry-onic absorption in frogs; and as far as we could tell lithium had an effect on embryogenesis but there was no teratology. Today, in the light of some later reports in humans, the teratology of lithium is more clear. The pur-ported increase in cardiac abnormality did not seem to be supported by later reports which indicated that the incidence of cardiac abnormalities with lithium is within the statistical distribution of the general population. Still, some teratological findings with lithium might be real.

TB: Did you participate in establishing the therapeutic window of lithium?

SG: Yes. We didn't go around and establish the therapeutic window. We essentially said that's what we thought it was. The idea that we should go around and establish it in controlled studies back in the early 1950s never entered our mind. There was no funding to ever contemplate such a study in Australia.

TB: Did you do any other clinical research with lithium?

SG: Oh, yes, we did many studies with lithium after the first one. In one of these studies we found increased retention of the lithium ion in the manic phase, and increased excretion of it when mania was resolved, followed by homeostasis. We published these findings in 1955 with the title "The excretion and retention of ingested lithium and its effect on the ionic balance of man," in the *Medical Journal of Australia*. I was also involved in the teratology paper and in another paper with lithium, which didn't have lithium in the title. It was a paper on the pharmacological treatment of shock dependency. We had bipolar patients and they were on maintenance ECT; we gave them lithium, not just for the episode, but also for prophylaxis, to replace ECT, and that's where the title came from. We could, essentially, treat shock dependency prophylactically by giving lithium for long-term.

TB: Any other studies?

SG: Yes.

TB: Could you say something about your other studies with lithium while in Melbourne?

SG: There were a whole lot of lithium studies that followed the first one. The other ones were related to findings that tended to indicate that we might have to limit the clinical indications for lithium. We thought first that it would be indicated for recurrent episodic psychotic activity. And that included what, some years later, Perris referred to as cycloid psychosis. The central thing we found with lithium is that its efficacy is restricted to pure bipolar disease, to the so-called typical manic depressive disorder as described in British texts.

TB: What other research did you do besides lithium in Australia?

SG: I did a whole lot of other research in Melbourne in the Department of Pharmacology. I got involved in looking at pharmacological antagonists to morphine, and we developed synthetic compounds in the department for this purpose. We tried them in animal models, for example in dogs, because the dog responds with dose dependent sedation to morphine. We actually developed a series of amiphenazole-like compounds, which were antagonists to morphine. We also developed some indole alkaloids that were also antagonists. Another morphine antagonist we identified was succinic acid. It's a dramatic antagonist to morphine-induced sedation and morphine coma. The last substance we tested in our animal model was THA, tetrahydroaminoacridane.

TB: Could you elaborate on your findings with THA?

SG: Well, we found that it was a morphine antagonist. It is clearly a cholineste-rase inhibitor. In the last ten years or so, the focus of research with THA was in the treatment of Alzheimer's dementia, based mainly on its cholinesterase inhibiting properties. At the time we worked with THA we also had a series of atropinergic agents available which could pro-duce aberrant behavioral states in dogs and induce atropine psychosis and coma in humans. The interesting finding with THA was that it was a potent antagonist to both morphine-induced sedation and atropine-induced aberrant behavioral states. It was also a potent antagonist to imipramine and amitriptyline delirium; and used therapeutically for these indications. Then later on, in 1960, we developed other aspects of its util-ity when we found that similar to succinic acid, it has a general alerting effect in many CNS depressed states.

TB: Could you elaborate on this research?

SG: Well, this research goes back to 1959, when I went to the University of Michigan to work in the – at the time famous – schizophrenia and psychopharmacology research project, headed by Ralph W. Gerard at Ann Arbor. Gerard was a neurophysiologist but he had ideas about how one could dissect schizophrenia by various basic science approaches. Of course it didn't work out that way, but it provided a very remarkable opportunity to do other research. What we were involved in was the use of chemical models for psychiatric disorders. We had available at that time a psychotogen, called Ditran, which was an anticholinergic agent and produced in dogs a hyperactive disturbed behavioral state. Based on my previous research with atropinergic agents in Australia we adminis-tered THA to dogs and found that it antagonized the Ditran-induced state and restored animals to normal behavior. So, we had an anticholinergic paradigm of what could be considered grossly aberrant behavior, and we had an antagonist. Ditran produced a psychopathological state where the individuals would have hallucinations, delusions and some disorien-tation, and its effect could be counteracted with the administration of THA. At the same time, other people were using phencyclidine, Sernyl, to induce a psychotogenic model state. We also had the opportunity to study Sernyl-induced psychotogenic model states. THA had an incon-sistent antagonistic effect of phencyclidine-induced psychopathology.

We had studied in Australia a series of yohimbine alkaloids, includ-ing yohimbine indole alkaloids, harmine derivatives, and ibogaine deriva-tives, in dogs, and found that all indole alkaloids antagonized morphine-induced sedation and coma, and also the psychotogenic states induced by anticholinergics. So when I got to the US, I had the opportunity of taking the yohimbine research from the animal model into the human and testing whether yohimbine has anxiogenic effects. After a series of experiments in animals, we injected yohimbine intravenously into humans and we saw a dose dependent anxiety state produced with all of the physiological concomitants. By increasing the dose of yohimbine we could produce panic. In both dogs and humans, there was an increase in blood pressure and pulse rate with all of the other autonomic effects that a patient with anxiety would have, sweating, etc. We had also shown that any of the anxiolytics available at the time would control this yohimbine-induced anxiety and panic state in humans. An interesting finding was that tricyclic antidepressants aggravated the anxiety. We did a lot of other experiments with this anxiogenic model and many years later, the group at Yale used the yohimbine model as a sensitizer in a whole lot of studies of panic states.

TB: If I understood you correctly, all this research started in Australia in animals?

SG: All of this started there. None of the indole stuff was done in Australia in humans. It was all done in animals. I was involved between Australia and the US in the development of a number of agents that could be used as chemically induced models of schizophrenic-like states, and yohimbine as a model of anxiety and panic. I was also involved in the development of antagonists to all these agents.

TB: Was all your research in Australia done in the department of pharmacology after you completed your residency in psychiatry.

SG: Yes. Actually psychiatry at the time was not a big thing in Australia. The departmental chairman in Sydney was a gentleman called Wolfgang Siegfried Dawson, who had written a textbook of psychiatry which would fit into your vest-pocket. That was the size of his textbook in psychiatry. In Melbourne, there was no chairman of psychiatry at that time. There were chiefs of psychiatry divisions at the teaching hospitals.

TB: I assume this was before Brian Davis became chairman.

SG: Oh, yes.

TB: Did you do any clinical work in psychiatry while you were in the Department of Pharmacology in Melbourne?

SG: I had an appointment as a consultant psychiatrist to two of the teaching hospitals.

TB: You went to the States for a year. Was your appointment at Ann Arbor in the department of psychiatry?

SG: I was in Michigan from 1959 to 1960, and during that year I was doing research in a schizophrenia and psychopharmacology project that Ralph Gerard was running. It was a project that was funded by the NIMH through Jonathan Cole's division. Actually, it was during that time that I met Jonathan Cole for the first time when he site visited our program that he funded.

TB: When you say Jonathan Cole's division at NIMH, are you referring to the Psychopharmacology Service Center?

SG: Right. He had with him, at the site visit in '59, Gerry Klerman and Reese Jones. So, I met Jonathan Cole and these other folks. And Jonathan was to become an important contact for me from then on, even after I went back to Australia for a year.

TB: What did you do during the year you were back in Australia?

SG: On my return to Australia in 1960, Dr. Shaw and I undertook a study on the effect of organo-phosphorus insecticides, which are non-reversible cholinesterase inhibitors that some scientists and farmers are exposed to. We found that some people in contact with such insecticides developed either a depressive or a schizophreniform psychiatric disorder. I was back in Australia only for a year, because on Jonathan Cole's suggestion, the people at the Missouri Institute of Psychiatry in St. Louis got in touch with me and invited me to join them.

TB: Was it George Ulett who invited you?

SG: George Ulett was there and also Max Fink; they were running the show and I joined them.

TB: Could you tell us something about the place and also about the research you did while there?

SG: It was a remarkable place. It was one of the premier physical facilities available for psychiatric research in the United States. George Ulett had an enormous vision for creating that research institute. Have you ever visited the place? Heinz Lehmann was there many times.

TB: I did visit, but later on.

SG: It was a remarkable place. I had 150 dedicated research beds when I got there. I had also the opportunity of becoming involved in finalizing the building. All of the animal laboratories were state of the art facilities. I stayed there for two years, approximately, and that gave me an opportunity to do a whole lot of animal work and a whole lot of clinical studies, as well. I also had the opportunity to do electroencephalographic (EEG) evaluations with Max Fink and Turan Itil, and study the central nervous system effects of the agents I worked with in Australia. So we could clearly document in a series of studies the dramatic slowing of the EEG induced by anticholinergic drugs in human. We administered Ditran and documented that it produced similar changes in the EEG which are seen in patients with neurological deficit, brain injury, and alcoholics with cognitive deficit. We also documented the antagonistic effect of THA to Ditran on the EEG, and noted that those patients with neurological damage get cognitive deficit after the administration of lower doses of the drug.

TB: So your later work with cholinesterase inhibitors was based on your research in animals in Melbourne and research in humans in St. Louis?

SG: Oh, yes. THA was the first cholinesterase inhibitor I worked with and we had our first studies in animals with THA in the late 1950s and early 1960s. It was many years later that based on our early research, THA was tried in the treatment of Alzheimer's dementia.

TB: So it was your finding in St. Louis that THA counteracts anticholinergic induced EEG changes combined with clinical observations that the substance could counteract the cognitive deficit produced by anticholinergic drugs that led to the research with cholinesterase inhibitors in Alzheimer's dementia.

How long did you stay in St. Louis?

SG: I was there about two years.

TB: Did you do any other research while there?

SG: There was a lot of activity in St. Louis; we had a very good group there, a bunch of laboratory pharmacologists and a bunch of clinicians. We had neuropsychologists and we had visiting psychiatrists that would come from other countries and work on our various projects. It was a very stimulating environment. And, as you know, later on, due to whatever political difficulties existed within the state of Missouri, it essentially died.

TB: Didn't this happen after you left?

SG: I left before it died.

TB: You left for NYU?

SG: Right.

TB: How did you get to NYU?

SG: I got a job there. Actually Arnie Friedhoff was responsible for recruiting me to NYU. Arnie had a very active program in psychopharmacology there, both preclinical and clinical. And, with his help, we had the opportunity of trying to replicate a combined pre-clinical and clinical program in psychopharmacology. I think I got there in about '63. It was a great setting; it provided all sorts of opportunities.

TB: Could you talk about your research at NYU?

SG: We had the opportunity there of having a research ward. We had laboratories and we had the opportunity of recruiting young research fellows into a psychopharmacology research unit in the department of psychiatry, with a lot of support from Arnie Friedhoff, and the chairman at the time, who was Sam Wortis, Joe Wortis' relative, not his brother. Sam Wortis was never an important figure in psychopharmacology himself, but he was sort of a main support individual for biological research in psychiatry in his department. I think it's not known to many people, but he was a very important figure, nationally as well, in supporting biological psychiatry in many ways, influenced in that direction by Arnie Friedhoff.

TB: Could you say something about the research in your unit at NYU?

SG: Well, I was there for a long time from 1963 until about 1980. That's almost seventeen years and, golly, we had a whole bunch of people. We managed to attract a lot of young research fellows, who really have all developed into very successful individuals. And I think it's very important to stress the value of the opportunity to mentor young people. It's really something that should be addressed in some form or way in a setting like the ACNP. They do have many fellowships in the ACNP for various groups, but that's not exactly the same as close physical mentoring, in one's department or division or facility. That seems to be the essential component. We started in New York a lithium program and a lithium clinic, at the time that Baron Shopsin joined. And we developed a very large program in bipolar disorders. Out of that program came a lot of work dealing with the specificity of lithium for the diagnostic entity of bipolar disorder; Baron Shopsin, together with others in the group, did a series of studies looking at lithium vs. neuroleptics vs. a control group in the treatment of schizoaffective disorder and schizophrenia vs. mania. The other person that joined us and worked in the same area of research was Gordon Johnson from Australia. He spent several years with us as a Fellow. Our research tended to support the idea that lithium was effective in controlled studies against a reference drug in mania. It was clearly better than placebo. Chlorpromazine was the active reference drug at the time. It was certainly effective, and had a faster onset of behavioral control in mania, but the opinion that resulted from those studies was that lithium had a much more significant effect on the core pathology than chlorpromazine did and patients could be discharged at about the same time, but their functional level appeared to be more intact with lithium than with the neuroleptic. These were the findings in the studies conducted by Johnson and Shopsin in mania.

Then, studies were done in a schizophrenia group and a schizoaffective group and there it appeared fairly clearly that in the schizoaffective group, lithium was dramatically less effective than the neuroleptic, either chlorpromazine or Haldol (haloperidol). These findings tended to support the specificity of lithium in the treatment of mania. In fact, not only was lithium less effective than neuroleptics but it appeared to increase pathology in the schizophrenic and the schizoaffective groups. Baron Shopsin then led a series of additional studies with lithium, where we pursued the finding that lithium has very major effects on thyroid function and caused hypothyroidism. And then, a whole lot of other research was conducted with endocrinologists to find out how lithium was producing hypothyroidism.

TB: Were these some of the earliest findings on the effects of lithium on the thyroid?

SG: I can't say that we were the first or the second in showing the effects of lithium on the thyroid but these findings were early on. Another very dramatic finding was that lithium produced leukocytosis. We published it in about 1970. It hung around as a potential harbinger of some horrible hematological disease, until these patients were followed up for longer periods of time, and other investigators in Europe, especially Schou and others, could assure everybody that lithium has no serious hematological effects. Later on, it was found that one could use lithium-induced leukocytosis in cancer chemotherapy to increase white cell count that was depressed by chemotherapeutic agents for cancer. So even if that was an adventitial finding, it was clearly, an important one. The actual mechanism of how lithium increases white cell count is unknown to this day. These research activities with lithium developed as a sort of separate research division from the other research activities we conducted with lithium at the same time. For example, we studied the ratio of intracellular and extracellular lithium and the importance of this ratio in the clinical use of the substance. We also developed an assay for measuring lithium in the saliva instead of the blood, and a statistic for translating the saliva value to the plasma value. Also, Gordon Johnson did a whole lot of EEG studies with lithium in bipolar disorder. He found that patients with cognitive or organic neurological damage were supersensitive to lithium's central nervous system adverse effects. He also correlated the lithium induced EEG changes with intracellular and extracellular ratio shifts of lithium. So we had a whole series of studies in our lithium program. We also had a schizophrenia research program with Burton Angrist.

TB: So you had a research program with lithium in bipolar disorder, and a research program in schizophrenia?

SG: We did have these programs, and we also started one of the early geriatric research programs at a time when thinking about Alzheimer dementia must have been pretty naive, because the first funding support we had from NIMH for geriatric research was for a very large and very expensive study on hyperbaric oxygen in the treatment of senile dementia of the Alzheimer type. Once we knew that we were going to get that level of support in geriatric research we had to recruit staff that would implement this very large and very expensive project. At NYU we already had a hyperbaric chamber which was not used very much, so they were very happy for us to use it. At that time I recruited Steve Ferris, who came as a neuropsychologist to the program, a bit later, Barry Reisberg, and later on, Mony DeLeon. All three are full professors now in the department of psychiatry. All three are now internationally recognized in the area of Alzheimer's research. And that was out of a mentoring experience; all three entered the field with no prior research experience in any area. I think this shows that all you need is bright people and a structure that permits intimate mentoring.

TB: You mentioned hyperbaric oxygen as one of the projects you had in your geriatric program. What did you find?

SG: It was clear at the end of this expensive exercise that hyperbaric oxygen was no better than placebo. But, it helped in establishing a very talented geriatric research group.

TB: What else did you do in your geriatric research program?

SG: That geriatric research program developed in many different areas, looking at potential therapeutic agents. And then, each of the people that I mentioned contributed to geriatric psychiatry with their particular knowledge and expertise. Mony DeLeon has gone on to become a major figure in looking at changes in the morphology of brain nuclei in Alzheimer's disease using magnetic resonance imaging (MRI) and identified the targeted changes in the hippocampus. Barry Reisberg has gone on to describe the phenomenological aspects of the deteriorating process and developed scales for documenting this. And Steve Ferris has become a major figure in the psychological measurements of changes in dementia in geriatric patients. The program provided the infrastructure for looking at potential therapeutic agents. THA was the first compound to get FDA approval as an agent in the treatment of dementia. It was the old compound, THA, which had some minimal effect on the symptoms of these patients, but no matter how modest its effect was, it changed the climate and moved research in the treatment of diseases in the aged from studies which made no sense, like the one we did with hyperbaric oxygen, to studies that would test and could support hypotheses like the cholinergic deficit hypothesis, as one contributing factor to the development of Alzheimer's disease. Regardless how minimal the effect of THA was, it changed our thinking in this area of research by turning attention on the possibility of trying to find drugs that would intervene with the process that leads to dementia. And that was very important, a major, major change in the watershed of looking at therapeutic concepts for this condition, considered completely untreatable.

TB: Was yours one of the first psychogeriatric units in the country?

SG: One of the early programs in the country was set up at NYU and the program has National Institute on Aging center support, till now. It was established early on and it has developed and grown enormously without me being there. It has done much better since I left.

TB: Could you say something about your program in schizophrenia?

SG: The schizophrenia program was quite diverse. We looked at lots of therapeutic agents, and we also looked at the concept whether there was a therapeutic window, a metabolic target with chlorpromazine in schizophrenia. Then we did quite a lot of research about metabolites of chlorpromazine that have therapeutic activity. We were the beneficiary of NIMH support for looking at plasma levels of chlorpromazine, its millions of metabolites and their therapeutic activity. We had a laboratory developed to do chemical assays for these compounds and we had several years of support in looking at the effects of these metabolites and clinical outcome. Again, our first effort in this area of research was not revolutionary. But soon after we started our program in schizophrenia Burt Angrist came along out of a residency program, and he was interested in starting research in this area. He joined as a research fellow, and we were looking around for a potential project for him. Based on my prior work with chemically induced models, we discussed the possible value of a dopaminergic model. We were at the time in the early sixties. There was important work done on amphetamine and psychosis, psychosis in amphetamine users, published by that time. We decided with Burt Angrist to do first a survey of patients admitted with amphetamine psychosis. Burt had a superior sensitivity to clinical phenomenology, and he would then follow these patients who were admitted through to their remission and document phenomenological changes from the acute phases of the psychosis to clearing and remission. He documented what might have been known before, that hallucinations went first, and then delusions and so on. He put the phenomenological changes on a very firm footing. Then, since with amphetamine we're not manipulating one but several transmitters, we carried out a whole series of experiments in which we had the opportunity of measuring metabolites of neurotransmitters on people who were admitted. Burt Angrist clearly showed that within a four to five day period, one could induce with amphetamine a psychosis that was not just a paranoid excited hyperactive state. You could produce a psychosis with negative symptoms as well. You could produce anergy, and, the whole clinical picture of schizophrenia. He raised the issue that this was in truth a very interesting analog of the disease itself, and then went along with many of the other hypotheses that supported the dopamine construct that was then the mainstay in the development of antipsychotic drugs. Then he took it further by looking at to what extent norepinephrine played a role vs. dopamine and its metabolites, and tracked the whole sequence of events to essentially target dopamine as the primary guilty component in this development. That whole program with Burt involved fit in, very much, with work that Arvid Carlsson was doing on the dissociation between dopamine and norepinephrine. So, that was really a very profitable venture. And there were many other people that were involved in our schizophrenia program. One of them was John Rotrosen, who joined the group early on. He is professor of psychiatry now at NYU, and a member of the ACNP.

TB: Didn't you have also a program in depression?

SG: Yes, we had a program on depression. Some of the work in this program was done with the scientific input of Menek Goldstein, and that was very interesting. Of course, it raised again the issue that's not one culprit, but then maybe there is one that's more important than another. We did some experiments, in which Baron Shopsin was involved and a lot of other people like Sherwin Wilk from Mount Sinai. So, essentially, what we were doing was that we treated endogenously depressed patients with either imipramine or a monoamine oxidase inhibitor, till there was a therapeutic response. Then all those patients that achieved a therapeutic response were assigned at random to either α-methylparatyrosine (AMPT) or parachlorophenylalanine (PCPA), thus inhibiting norepinephrine metabolism in one and serotonin metabolism in the other. The dramatic effect simply was that the group in which we inhibited norepinephrine stayed fine, whereas in the ones we inhibited serotonin all relapsed within twenty-four to forty-eight hours. These findings, of course, were later confirmed by Aghajanian and De Montigny at Yale doing neurophysiological studies. Later on, the Yale group by using their tryptophan cocktail replicated and extended our initial findings about the significant role of serotonin in depression. The role of serotonin in the therapeutic response has become clear, but to what extent the role of serotonin was primal in the etiology of depression was not clarified. But the findings in our studies were of importance in the development of an understanding about the significant role of serotonin in depression, because at the time, as I'm sure you will remember, there was the catecholamine hypothesis that simply put norepinephrine up in mania and norepinephrine down in depression. Our findings did not entirely support that conclusion.

TB: Your findings were more in keeping with theories of depression advanced in Europe.

SG: Well, actually . . . .

TB: So, these were the activities in the famous Sam Gershon unit at NYU?

SG: Right. The psychopharmacology group was not only a vehicle for research. It was also a production line for very talented people to become successful.

TB: And all of them seem to remember their experience working with you very happily. They talk about the years when these activities took place as The Golden Age.

SG: Well, it was a very pleasant time. Everybody could interact with everybody in a free environment.

TB: Is there anything else you would like to add about your research at NYU?

SG: These were the essential things. In essence, there was a psychopharmacology research group at NYU, it did have these categories of activity and it produced a lot of very smart people.

TB: Then you moved.

SG: Yes, I moved to Detroit, to Wayne University.

TB: Could you say something about your activities in Detroit?

SG: Well, I went there as a bureaucrat, as the chairman of the Department of Psychiatry. They had that remarkable facility, the Lafayette Psychiatric Research Clinic there, and that gave me an opportunity to bring in a group of people that could be actively involved. We had a pre-clinical and a clinical geriatric program at Wayne. Nunzio Pomara came with me from NYU, and also Mike Stanley to become head of the pharmacology laboratories. We recruited about a dozen PhDs to run laboratory programs. We had very generous support for visiting research fellows from overseas. One of them was Bernard Lerer, who came for two years, and in the first year he got the second prize of the Bennett Award for biological research and in the second year, he got the first prize of the Bennett Award for his research.

TB: What did he do?

SG: He was doing work on a series of things with Mike Stanley and he was also involved with bipolar disease and carbamazepine. He did studies on cholinergic mechanisms and ECT. He was involved in a wide range of activity, but each of the prizes, of course, was for a focused and directed research project.

TB: Is there anything else you would like to add about your activities at Wayne?

SG: Nothing else except the fact that it again provided an opportunity for the development of research activities in the well-supported atmosphere of a state funded clinical research program. As you know, the Lafayette Clinic is no longer in existence. It suffered the fate of many state funded research programs throughout the whole US. The one in St. Louis, The Missouri Institute of Psychiatry, was essentially closed down. Lafayette Clinic was closed down and that's another separate problem.

TB: Where did you go from Wayne?

SG: I went to Pittsburgh to join the master organizer of the age, Tom Detre, as the associate vice chancellor for research for health sciences. And with

Tom as support, we then carried out his vision of growth in the medical research programs at the University. I had the opportunity to put in place some new directions.

TB: Like what?

SG: It's important to stress that without Tom's involvement, nothing would have been possible. He saw the value of having a clinical pharmacology program. Clinical pharmacology in the US was not a major activity. It certainly had its strongest activity in the United Kingdom. It had activities in Europe, but was mainly active in the United Kingdom. With Tom's assistance, we got support to develop a clinical pharmacology program at Pittsburgh. We recruited a director, an Englishman, Bob Branch, who came and developed an important clinical pharmacology program. He became director of the CRC (clinical research center) for the medical school. And again with the support and vision of Tom Detre we could create an imaging center, which as you know, is a very expensive toy. But it was created and there is now a positron emission tomography (PET) Center in the medical center, a nuclear magentic resonance imaging (NMR) Center and an NMR Spectroscopy Center that is located on two separate floors in the medical school. It is important to recognize the fact that it was put in place at a time when in many places the importance of such a center was debated. The importance of an imaging center is highlighted by the fact that at this meeting there was a major session dedicated to imaging research.

TB: What are you doing now?

SG: Now, I'm an elderly gentleman and removed from most administrative activities. I'm a professor of psychiatry. I have continued, up to recently, to be the director of an adolescent alcohol research center, which is funded by the National Institute of Alcohol Abuse and Alcoholism (NIAA), that I will hand over to a younger and more creative gentleman.

TB: But at this point in time you are still the director of that center?

SG: Well, it's in transition right now.

TB: You have been very active since the 1950s.

SG: Early fifties.

TB: During the years you have published widely. Do you remember what your first publication was?

SG: My first publication was on the embryological effect of lithium. Then I published on morphine antagonists, on succinic acid, a morphine antagonist.

TB: Didn't you collaborate while still in Australia with Barney Carroll?

SG: Right, Barney Carroll joined me to do a science degree in pharmacology in the middle of his medical training. We looked at succinic acid in carbon dioxide poisoning and found that it has beneficial effects. Barney did his thesis on that. Dr. Carroll came to the United States, subsequently, and became chairman of psychiatry at Duke.

TB: Didn't you work in the same period also with barbiturates?

SG: That's right. We looked in addition to antagonists to morphine, at pharmacological antagonists to barbiturates. At that time, barbiturate poisoning and barbiturate suicide were a big deal. It isn't now, but it was then, and it was important to develop analeptic treatments for barbiturate poisoning. And, we did, in fact, develop Bemegride (3-ethyl-3-methyl-glutaramide), a suitable agent for the treatment of barbiturate poisoning. It was also marketed as a mixture with barbiturate pills. It is not specific against barbiturates; it has analeptic properties but it has not been studied beyond barbiturates.

TB: How many papers have you published approximately?

SG: I'd say about six hundred and fifty.

TB: What was the last one?

SG: The most recent ones were dealing with inositol. Lithium is an inhibitor of inositol phosphatase and affects inositol metabolism. A series of experiments were done at Pittsburgh in this area of research with a research fellow, Dr. Levine, who came to us from Israel. We found in our clinical research that inositol has an effect on treatment resistant depression, but the sample size of our study was too small to produce more than a trend.

TB: So, this was your last publication?

SG: Well, don't say the last. That's a horrible thing to say; most recent.

TB: Most recent, I'm sorry. Is there anything we left out that you would like to add?

SG: No, other than the fact that my experiences in the US all produced opportunities for growth. And the people I met in the US, from Jonathan Cole on, all promoted growth and the PSC was the engine of growth in psychopharmacology in the US. I'm sure you're the beneficiary of some of that fallout in Canada. And, it should be clear that individuals can make an important difference and that goes right down to the sort of ability to mentor other investigators and do it on a personal level. It isn't the institution or the money, alone, that creates these things. It's a matter of individuals all along the way making contributions far beyond what an institution alone can do.

TB: What would you say was your most important contribution?

SG: Oh, we listed some of the actual scientific activities, which all have a different value, but the most rewarding, really, was to work with young talented people and have a mutual interchange of excitement and growth. That really was the most rewarding, following all of these experiences.

TB: Thank you very much for sharing all this information with us.

SG: Very well, terrific.

TB: And I hope you will continue with your work, training people and doing research even if retired from your administrative activities.

SG: Yes, I will continue with a sort of research.

TB: I hope you will continue for many years to come.

SG: Thank you very much.

TB: Thank you.

HANNS F. HIPPIUS

Interviewed by Andrea Tone
Paris, France, July 5, 2004

AT: Good morning. My name is Andrea Tone, we're at the Paris CINP Congress in 2004, and, today it is my pleasure to interview Hanns Hippius.* Thank you for joining us. Can I start by asking you about your background in Germany and how you became interested in psychiatry?

HH: I was born in the middle of Germany in Thuringia in 1925, and after the war I studied medicine and chemistry; that is my background to psychopharmacology. After finishing my studies in medicine at the University of Marburg in Germany, I was an assistant for two years in immunology in the Institute of Experimental Medicine in Marburg. And then I moved to Berlin to the Free University of Berlin and was engaged in research, mainly in epilepsy. It was just a year before chlorpromazine was introduced.

AT: That was in 1953?

HH: I came to Berlin in '52. At the time we didn't have much contact with other countries, because people still remembered what happened in psychiatry during the Nazi regime in Germany. When I was an assistant we had difficulties in getting information from the rest of the world. We spoke only German and no other languages. When I learned from research done in other countries that chlorpromazine has an effect on psychotic illness I became interested in doing some basic research with the drug. It preceded my interest in clinical investigations and the research I was to be involved in throughout my professional career.

AT: Let me take you back a bit. You have said in previous interviews that your father, who I believe was a chemist, was conflicted about you going into medicine. Why did you choose medicine, and at what point did you decide conclusively that you wanted to pursue psychiatry?

HH: My father was a teacher, and he advised me to study physics and chemistry, but I was not very successful with my first steps in those fields and decided to enter medical school. I studied medicine first in Marburg and, then in Berlin, and was fascinated with the basic sciences of medicine. But I had also other interests, e.g., in fine arts, and while studying medicine I also took courses in those other fields. At the time it was possible to do that. After I graduated in medicine I thought of doing first some research in the basic sciences and was involved for a couple of years with research in immunology in animals. Then I decided to spend a couple of years at the Free University of Berlin and it was during that time that I

---

* Hanns Ferdinand Hippius was born in Mühlhausen, Germany, in 1925, and graduated in medicine at the University of Marburg in 1950. In 1953 he began training in psychiatry at the Free University of Berlin, where he remained until becoming professor of psychiatry in Munich and head of the department in 1971.

became interested in doing biochemical research in psychiatric patients. In 1953 I began with my training in psychiatry. My idea at the time was to combine psychiatry with my other interests. But I became fascinated by psychiatry and decided to continue my activities in the field. And I would do the same again but with much less prior hesitation.

AT: Was German psychiatry, at this time, in any way resistant to the introduction of chlorpromazine, and if so in what way?

HH: Yes, it was. It was a difficult situation because of what happened during the war with psychiatric patients. As a result, after the war, psychiatric patients were completely neglected. Psychiatric hospitals were run down and had to be rebuilt and renovated. I was very much involved in getting that done. The German government had appointed a special committee of 25 members to attend to those matters and I was a member of that committee.

AT: Can you tell us more about that? That's very interesting.

HH: Between 1945 and the end of the 1960s, those entering the field of psychiatry were very displeased with the situation they saw in state mental hospitals. It was a horrible scene. After the war for some time the university departments in psychiatry were inactive. People were hesitant to do anything because of what happened in the past. The professors were skeptical about treatment with the new drugs. They were very hesitant to treat psychotic patients with drugs. Immediately after the war, people in psychiatry were interested in psychoanalysis, psychotherapy, and social psychiatry. I understand that people who were responsible for psychiatry immediately after the war had to be very careful and why they were hesitant using psychotropic drugs. I'm glad that I was not in their position. But we, the younger generation of psychiatrists, started to do research. We had done what we could to revive psychiatry in the old German tradition. But we also looked at what was happening in psychiatry in the United States. In 1975 our committee delivered to the government a report and proposal of changes we thought would be needed in psychiatry, and after that was accepted everything moved ahead smoothly. In January 1971 I moved from Berlin to Munich. It was an opportunity for me to do something that I thought was needed in psychiatry. I was able to get people interested in my approach and I had many pupils there. I'm proud that many of my pupils are now in charge of university departments in Germany, Switzerland, Austria, and other countries all over the world.

AT: With that impressive legacy, to what extent would you say there is such a thing as a German psychiatric tradition today, or how much have historical differences been glossed over or internationalized?

HH: I believe in the German tradition more and more. For instance, we will celebrate the centennial of the department of psychiatry at the University of Munich. It was the department of Emil Kraepelin. It is the department where Alois Alzheimer worked. In 1955, I was invited to Paris to attend the first symposium on chlorpromazine. Two years later I went for the first time to the United States. The practice of psychiatry everywhere is based on Kraepelin's work and also to a lesser extent on Alzheimer's work. I am convinced that German psychiatry has influenced international psychiatry. But, it is also important that psychiatry in Germany was influenced by the US in the areas of psychotherapy and psychoanalysis.

AT: Given your enthusiasm for psychotropic drugs, what role do you see therapy and psychoanalysis playing in the treatment of patients?

HH: In the first period after the introduction of psychotropic drugs it was believed that it would not be necessary to combine psychotropic drugs with psychotherapy. I am convinced now that this was wrong. We need to combine the two to get the best for individual patients.

AT: You have expressed some misgivings about the current diagnostic classification, and that you think we need to go further and not just look at target symptoms, as a laundry list of symptoms. Could you say a little bit more about that and how that might work in practice?

HH: At the time I had my training in psychiatry we were primarily interested in Kraepelin. But by the late 1950s there was steadily increasing interest in Ernst Kretschmer and in a dimensional approach to psychiatry. Kraepelin began with his work in the nineteenth century and he was influenced by the concept of illness that has a cause and is manifest in a typical syndrome. And in the late 1950s we felt that that concept was too narrow. Kraepelin came to Munich in 1904 and established in Munich the so-called Deutsche Forschungsanstalt für Psychiatrie. Kraepelin was not rigid and was open to change. His textbook has nine editions and it is fascinating to read his thoughts. He was an empiricist in his research. He described exactly what he saw. At a certain point in time I became skeptical about some of Kraepelin's work but as time passed I recognized that he was the founder of biological psychiatry. He was very much interested in psychological studies but he had experts doing research in all the different areas of psychiatry at his clinic. Kraepelin in the late 19th century published a small book that dealt with the effect of drugs on psychometric performance. The title of the book is *Ueber die Beeinflussung einfacher Vorgänge durch Arzneimittel*. It was published in 1892. The roots of psychopharmacology are in that book. I am proud that I had the Kraepelin chair for many years. It is true that he described only the symptomatology of mental diseases without any consideration of the brain. But with hindsight one can understand this. My only criticism of Kraepelin is that his idea that of nosological entities was too narrow. Kraepelin himself, after founding the Research Institute in Munich, abandoned his early concepts. He died in 1926, and I'm convinced that if he had lived longer, he would have got to a multidimensional approach.

AT: I have a final question for you. I've interviewed a lot of psychiatrists now. Not all of them have the same passion for history that you have. You have it; Tom Ban has it; David Healy has it. Why the interest in history?

HH: I was already interested in history when I was a young boy. And after the war, I was interested in the history of the Nazi era, how those terrible things could happen. Then, I worked at the Free University that was established by the United States. The other university in Berlin was in East Berlin.

AT: What would you say, looking back, the chief contribution of biological psychiatry has been? Some people say it's overemphasized, because we've spent too much time clinging to or identifying brain chemistry.

HH: In the US, psychoanalytic psychiatry dominated the field when the first effective drugs in psychiatry were introduced. It was important to move ahead with research in all the different areas of psychiatry. In Germany there was considerable hesitation about accepting biological psychiatry in the 1950s. Social conditions have a major impact on psychiatry and there was great interest in social psychiatry, but it was important to combine biological and social psychiatry. And of course, general psychopathology, developed in Germany, and the French clinical tradition in psychiatry, should not be forgotten.

AT: Can you think of anything else you would like to add to the interview that I haven't asked?

HH: No. It was very enjoyable.

AT: Yes, I also enjoyed it very much.

LEO E. HOLLISTER

Interviewed by Frank J. Ayd, Jr.
San Juan, Puerto Rico, December 11, 1996

FA: Good day. I'm Dr. Frank J. Ayd, Jr. from Baltimore, Maryland. I'm an active member of the American College of Neuropsychopharmacology. It's my pleasure and my honor to interview this morning an old friend who has been active in psychopharmacology and was, at one time, the president of the American College of Neuropsychopharmacology. Leo Hollister* is his name. He's been around a long time. Everyone knows who Leo is and everybody is familiar with most of what he's done, but not all, because he's done so much. So, Leo, let's start off with a little background. Where did you go to medical school?

LH: I went to the University of Cincinnati, largely because I couldn't afford to go out of town. I lived in Cincinnati. But the motivation of going to medical school, I think, began during my high school years of reading some of the publications of Paul De Kruif. He was a wonderful journalist, who wrote books called *Men Against Death* and *Microbe Hunters* and other rather inspiring tales of the accomplishments of medical research and medical progress. I think De Kruif probably had much more influence than anyone really believed, because I've talked to a lot of people who say they had the same experience. Did you have that?

FA: No, I personally, didn't, but I know plenty of people do. In fact the *British Medical Journal,* recently, and *Lancet*, recently, had something about literature and medicine and they gave a lot of credit to De Kruif for, in a sense, converting a lot of people to become medical students, and even to go into certain specialties right from the very beginning.

LH: Yes. Well, that was my motivation. I didn't have a whole lot of money, though, to support my medical career. And it turned out that two jobs I got in the course of getting medical education, in retrospect, seemed to have had a profound influence on the way my career has developed. During the pre-medical years, I got a job in a chain drug store nearby where I lived. I was kind of a general factotum, but most of the other employees were pharmacy students and there was a registered pharmacist on duty all the time. So I got interested in drugs through that kind of contact. And then, after I got to medical school, I was running short of funds and word got around to the dean that I was considering dropping

---

* Leo Hollister was born in Cincinnati, Ohio, in 1920, and graduated in medicine from the University of Cincinnati in 1943. He trained in internal medicine at Boston City Hospital and the Veterans Administration Hospital in San Francisco. In 1953 he became chief of the medical service of the Veterans Administration Hospital in Palo Alto, and remained there until taking a post in 1986 as professor of psychiatry and pharmacology at the University of Texas Medical School in Houston. Hollister died in 2000.

out and joining a program for training naval aviators, which, thank God, I didn't get into, because in those days your life expectancy wasn't very great as a naval aviator. The dean called me in and found out what the problem was and he said, "I'll try to find you a job." He found me a job as a technician in the neuropathology laboratory, where I came under the influence of a very great neurologist, Charles Erin, a neurosurgeon, Joe Evans, and a whole group of people. Al Sabin used to come there and it was an inspiring experience, because the people from internal medicine, from psychiatry and from neurology attended the Neuropathology Conferences in Cincinnati, and that was almost unheard of to have three disciplines like this not only attending the same conference, but also collaborating in research. So, I think that's where I got the influence of the nervous system and the complexity of it and the desire to learn more about it.

FA: Then after you left medical school, what did you do?

LH: Well, after I left medical school, I finally became an internist, and one of the residents in my first year of training in internal medicine was Mort Reiser, who ultimately became Chairman of Psychiatry for many years at Yale. Mort had gotten interested in psychosomatic medicine, but I was interested primarily in general medicine, particularly hypertension. And, again, this was something of a probable influence in my career. Over the years, as an intern, I was trying all kinds of things to treat these hypertensives. In those days hypertension was a very serious matter. We could hardly budge the blood pressure, and sometimes they'd have a malignant hypertension and we knew damn well they were going to be dead within a few months. So I was trying a lot of things to remedy that, and eventually that is what got me into psychopharmacology.

FA: All right, Leo, where was this training going on?

LH: Well, I had an internship in medicine at Boston City Hospital, and then I went back for an assistant residency in medicine at Cincinnati before going into the Navy. Then, after discharge from the Navy, I completed my training in internal medicine at the Veterans' Administration (VA) Hospital in San Francisco, which was then affiliated with both the University of California San Francisco and Stanford. I got recalled into military service during the Korean War and decided that if we were going to have wars every five years, I would not want to try to establish a practice, but rather go into a salaried position with the VA. It turned out that the initial position I had, which was in San Francisco, was far from where I lived near Palo Alto, whereas a chap from the Palo Alto VA lived in San Francisco. So we traded jobs and I became an internist in a psychiatric hospital in Menlo Park, California. The previous guy left about 250 unanswered medical consultations, which I tried to liquidate as fast as possible, but during the course of doing that, I learned that most of those who were in the hospital had hypertension. That came in handy, because – I guess this was in 1953 – a detail man from CIBA came and said, "We have a drug that we think is pretty good for hypertension," and I said, "Gee, I've tried them all and nothing seems to work very well; let me try this one." To give you some idea of how simple matters were in those days, he walked out to his car; he opened the trunk, and pulled out some reserpine and gave it to me. Within three days, I had new patients under treatment. So, about two or three months later, he came by and said, "How're you doing?" And, I said, "Gee, that's just fine. It works." He said, "Well now, we've got word that it might be useful in psychiatric patients, this being a psychiatric hospital." And, I said, "Well, I don't know anything about psychiatry. I'll have to find what the psychiatrists think about that." I went to the Chief of Psychiatry and told him the story and he said, "Leo, we've had drugs come and go, and you know, they never amount to much. I wouldn't waste my time." So I asked some of the psychiatric staff, some of whom were golfing buddies. They said they wouldn't mind trying this under my direction, and we said, "Sure, we go ahead." And that's how I got into psychopharmacology. It was through reserpine being used as an antihypertensive, and then later on as an antipsychotic drug.

FA: And, that was 1953?

LH: That was in 1953. In 1954, I became aware of chlorpromazine and, in the same simple manner as I did with reserpine I was able to get hands on that. Now, it turned out that CIBA had some interest in getting studies started with reserpine in California and they sent out a very admirable physician, named Dick Richards. Richards was a big guide in the proper use of reserpine, because I think in the initial studies that Nate Kline did, the dosages were very small, and by that time, they'd come to the conclusion that they should be larger. So we used the larger doses. Right off the bat I figured we should do double-blind controlled trials, which we did with both reserpine and chlorpromazine, using a dosage schedule where the initial doses are given parenterally, and then followed by oral doses. The parenteral dose is sort of loading them up, and then the oral is maintaining them. This worked pretty well. By the end of 1954, they were having the annual meeting of the American Association for the Advancement of Science in Berkeley, which usually occurred during Christmas week, and I was invited to present my findings at that. That was the very first meeting that I ever attended in this field. I think it was organized by Jon Cole, who was a protégé of Ralph Gerard. That was an interesting meeting. I met a lot of people in the field, John Kinross-Wright, Nate Kline and

Murray Jarvik, and a few others whose names escape me now. My initial meeting with Nate was very strange. I was sitting with Dick Richards and Nate came in. Dick got up to greet him, and did so with some difficulty, because he had had polio in one lower extremity and was sort of lame. I got up and we said hello to Nate, but Nate was very high hatted, you know, he didn't give us much heed, and proceeded on up to the front of the auditorium. I turned to Dick and said, "Is that guy going to get the Nobel Prize today, because he used your drug?" Well, it turned out it wasn't a bad hunch, because two years later, he got the Lasker Award for doing just that.

FA: Leo, if you did a controlled trial with chlorpromazine in 1954, it would be nice to know, if you can recall, what month? The reason I ask that is, I had tried to find out recently, for the talk I'm going to give tomorrow night actually, what it was like "back then," when we first started. Who did the first controlled study? And, what I learned was that Joel Elkes did a controlled....

LH: Crossover study.

FA: Yes, that's right.

LH: Joel did a crossover study, but ours was a parallel group design, the kind that is used even today. I started with reserpine. I would say in the first quarter of 1953, and with chlorpromazine, say, about mid-year, but it's sort of hard to pin these things down, because it wasn't an original idea, by any means. Harry Gold at Cornell had promoted that design for years. The VA and the Armed Forces had done a controlled study with anti-tubercular drugs around 1946–47. So it wasn't a novel idea.

FA: No, but it was the beginning of psychopharmacology. That's why I was trying to find out, precisely, who did it and when and where. Joel did his in England, in Birmingham.

LH: Now, as I understand it, his was a crossover study.

FA: That's correct.

LH: A variant of crossover design; he substituted placebo in patients who were already on a drug.

FA: But that was in the spring, as I understand it, of 1954. I'm going to con-firm that when I see Joel, at this meeting. All right! Now you, from the very beginning, got very active, but you started to write somewhat later.

LH: I was incredibly naive in those days. I thought, well, if you published something, it was there forever. It was written in stone and you didn't need to say it again. So, this conference at Berkeley at the end of 1954 was supposed to be published, and ultimately was, with Jon Cole and Ralph Gerard as editors of a book called *Psychopharmacology*, but the book didn't appear until 1957, and I don't imagine there are more than several hundred copies extant. So what I was doing was essentially kept a secret. I continued to do the work and expand the study with both of those drugs. But I guess around April or May of 1955, the New York Academy of Sciences (NYAS), under the direction of CIBA, had a second conference on reserpine. Now this time they focused on the psychiatric aspect. The first one was more on hypertension. I was invited to that program. Nate was on the program. Tony Sainz, whom I've lost track of completely....

FA: Tony is dead. He died several years ago....

LH: ...and, I think Fritz Freyhan was on the program, and some of the other early people in the field.

FA: I was there. I didn't give a paper, but I was there.

LH: Oh, you were?

FA: Oh, yes, I was there, definitely.

LH: Well, for some reason or other, and I'm not sure just why, the paper I gave attracted the attention of the press and I was interviewed by all kinds of wire services, and the next thing I knew, every newspaper in the country was telling about this wonderful new drug for schizophrenia that Leo Hollister in Palo Alto had. And I was absolutely overwhelmed by the power of the press and how it influenced people with dire illnesses to seek help, because all of a sudden I was getting stacks of mail saying, "Can I bring my son, daughter, father or whatever, out to California and get this drug?" I made a policy of personally responding to every one of them, although some were rather formal letters. I said that there were no secrets in medicine, and I was sure the drug would be available in their locality and they should talk to their local psychiatric chapter and see what they could find. But it was really quite humbling to see the enormous power that the press had to stimulate interest in possible treatment for a very serious illness. I suppose that still exists today.

FA: Well, I'm fairly certain it does. That happened to me in 1955, when I gave my first paper on chlorpromazine at an American Psychiatric Association meeting. It was picked up by the press and by the time I got home that evening, it was on the front page of the *Evening Sun* in Baltimore, and all of a sudden I became a local hero. And the patients kept calling for days afterwards, wanting to make appointments and what not. That's a thing that can generate a lot of professional jealously.

LH: Well, I think, in that sense, that there was professional jealousy on Nate's part, because he thought that he was going to be the dominant person at that meeting. And when he was totally ignored, and this guy that nobody ever heard of before, Leo Hollister, who was not even a psychiatrist, caught all that publicity, I think that ruffled Nate's feathers. We always had a kind of a rocky relationship after that, sometimes friendly, sometimes a little fractious, but that's the way Nate was with most people.

FA: That's right. Now, tell me, have you become board certified in anything besides internal medicine?

LH: Well, I was board certified in internal medicine in 1950, and then re-certified in 1971. I never did bother to get formal training in psychiatry, but I tried to be self-taught and keep my ears open, go to the conferences and learn things, review records, and the same way with pharmacology. I never had any formal training in either one of them, and sometimes I tell the students – not to brag, but to try to give them a sense of the fact that you can continue your education beyond the formal years – by saying that I'm the only person I know who's been a professor of pharmacology and psychiatry in two different medical schools who had no formal training in either discipline.

FA: That's right. That's exactly the experience I had. I've had no training, per se, in pharmacology, but by attending the meetings, reading, and asking questions, I acquired a considerable knowledge, to the point that many people thought I was trained in pharmacology.

LH: I don't see anything wrong with it, and these days, with all the cross-disciplinary stuff going on, you almost have to do that. Especially in the basic sciences, it's hard to tell who's a biochemist, who's a molecular biologist, who's a structural biologist. What people do is often different from the label they wear.

FA: Now, Leo, you mentioned your early publications. I know you've published many articles and contributed to a number of books, and I believe you may have published one or two books on your own. If you could tell us about that part of your life, I'd like to record that.

LH: Well, just as I did with the conference in Berkeley, I thought the one in New York was going to be published in the *Annals* of the Academy and I didn't need to say anything more about it. That was published, I think, in 1957, and again I don't think the *Annals* had very wide circulation. So for the first three or four years of my career, I was what you might call a stealth candidate, because I was doing this work but nobody knew about it, other than those attending these two meetings and a few others. As far as written publications were concerned, I was way behind. Over the course of the years, we looked at most of the newer antipsychotic drugs that came along. We looked at Stelazine (trifluoperazine) and again in this case used a design a little bit akin to what we used with chlorpromazine. We treated patients with Stelazine and in some of them we substituted the Stelazine for phenobarbital as an active placebo, and in some others we discontinued the treatment to see how they did. And of course, the ones who were discontinued had had a higher relapse rate. That told us that Stelazine was doing okay. We looked at prochlorperazine, which at first was thought to be an antipsychotic drug, but by that time Smith, Kline & French (SK&F) had both Thorazine (chlorpromazine) and Stelazine, and didn't need another phenothiazine antipsychotic, so they promoted it primarily as an antiemetic.

FA: One of the reasons for that, Leo, I think, for the record, is that prochlorperazine had a capacity to evoke acute dystonic reactions, particularly if it was given in a suppository form, and it was available in that formulation. A lot of people just were shocked because they had not seen this with chlorpromazine.

LH: I remember that quite well. When we first started treating patients with prochlorperazine, as I told you, the technique was to give loading doses parenterally, and then follow it with oral doses. I had three relatively young patients there. I think they were all, certainly, no more than mid-thirties. These are the kind of patients who are most susceptible to dystonic reactions. So we started them off in the morning with shots of prochlorperazine, and by that afternoon, when I was at the nursing desk, writing some orders, one of these patients came up and said, "I-I-I can't talk." I told the nurse, "Well, I don't think he's crazy." I saw it as hysteria, so I just started giving him phenobarbital or something. But then after I got home, my collaborator in the study called me up and she said, "You know, those other two patients we started on that drug today are doing the same thing." And that was my first experience with acute dystonic reaction.

FA: Well, my first experience was with a young girl, who was a manic, and we were trying to keep her out of the hospital. So I kept boosting the dose of chlorpromazine on her, and lo and behold the parents called up and said, "She's twisted like a pretzel; she's twisted like a pretzel!" They brought her over, and it was so dramatic that I called a friend, who was a professional photographer, movie photographer, and he came over and we filmed her. And then, I took it up to SK&F and showed it to them. They said they'd never seen this before. I said, "Well, here it is." And actually, what I did was I gave that girl phenobarbital also, and that alleviated the problem. But SK&F arranged for me to go down to Atlantic City to the American Neurological Association meeting and they got a group of neurologists together, because they really wanted to know what this was. And I showed this film and the consensus was: hysteria. That was the consensus vote of the neurologists, and they too had not seen this before. So, very early, we learned about some of the potential adverse effects of these drugs.

LH: One of the curses of living in a place that's rich in medical literature and has a wonderful medical library is that you can find almost everything that's been happening in the world. So I went over and looked it up and there was a beautiful article in a German neurological journal, the *Nervenarzt*, about Largactil (chlorpromazine) and tardive dyskinesia. They had pictures and everything, and we were told the whole story. I think that article could be written and published today and would show everything you needed to know. "Gosh," I thought, "the *Nervenarzt* already reported this reaction; there is no need for me to report these three cases," and I never did. Well, ten years later, there were case reports, of course, coming out about dystonic reactions from antipsychotic drugs.

FA: We're still having them come out now, dystonic reactions, with the atypical antipsychotics, you know.

LH: Yeah, it doesn't take much more than four milligrams a day of risperidone to induce a dystonic reaction.

FA: Leo, during the period, when we started off we had reserpine, and then we got chlorpromazine. Then we got a number of phenothiazines, but we still had the problem of the neurotic patient. And as you know, the first so-called anxiolytic was meprobamate, and I wonder, did you ever do a study of meprobamate yourself?

LH: Well, we didn't have very many anxious patients in our hospital, because you don't get hospitalized for anxiety, but we did have some psychotics, so I tried fairly large doses of meprobamate in them and we did find some calming effect, but not really an antipsychotic effect. We reported that at another NYAS meeting on meprobamate, but I would have preferred not to have published that one, because I think it created the impression that meprobamate might be useful in psychotic patients; whereas it was essentially acting as a sedative.

FA: As a sedative drug, right.

LH: So that was not one that I was proud of. It was a curious way I got into the field of substance abuse. Sidney Raffel, who was the Chairman of the Department of Microbiology at Stanford and a good friend of ours, said, "We've been looking at drugs for action on microbacteria in tuberculosis and we find that chlorpromazine in concentrations of five micrograms per milliliter kills it." In those days, they didn't have very many anti-tubercular drugs that would actually kill the bacteria. They'd done some *in vitro* studies, which were ready to be published, so I said, "Let's do a clinical study." In a nearby tuberculosis sanatorium we added 300 milligrams of chlorpromazine or placebo to the ongoing treatment of about thirty-some patients. In those days, you usually followed the tubercular patients every three months to see their progress in the sputum and the X-ray. After six months went by, we saw really no differences between the two groups, so we decided that either we weren't giving the necessary concentrations of the drug, or something was wrong. We decided to stop, and within twenty-four hours, I think, seven out of the fifteen patients who were on chlorpromazine, experienced nausea, vomiting, jitteriness, sleeplessness, the whole withdrawal reaction.

FA: Withdrawal reaction.

LH: None of the patients on placebo showed this. So in a sense this was the first demonstration, by using a placebo control, of a withdrawal reaction to a drug; and secondly, it was the first demonstration of what might be called therapeutic dose dependency, that therapeutic doses of drugs could probably produce this kind of dependence. Well, again, with my way of publishing in those days, this was described in about a paragraph or two in the paper in which we published the results of the main study. We never did publish it separately and, of course, it was published in the *American Review of Respiratory Diseases*, which was not a widely read psychiatric journal.

FA: That's for sure.

LH: So that was the first withdrawal reaction we studied. Later, we followed withdrawal reactions to meprobamate and compared them with a preparation in which meprobamate and promazine were combined. Our hypothesis was that possibly the combination with promazine would mitigate the withdrawal reaction, whereas in fact, it was the opposite, it made it worse.

FA: Because both of them were pretty anticholinergic.

LH: Yes.

FA: Promazine and chlorpromazine are fairly potent anticholinergics.

LH: In 1959, I think it was, just before they launched Librium (chlordiazepoxide), Roche had a private meeting of the investigators at Princeton, New Jersey, and I was invited just as a participant observer, because I had not worked with the drug. And when I heard all the glowing reports about how people brightened up on Librium, I said, "Gee whiz, if this is as good as they say it's going to be a beaut." Again, they hadn't tried big doses of Librium in psychotic patients, and I decided it would be an excuse to use large doses. So we started treating some psychiatric patients with Librium with doses up from 300 to 600 milligrams a day, and then, under very closely controlled circumstances but without their knowledge, we switched the patients to placebo, and followed them by recording their electroencephalographs, clinical observations, and measuring blood levels. And much to our surprise, when we stopped the Librium, nothing much happened for a day or two, and then about the third day, they began to develop withdrawal reactions, which peaked around the fifth day; two patients had seizures on the eighth day, as compared the second or third day as usual. Well, our blood levels were incomplete, because I had no idea of measuring it at the eighth or ninth day, but it indicated that the half-life would be such that by the eighth day, you'd be down to zero level, and the attenuation of the withdrawal reaction was due to the slow disappearance of the drug. I think that was one of the first withdrawal studies to indicate that the half-life of a drug has a bearing on both the onset and the severity of the reaction. And that concept, I think, has held true over the years. So that's how we got into withdrawal reactions, largely through the anxiolytics.

FA: Right. And that's because the benzodiazepines had become available.

LH: Oh, yes. Of course, they were enormously successful. Then diazepam came out a couple of years later, I guess, in 1963. We were doing a study on diazepam in schizophrenics, as part of a collaborative group that I'd set up, and the Salt Lake City group decided they would goose them all up to the maximum dose of 120 milligrams a day, and suddenly discontinue it. And they had precisely the experience that we had with Librium; that is, delayed onset withdrawal reaction with late seizures.

FA: Late seizures.

LH: So, apparently diazepam was rather similar in that respect to chlordiazepoxide. Well, personally, I thought, with these two studies I was publishing at the same time that the drugs came out, they would be warnings that this could happen. I fully expected that Roche would have a warning on withdrawal reaction. It was several years later....

FA: One of the reasons was, of course, that the drug has a long half-life and people were not giving the doses that you gave. They are uncommon....

LH: They were giving smaller doses and the drug has a long half-life. I guess, around the 1970s the issue of benzodiazepine withdrawal became alive again, but I don't think there's ever been a major problem with it.

FA: Well, it depends on the patient, how much he's had in terms of total daily dose, and also for how long....

LH: Well, I was looking for patients who were chronically on diazepam, because I wanted to see what it was like in nature. So I sent Hamp (Gillespie), my associate, over to the psychiatric clinic, and I said, "Find out how many patients that are being seen that are on diazepam for several months." He came back and said, "Oh, two or three." I said, "Well, try the medical clinic," and he came back with the same thing. Then we hit a bonanza in the neurosurgical clinic, because they were using diazepam for people with back pain, and using substantial doses over long periods of time. So, oddly enough, we had, a collaboration then with the neurosurgical group, and we studied over a hundred patients who had been on chronic diazepam for an average of about five years and on fairly substantial doses. We measured the plasma concentration, and much to our surprise, the plasma concentration withdrawals were lower than they should have been for the dose they were getting, which meant that the patients weren't taking the full dose prescribed. This was more often the case than not, and a few, whose concentrations were high – we found later on – were due to the fact that the proper interval between the last dose and blood drawing hadn't been fulfilled. When we repeated it with the proper time interval, the apparent high levels had disappeared. So there was no evidence of abuse in these patients, who had been exposed to it for a long time. Well, of course, neurosurgical patients might be quite different from anxious patients, so I can't be sure that would apply to all of the anxious patients.

FA: Well, the majority of people who have really abused benzodiazepines were multiple substance abusers.

LH: And possibly finding a benzodiazepine abuser who doesn't use alcohol or other drugs is difficult.

FA: Absolutely, that's right.

All right! Now tell me, you've mentioned some of the articles you wrote. You also mentioned that you'd published a book or two.

LH: Well, I didn't publish a book until somewhere in the 1960s, I guess, just a little paperbound volume that reviewed the evidence for the effectiveness of some of the psychotropic drugs from the VA cooperative study. It turned out that one of the drug companies bought a great supply of the book and provided them free, so, it was very widely circulated. I was delighted, because you never make a whole lot of money writing books. And I was delighted to have people come up to me from time to time and say, "I've read your book and it was very helpful to me in learning about the drugs and using them." So that was a fair success.

One of the drugs that we studied early, I guess, it was still in the 1950s, was Mellaril (thioridazine), which today, begins to look like the first of the atypical antipsychotics, doesn't it?

FA: Exactly.

LH: A lot of people doubted whether it would be an effective antipsychotic drug, because it had such weak D_2 antagonism, and it also blocks serotonin receptors. Of course, those are probably the most potent anticholinergics. What was interesting is the fact that it was an antipsychotic, and the dystonic reactions and Parkinson syndrome with Mellaril were much, much less than with the other antipsychotics.

FA: That's right.

LH: Regardless Joe Correll and George Simpson, I think, published a joint letter saying, you can still get tardive dyskinesia with it....

FA: That's correct....

LH: ... because the company was making the claim that you couldn't. But, you know, that was an interesting jaunt.

FA: Now, besides the benzodiazepines and meprobamate, and the different phenothiazines, we got into the tricylic antidepressants. When did you start working with them?

LH: Well, again in the VA population, we didn't have a whole lot of depression, so I didn't have a very great reason to get into that field. We did get iproniazid from Roche and, as luck would have it, I think out of the first ten patients, we had three who had hepatitis, so that cooled me off a little on it. And of course, iproniazid subsequently died because of that; although many people said it was the best antidepressant that we'd ever had. But we didn't follow up on it until later. Now in 1959, I think it was, the VA decided since they had the largest number of psychiatric beds in the US that they'd better get interested in studying these drugs and that started the VA Cooperative Studies Program. I was not invited to the first organizational meeting but they invited me to the second, and from there on, I became one of the prime movers in organizing these large scale cooperative trials, which I think were very successful, and which I truly believe have never been given the credit that they deserve because they were the first, and set the model for studies done by state systems. California did one, New York and, I guess, Fritz Freyhan in Delaware. And then, subsequently we had the National Institute of Mental Health Psychopharmacology Service Center there in the field with a study and I was invited by them. I think they copped off with most of the jewelry, largely because they were financing everything in those days, and you always like to pay attention to the people who have the pocketbook. So one of the stories that I think isn't dealt with enough is the way the VA started the whole thing. In retrospect, I call this a massive scientific overkill, because even my early controlled trials were not very necessary. All I had to do was, give these drugs to a patient and watch him. You knew damn well something was happening. But at that time, the Zeitgeist in psychiatry was such that nobody wanted to believe it. You know, psychoanalysis was dominant, so I think that these controlled studies served a useful purpose, because they overcame the reluctance to accept these drugs. Of course, now, opinion on this has gone completely in the opposite direction. But in the 1950s and early '60s, almost every chairman of a department of psychiatry in the country was an analyst or analytically oriented. Today it's a biological psychiatrist or a biologically oriented psychiatrist.

FA: Right. There's been a lot of change in psychiatry.

LH: So the VA cooperative studies were good.

FA: They were very important.

LH: I was able to get funding from the Psychopharmacology Service Center (PSC) to set up kind of a separate group, along with John Overall, and we studied a series of drugs including antidepressants for the next several years. Working with John was a great pleasure, because he knew a great deal about experimental design, about statistical analysis, psychometric ratings, of which I knew very little, and I knew something about the clinical side and the use of drugs. So we formed a nice joint group where our expertise kind of complimented each other, and that was a very productive time. We did waste a lot of time, however, because we were then searching for what we might call the right drug for the right patient. The problem was that every time you thought you'd found it, if you checked it back, which we tried to do, we learned that other people couldn't find it. So we were frustrated in that effort. Now it makes sense that these drugs are acting on a specific kind of psychosis. So that was my early career in psychopharmacology. By that time, of course, I had become fairly well known. I was one of the first members of ACNP, but I never attended a meeting of the ACNP for the first two years, which should have gotten me kicked out, according to the rules. Ted Rothman had to prevail on me to get me to join, because it appeared to me there were enough organizations now, and we didn't need another one, about which I was dead wrong. So I did attend the third meeting, and as we were checking out of the hotel, I walked over to Ted and I said, "Ted, I was dead wrong. This is a great organization. I'm awfully glad you persuaded me to join." Since then, I've never missed a meeting.

FA: I know that. That was in Washington, that year.

LH: That was the meeting in Washington.

FA: Was that the one where we had the blizzard?

LH: Yes.

FA: I had flown in from Rome for that, and we only had a handful of people there because of the blizzard.

LH: Well, I never attended any of the meetings of the Collegium Internationale Neuro-Psychopharmacologicum (CINP) until 1964, in Birmingham. I remember very well we had lunch together in Birmingham and you were coming from the Vatican then also.

FA: That's correct.

LH: I told you, my secretary told me last Christmas, "There's a card here from the Vatican," and I said, "Well, that must be from my friend, Frank Ayd, and if there's not a signed picture of the Pope, I'm going to be disappointed." You didn't say a word. The next Christmas, there was that photograph of you and the Pope with your whole family.

FA: The CINP is an organization that you know something about, in terms of its early days, and you also became a president of the CINP, right?

LH: Yes, that was quite a surprise to me. I didn't anticipate it at all. It was at the meeting in Paris in 1974 and I understand that they had the idea that they should increase their bonds with the ACNP. At that time, I had become ACNP president, so they figured if they had somebody there from the ACNP that would increase their bond. My understanding is that Nate Kline argued fiercely against my being given that job. Of course, in those days, it was given and it still is, I guess. You're really not elected, but selected. But they did give it to me anyway and I became president. I had a tremendous influence, much more so than usual presidents do, in selecting my successors. I got Arvid Carlsson as one successor, as well as Paul Janssen, Paul Kielholz and Ole Rafaelsen. I think that getting both Arvid and Paul as presidents was the right thing to do. They're giants in the whole field, far more so than I am or any other presidents we've ever had.

FA: There were a lot of politics, and if you got the right people behind you, then you had a chance of becoming a president.

LH: Speaking of presidents, though, I really think that you have been slighted. You should have been president of this organization and you damn well could have been president of the CINP. I was very happy to see your photograph with all the presidents, as a founding member, and I think that gives you the same rank.

FA: Oh, I'm pleased. I never aspired politically, you know, and I don't think you have either. If someone had asked me, I would have said yes, but I never said no to any request I've had from the College.

LH: Well, how I became president of the ACNP is kind of a strange thing. The council had a nominating committee, of which Doug Goldman was the Chairman, and Doug had come to me and said, "I'm the Chairman of this nominating committee, and I'd like to see Ted Rothman nominated as president. Do you have any objection?" I said, "No, how could I have any objection, because Ted got me into this organization." Well, he gave his report and the council was upset because they thought he was going to nominate me. So Dick Wittenborn, I think it was, came to me and said, "Say, is it true that you don't want to be president of this organization?" I said "No." I told him the story, and eventually got into a little hairy situation, because I was very good friends of both Ted and Doug. And here it looked as though I was trying to intervene over Doug's decision and over Ted's ascendancy, so I didn't feel too good about that. But ultimately Ted was given the Paul Hoch Award and I think we all recognized his importance in the founding of this organization.

FA: Oh, yes, absolutely. He was really the man who did the negotiations in the beginning, no question about that.

All right, now, if somebody would asked you what was the important thing you did in psychopharmacology, what would be your answer?

LH: Boy, that would be tough because, you know when you look back, you become extremely marred. You say, now really what did I do that's so important? What did I do to change the course? I suppose I would have to answer, in a more general sense rather than in any specific accomplishment.

FA: The role you played in getting controlled studies done?

LH: Our controlled studies in the 1950s may have not been the first, but at least set a precedent, and then the VA studies following this. So even though I think they were probably overkill in a way, they did set a pattern by which we know we can get effective drugs and relatively safe ones. We haven't had too many misadventures in this field on the market, and it helped overcome the reluctance of organized psychiatry at that time to admit that drugs could be useful. If anything, it was more in this general sense than any specific thing I did. I still enjoy proving the efficacy of these drugs. Yet I haven't done that for years, because now most drug companies have in-house people who can write protocols, statistically analyze all the data, and there are professional contract organizations to do clinical trials. All the investigators do is collect data. You know, it's kind of a dull business. It's become formalized, not in the way that I think it should be. I think we ought to experiment with different designs beyond the parallel group controlled trials. And there are other things that we might very well try that might shorten the course of developing the drugs and reduce the tremendous expense.

FA: In the beginning, when you started in psychopharmacology, there was no pharmacokinetics, correct?

LH: Well, I never was a pharmacokineticist; although I would say we did blood levels in the meprobamate withdrawal study, and also in the Librium withdrawal study. But the methods that were available then were very crude and measured all kinds of metabolites, which in case of benzodiazepines was probably okay. But I never did go into pharmacokinetics.

FA: My point is that pharmacokinetics came sort of late. The trials had already started, and the way of measuring what was really happening was purely clinical, and it had nothing to do with our ability to know how much was absorbed, where it went and all the other things.

LH: I've never been very keen about measuring plasma concentrations of these drugs in the clinic. You know, first of all, almost every drug had very wide therapeutic ranges. For haloperidol it could be anywhere from two to twenty mgs. a day. What does a ten-fold range tell you? It doesn't say a damn thing. We did a study some years back that tested that with nortriptyline, because it was the drug that had been widely studied with the plasma concentration related to clinical response. What we did was, we looked at patients treated by the clinician the way they wanted to, but with half of them, chosen randomly, we fed back the information about where the plasma concentrations were and the other half, we didn't. And then, the two questions were, did having the knowledge of the plasma concentration result in their staying within the therapeutic range more often than not, and did it make any difference? Both answers were no. So why spend people's money measuring plasma concentrations. It seems they really don't help much.

FA: That's right. Now, in the early days of psychopharmacology, aside from the Rorschach and the Minnesota Multiphasic Personality Inventory and, say, the Weschler intelligence tests and few other tests that would measure organicity, what other assessment instruments did we have? I'm asking that, Leo, because a lot of young people have a very difficult time visualizing what it was like thirty-five years ago.

LH: Well, in our initial studies, we didn't use any rating scales. We just sort of arbitrarily divided the patients into markedly improved, moderately improved, slightly improved, or unimproved. It was all clinical data and I think that worked pretty well. You know, if you watch your patients, you can learn a lot.

FA: By that, are you advising the young people or the young doctors, who may be watching this videotape in the future, to be a clinician and an observant person and don't worry?

LH: Be a clinician; watch the patients; listen to them. You know, I'd always been mystified by the great concern about negative symptoms and drugs that are specific for negative symptoms, as if the other drugs didn't do a damn thing for them. So, some years back I went to John Overall and while we had dinner, I said, "Look, John, we've got data all along and we're showing that negative symptoms respond as well as the positive symptoms." John wasn't interested, and he'd thrown away a lot of the raw data, so he would have had only abstracted data to work from. But early on, I remember calling one of my golfing buddies, who was one of my prime collaborators, and asking him, "Would you like to have some more patients on these new drugs?" And he said, "Leo, I've got so many patients talking to me who never talked to me before, that it's all I can do to keep up with them, and now you want to talk about negative symptoms." So, you know, there were effects on negative symptoms. Maybe the newer drugs are better, I don't know.

FA: We've had no comparisons yet.

LH: I'm, maybe, a little too skeptical in that part. But there certainly wasn't an absence of response of negative symptoms, by a long shot. People who were mute – you know, in those days, we had people who had never talked for years – and in a couple of weeks, they'd be conversing with you. I remember one of our patients I inherited when I first started was a young chap, an Armenian chap, who would curl up in a fetal position, wouldn't respond to anything, just about the most regressed schizophrenic I've ever seen. And I tried every damn thing. I gave him electroshock, insulin, and other things, and it wouldn't budge him. And when reserpine came along, he perked up a bit, eventually left the hospital. And when Sputnik went up in 1957, in the *Encyclopedia Britannica*, there's a picture of Sputnik by my Armenian friend. He got into photography. He got a good picture and got in the *Encyclopedia Britannica*. Well, twenty-something years later, I was making rounds in the intensive care unit of a medical service, and I heard my name. And I looked over and there he was. He'd had a coronary. He knew me, remembered everything, but he had been so crazy. So these were the kinds of things that I think were really quite impressive.

FA: Right. I think that's because in my opinion, we were more interested in the patient as a person, than we were in the disease the patient had. And that, I think, should still be the moving force.

LH: And, the other thing is, when I see a patient, I say "Well, here's what we are going to do first." But then, I have the second, third, fourth choices in my mind, or even on paper, as what we do next when the first one doesn't work. You have to plan what your alternatives are, because you're never sure. Each one is so individual. If you're lucky, you hit it well on the first time, but if you're not, then, you have to try other things.

FA: Right.

LH: But, getting back to rating scales, the first popular rating scale, I think, was the Lorr scale, what Morey Lorr came up with in the VA, and called the Inpatient Multidimensional Psychiatric Scale or IMPS. That was a rather detailed scale, used a lot to describe the different domains of psychopathology. And it wasn't a bad scale. Then John Overall and Don Gorham shortened it, condensed it, and came up with a Brief Psychiatric Rating Scale (BPRS).

FA: When were these scales introduced?

LH: I think the IMPS came out in the mid-1950s. I know we had it for our first VA studies. The BPRS, I think, came out around '59 or '60.

FA: So it was just before we organized ACNP.

LH: And of course, since then there have been scads of scales.

FA: Oh, yes, yes.

LH: In fact, I remember, Jim Clinton and some of the psychometricians in the VA were interested in developing a scale for depression, and they asked a whole lot of questions about what depressives might show. And when they boiled it down they found only thirty-two discrete statements that you could make about depression. I think that's the extent of it, rather, than probably thirty-one scales, based on various combinations of everything.

FA: That's correct.

LH: But you don't need scales, unless you're trying to impress the Food and Drug Administration (FDA). If you know what your patients have been doing and have some sense of their past history, you can tell when they're changing. That's the way you operated, isn't it?

FA: That's exactly how I operated. Yes, it's the only way I could operate. I was in private practice. I was not in an institution and it was observation, knowing the patient, forming a relationship with the patient. I don't know if I ever told you this story, but early with chlorpromazine, I had this elderly woman who was a chronically agitated depressive and she suffered. She really did suffer and I tried everything. I even, unfortunately, produced a little bromide intoxication in her. Chlorpromazine came along and I started her on it, and she came back two weeks later, walked in and she's jaundiced. I said, "Oh, my God, Mary, how long have you been like this?" She said, "Oh, about ten days." I said, "You stopped your medicine, didn't you"? "No, doctor, you've tried so hard to help me, and I do feel better. I'm not as agitated." So, you learn from that. You could keep up with chlorpromazine and not necessarily make the jaundice worse.

LH: I published a paper in the *American Journal of Medicine* in 1957, on "Allergy to Chlorpromazine Manifested by Jaundice." I think I reported seventeen cases and I don't know what internal clock told me that that was enough, because if I'd looked for twenty-five, I would still not have published the paper, because all of a sudden the jaundice in the patients vanished. But that's true; some patients sometimes inadvertently go right through with the drug and still resolve a cholestatic jaundice as they develop. I guess if that had happened today, in today's climate, you get three percent of such patients and you might kill a drug.

FA: Absolutely, sure.

LH: I am not so sure about Sertindol (mesoridazine). It prolongs QT interval and there is sudden death that of course worries me a little bit. But we had the same thing with Mellaril.

FJ: All right.

Now, another question, Leo: Since you've been in this field for so long you know who the ballplayers are. Who among the North American psychopharmacologists would you list as those who made major contributions to the advancement of psychopharmacology?

LH: Oh, dear. Well, I think you certainly are on the list. You've been in the field longer than I have, or at least as long, and have produced an enormous amount of information that has been clinically useful. Jon Cole certainly is also one. I suppose before that, Nate Kline was an enormous influence on a political level; he got Congress to provide funding; he established hospitals in other countries, and with his usual flair for publicity, he put psychopharmacology on the map. We can't deny that he was a major influence. I think Jon Cole, starting the PSC was important in getting things started and funding groups to look at drugs. And, probably, had he lived long enough, Fritz Freyhan would have certainly been that way, and also, probably Paul Hoch. But as far as the basic pharmacology is concerned, there I haven't been as impressed with the people in North America as I have been with the people in Europe. I think Hornykiewicz, for instance, in showing that dopamine was not only a neurotransmitter but was intimately connected with Parkinson's disease, was a major influence. Levodopa treatment of Parkinson's disease was a major accomplishment. Arvid Carlsson, who established the role of dopamine in schizophrenia, also was a major influence. And, of course, I remember vividly one night at Paul Janssen's house, after a few drinks and coffee, Arvid got Paul talking about how his company got started. I sat in the middle, and I only wished we'd had a tape recorder to get this all on the record, because it was an enormously interesting history. But, you know, he's got the most productive pharmaceutical company in history. It's not only psychotherapeutic drugs it's the whole field....

FA: The whole field.

LH: Yes, and it's a remarkable institution. He's almost the Henry Ford of psychotherapeutic drug development, because he established a system that goes from chemistry right up to screening tests and so on. So he was an important person. I'm trying to think of an American pharmacologist who was important.

FA: Let me throw in the name to see what you think of Gerry Klerman, a clinician?

LH: Oh, Gerry was of course important. I first knew him when he was a Fellow with Jon Cole, a very bright, ambitious fellow full of energy and wonderful personality, always had something to make you laugh. You know, Gerry became quite influential later on. I guess the only reason he wasn't the president of this organization was that he was the head of the NIMH. He had some big government job and they figured it a conflict of interest. But he did a remarkable thing. And I remember, shortly after his death, I wrote to Myrna Weissman and told her what an angel she had been in his last years, because he remained very productive right up till the time of his death, and this was largely due to her keeping him going. Again, when I go back to basic pharmacologists, I suppose, Bernard Brodie and Julius Axelrod are the two big guys. It must have broken Brodie's heart when Axelrod got the Nobel Prize and he didn't, because they were both excellent candidates. Axelrod's contribution of the inactivation of neurotransmitters by uptake was a completely new concept. And of course Brodie was the father of biochemical pharmacology and established the concept of active metabolites of drugs, and he had a whole lot of other seminal ideas. Mimo Costa, I think, has had a distinguished career in pharmacology and psychopharmacology. Most of the names that come to me are people who were at the National Institutes of Health in those early days.

FA: Another one that you haven't mentioned is Sol Snyder.

LH: Oh, yes, Sol. I remember, I was at a meeting in Washington, one of the things where I used to go every fortnight, and Milton Jaffe, who was then with the FDA, I think, said, "We've got a problem with a drug out in San Francisco, called STP (2,5-dimethyl-4-methyl-amphetamine), and we don't know what in the hell is going on with it. We've given a contract to Sol Snyder to study it, but he says it's going to be a while before he gets the answer." So, I said, "Milton, have you got some of this stuff?" And, he said, "Sure, I've got some in my desk drawer." I said, "Give it to me." This was about two hours before I caught the plane back on a Friday afternoon, and by Tuesday, we had the first subject run, because I had a protocol set up for something that we were going to do with lysergic acid diethylamide (LSD) and just worked this one into it. Within a few weeks, we had the whole answer on STP. It was an amphetamine homologue that had mescaline-like qualities. It was in the same ballpark as mescaline, in terms of potency. You could build up tolerance to it. And Sol had done some things too with it. Sol had a contract with *Science*, so we got our preliminary report published in *Science*. I met Sol first when I visited him in his office at Hopkins. He has been on the forefront of almost everything from the dopamine receptors to the opiate receptors. He was always at a close place in the horse race even if not a winner. It was the same way with nitric oxide. Sol had an extraordinarily distinguished career.

Some years back, a friend got me on the list of people who could nominate Nobel Prize winners. I took advantage of it for several years, because you can make more than one nomination for it. So I was nominating all of my pharmacologist friends, and I had Paul Janssen linked up with Hitchings and Black. I thought that was a wonderful trio. Hitchings and Black made it, but Paul didn't. I talked to him about it and he said that maybe the Nobel Committee figured he was making so much money that he didn't need the prize. But he certainly could have very well had it, with all of his contributions in drug development. I don't think his were as novel as Hitchings' or Black's, but his was perhaps the greatest extension of structural activity relationships that's ever been done.

FA: Another question, because I want to move on, and that is if you could in a capsule describe for the young doctors who will be seeing this videotape, what was it like in psychiatry when we started with psychopharmacology?

LH: Well, first of all, psychiatry was pretty well dominated by psychoanalytic thinking in those days, I guess *DSM-I* days.

FA: Yes, it was.

LH: They didn't call it schizophrenia; they called it schizophrenic reactions, the idea being that with reactions, there's some set of life circumstances. So advances in psychoanalysis would explain these illnesses. The introduction of biological terms has been a major event. Now, maybe, we've gone too far. My friend Mort Reiser wrote a paper called "The Mindless Brain." We're so focused on the brain that we're not thinking much of the mind. But I don't have any trouble with that. I think mind is an abstraction like circulation or digestion or respiration. It describes an abstraction of a great many different functions. The second thing was that not a whole lot of attention was paid to diagnosis. I think diagnosis came, really into its own with the *DSM-III*. If you look back, in those early papers in the proceedings of the Berkeley meeting or the NYAS meeting, people were talking about treating a hundred and fifty or two hundred psychiatric patients with no diagnosis at all. Because of my training in internal medicine, I was more likely to specify the diagnosis of the patient than those with a psychiatric background. But now diagnosis has become important. I'm not sure that we've got diagnosis nailed down, but at least we have a common language, so that people can define their terms, and so as for Alice in Wonderland, the words mean what I want them to mean, so we arbitrarily make our diagnoses.

Of course in those days, mental hospitals were barbaric by today's standards; we had patients in the Palo Alto VA who had been there for fifty years, since World War I, never left the hospital, stayed there until they died. We had about a thousand patients and most of them were very, very quiet. We had a wonderful social service department, which managed to get many of the patients into local foster care homes and that was a great advance. But even before the drugs came along, I remember a congressional committee came and said, "What's your estimate of how many patients we could get out of here if we had funds for their care outside?" Well, I said, "Well, fifty percent, at least" Ultimately, that became the case. But the mental hospital became a way of life. Hardly a day went by that there wasn't some assault by a patient on a member of the treatment team. I never was assaulted, because I did two things. I always wore a light coat and I always sat close to the patients, so they did not have enough leverage to hit me very hard. I always nestled up close, and you get outside of a good swing. But there was an ever-present danger. Patients weren't allowed to have any kind of sharp objects, so you ate your food with a spoon. There were no seats on the toilets, because the toilet seats could be ripped up and used as weapons, so you sat on the cold porcelain. Bath days were public occasions, where everybody went in the shower nude and dried off on the ward. It was just unthinkable by today's standards of care. And that was in the VA hospital, which at that time was spending about twice as much per capita as the average state hospital, so you can imagine what it was like in the state hospitals. We don't think any longer in terms of treating patients with schizophrenia for years, but rather for days, and the whole outlook has changed to a much more favorable prognosis. I'm not sure that eliminating mental hospitals entirely was a good idea, because a lot of times we just change the scenario from sitting in front of the television set in the mental hospital to sitting in front of the television set in a skid row hotel. So it might not be a whole lot better for some patients, but by and large I think things have improved immensely.

FA: Okay, now, predict what you see for the future of psychopharmacology and, also the ACNP.

LH: Well, the ACNP, in recent years, has become a kind of secondary society for neuroscience, at least, in terms of the program content. Neuroscience advances have been so enormous, especially in molecular pharmacology and all the explicit techniques that are now used for genetic analysis. So as we have your lexicon for psychiatric terms, we need now a lexicon for the terms in molecular biology, and this hurts some of our members. There's been an eclipse in the clinical emphasis. Now, whether this will continue indefinitely or not, I don't know, but I think maybe we as clinicians, need to try to develop some new approaches of our own in evaluating these drugs and seeing if we can find some ways to reduce the time and the cost of getting them on the market. What most people don't realize is that these new drugs are terribly expensive. It costs you eight dollars a day to be on Risperdal (risperidone). It'll cost you about eight cents a day to be on haloperidol, a vast difference. Now there are all kinds of pharmacoeconomic studies being promoted these days, but they show that they come out even. I had a little trouble believing that, and it doesn't matter anyway because hospital pharmacies don't have the money to spend on these drugs and patients can't get them, so we've got to find a way to reduce that cost. As far as psychopharmacology itself is concerned, it looks as though we're beginning to move into an era of designer drugs in the true sense of the word. We are looking for drugs for either specific pharmacological profiles or, even more importantly, with structures that would fit different transporters or receptors. So we may be able to have even more specific drugs than we now have. Beyond that, there's a possibility that we can even influence some of the genetic factors that would play a role. It's a terribly exciting time that we're in. It's kind of frustrating to us old timers, who have to learn all the new stuff. I always give up or I feel depressed about what I don't know, but, by the same token, that's a good sign.

FA: It is a very good sign. As a matter of fact, I share with you the belief that this is an extremely exciting time. You know, there is a lot yet to be learned.

LH: I think you would agree with me that we've had a wonderful life.

FA: Oh, yes.

LH: I feel so privileged to have known so many bright, productive people and have become friends with them, acquaintances with them, and to have had the intellectual stimulation of being in this field over the years. I often have wondered what would have happened had I stayed in hypertension, because that's been an exciting area, too. But you can't change history. History has only one side and you can't tell what the alternative would have been; but nonetheless it's been a real privilege to be a member of the ACNP and to know the members in it, to be friends with people like you, and I have no regrets.

FA: I have none, either, Leo, and I thank you for letting me be your interviewer.

LH: Well, it was turn about, fair play.

FA: Fair play, yes. Leo interviewed me, two years ago, wasn't it? Yes, I think it was two years ago. But, actually, on behalf of the ACNP members, I want to thank you for what you did for us; you did for us a lot.

LH: I'll just say, in retrospect, you're not very impressed with what you accomplish, and wish you could have done more, but we do what we can.

FA: That's right. Well, that's it.

ALBERT A. KURLAND

Interviewed by Leo E. Hollister
Washington, District of Columbia, April 15, 1997

LH: It is Tuesday, April 15, 1997, and we're in Washington, DC, continuing a series of interviews on the early history of psychopharmacology, sponsored by the American College of Neuropsychopharmacology (ACNP). Today's guest is one of the pioneers in the field of clinical psychopharmacology, Dr. Al Kurland,* who lives nearby in Baltimore, and we welcome Al to this series.

AK: Thank you.

LH: We're always interested in how people decided to go into psychiatry, and how they ever decided to go into psychopharmacology. Can you tell us how you got started?

AK: It may sound like ancient history, but I have to go back to the year 1941. I had just completed a year's internship at the Sinai Hospital in Baltimore, and I decided to get my selective service out of the way before I continued with my education. So in July 1941, I was in the armed services and was assigned to an infantry unit of some type and shipped off to maneuvers in the Carolinas. On December 7th, late in the evening, I discovered that Pearl Harbor had happened and when I heard that, my immediate reaction was, how did I ever get in this mess and how will I ever get out? And events followed very quickly thereafter. I was only recently married. Then, in a few months I was on a ship bound for overseas. I didn't get back for a couple of years, and during my service, I discovered many things. First of all I discovered that I didn't like ships. I got sick on whatever kind of ship they put me on, whether it was a big ship or a small ship or a landing craft or whatever. And on many of these occasions, I was not certain that I was concerned about which side won. But anyway, I managed to survive a couple of years of that, and in the course of my activities, I was promoted to being in charge of a battalion.

LH: You were a medical officer?

AK: I was medical officer at that time, and I saw an extensive amount of combat. Apparently, my activities were recognized to a certain extent. After awhile, they thought that maybe I had enough of it and decided to rotate me back to the States. That was after a couple of years. And they asked me what I would like to do when I went back. I hadn't thought about it

---

* Albert Kurland was born in Wilkes-Barre, Pennsylvania, in 1914, and graduated in medicine in 1940 from the University of Maryland. After training in Army facilities during the war, in 1949 he became a staff psychiatrist at Maryland's Spring Grove State Hospital. He became director of research in 1953 and in 1969 was appointed director of the Maryland Psychiatric Research Center. In 1979 he was appointed research professor of psychiatry at the University of Maryland, School of Medicine. Kurland died in 2008.

very much, but when they said "we're going to send you to Carlisle to get some combat training," I said, "Hey, you guys pulled the wrong switch."

LH: You'd already had that.

AK: I said, "I already had that. I don't need a post-graduate training, can you think of something else that might be more appealing to me?" So, they said, "well, what would you like to do?" I said, "Well, I saw in combat an awful lot of stress. I saw a lot of stress reactions. I saw troops killed by friendly fire, and then the troopers shoot themselves. I saw all kinds of dreadful things." I said, "Look, I'd like to go to a neuropsychiatric unit, if possible to learn something about this situation, and, maybe, I might be able to find ways and means of being helpful in this area." Anyway, I was assigned to the Army General Hospital at Valley Forge to a neuropsychiatric service. It was a very awakening experience. It also brought to my attention a number of issues that had to be addressed, at least from my standpoint, in learning more about.

LH: Now, was this one of the 90 Day Wonder training groups?

AK: Well, I don't know what you would call it, because wherever I seemed to go, I always seemed to be learning something. They sent me up to a general hospital on Long Island. I guess it was Mason General Hospital. The Army had a course for training people in neuropsychiatry. I went up there, and then got to the hospital. And they came along one day and said, "Hey, you've been in the armed service for a couple of years now. You're due to get out. Would you like to stay in and get promoted?" I said, "I'd like to get out and not be promoted, because I've got a lot of things to catch up." Four years in the service put me pretty far behind in keeping up with the work I wanted to do. I arranged to get a Fellowship in Neuropsychiatric Research at the Sinai Hospital when I came out. So I started on that. Then, as I was working, I also got a part time job in an outpatient Veterans' Administration (VA) psychiatric clinic. At that time, there was considerable interest in psychiatric circles in psychoanalysis, so I thought, well, maybe I'd go and learn something about this. I exposed myself to a couple of years to analysis, and as I went along, I discovered that I was not considered a suitable candidate for psychoanalysis.

LH: Too analytical.

AK: Too analytical, all right. So then, a couple of years had gone by, and I wanted to get myself certified in psychiatry. They said, "well you've never had any experience in a psychiatric hospital, you ought to go there for maybe a year or two." I had heard all kinds of dreadful stories about psychiatric hospitals. Remember, this is before the chemotherapy revolution took place. This is prior to 1951.

LH: In the 1940s.

AK: I went into the Army when the war started. It was 1941, right?

LH: Yes.

AK: I came out in 1945, 1946, and then I started getting back into training again. I had the Fellowship, I went to work in the clinic, I went into psychoanalysis, and then, I needed to get this hospital training. So it was about 1949 or '50 that I got out to the State Hospital at Spring Grove. My assumption was that I was only going to spend a year to get my training there, and then move on. I go out to Spring Grove, and I go to the Superintendent, and he says, "I'm going to give you an assignment". I said, "Well, all right." The hospital at that time had over 2,700 patients. It had about 23 psychiatrists, and they had a budget for medication of about ten thousand dollars.

LH: A year?

AK: A year. That was for 2,700 patients. So, the Superintendent says to me, "You're going to be assigned to the unit for the criminally insane, there's 65 beds and you take care of them." So I say, "Well, I don't know anything about the criminally insane." He says, "Don't worry. If you need any consultation you can go to any one of our psychiatrists and ask them." I do the mathematics in my mind very quickly: there are 23 psychiatrists and 2,700 patients. I've got 65 patients and if I try to get a consultation, the chances are they won't have much time for me, because they've other things to worry about. So I go to work that I will be able to learn only by doing things. To do the best I could, I figured, "I've got to find something to activate myself." I started thinking of things I'd like to do, and I went to the Superintendent and said, "Look, I'd like to do some investigational work". He listens very quietly, very politely, and he says, "You can do this under three conditions." I say, "What are the conditions?" "First of all, you do this in your extracurricular time, okay? Secondly, you do not get the administration involved in any problems; and, thirdly, you don't ask for any funds."

LH: That's a good auspicious start!

AK: I figured, well, this is ground zero. But, anyway I went to work and started to study whatever I could latch onto. And then, I heard a rumor that a drug had appeared on the scene, Thorazine (chlorpromazine). It had taken about two years to cross the Atlantic. This was about 1954. Heinz Lehmann up in Canada had been working with it and just published a report on it. Have you ever heard the story about how Heinz Lehmann got involved with Thorazine? Are you familiar with that story?

LH: No.

AK: It's an interesting story. They had a detail man from Rhône-Poulenc come over to Canada, and Heinz Lehmann was working in a Canadian psychiatric hospital. So they tried to have an interview with him and tell him about this medication but he was too busy to see them. He says, "Leave the papers on my desk and I'll read them at my leisure." So, he picks it up Saturday, takes it home. Now, Saturday was his day for reading; he always did that in his tub. While he was relaxing and reading the article about Thorazine he said, "Well, that sounds like an interesting idea. I'm going to check it out." He goes to his wards, selects 25 nurses and 25 patients and he gives 25 of them Nembutal (pentobarbital), one of the barbiturates, and then he gives another 25 patients the Thorazine. He immediately realizes that there's a very important difference in what he's observing, because the effects of Thorazine are quite obvious. It brings a tranquilization, but it doesn't do anything to the consciousness in contrast to the barbiturate. Within three weeks, he carries out the study, gets a publication, and the dawn begins to break. Can you imagine trying to do a study today, getting something like that set up, underway and finished in three weeks? Impossible!

LH: You'd have to have a year of lead-time.

AK: All right. So people start hearing about this new drug, and the superintendent says to me one day, "Look, you know, I heard about this Thorazine. Someone has told me that they gave it to a patient in one of the hospitals here and it seems pretty good." So I said, "Well, I'll go ahead and try to get some." I get hold of somebody at Smith, Kline & French (SK&F) and say, "Could I have some of this to try it on a patient?" "We don't have any more supplies, but if you want to buy it, we'll sell it to you." So what am I going to do? I go back to the Superintendent and say, "Look, they'll sell it to us, but where are we going to get the money"? He says, "Well, I don't have anything in my budget." So I say, "Well, look, will you let me go to the relatives and see if I can solicit some funds from them to pay for it?" He says, "Sure, go ahead. I have no objection to that." I went to relatives and solicited funds from them, and got the Thorazine, and when I got the Thorazine and started to use it, I began to see that we've got something dramatic happening. So I went home to my wife and said, "Hey, look, there's an amazing drug coming along. Maybe we ought to buy some stock in this company." She says to me, "You're crazy. We just moved into this house. We've got a big mortgage, and we can hardly make the payments on it and you want to buy stock. Forget it." So I said, "All right, I forget it."

But I began to get involved with Thorazine in my patients. This was very early. I built up a series. I went through all the rigmarole. Even in those days, to get informed consent and clear it with the administration took some time. It wasn't as elaborate as later, but, anyway, I got underway with my studies and while I was working in this area, we got a call at the hospital from the National Institute of Mental Health (NIMH). You know, the NIMH had just been established about 1956 or 1957, somewhere around that time. I don't know the exact time. But, anyway, there was a chap there by the name of Savage. You probably know Charlie Savage. He was working at the NIMH, and there was a chap by the name of Lou Cholden, who was also at the NIMH. Cholden had come from the Menninger Clinic, and Charles had also been involved in analysis. And he'd been out in California, somewhere. They had heard about lysergic acid diethylamide (LSD) and they wanted to see just exactly what this drug was doing. Now Charles Savage had done some earlier work with LSD. This was in 1947; remember Hofmann came out with LSD in 1943. Savage tried to give it to depressed individuals on a chemotherapeutic basis but it didn't work. They were studying to see if they could give it to chronically ill psychotic patients and found out if it did anything to them; the individuals developed a tolerance. The superintendent calls me and says, "Hey, you're interested in research. I've got these two people from the NIMH. Would you like to show them around, sort of be their guide in the setting, help them find the patients, help them in whatever way you can?" I said, "Sure." I became an understudy to them. I saw what was going on with the patients and I went along with them. They discovered Nembutal tolerance, and that did not seem to be anything dramatic for them, so they went back to Washington.

In the meantime, with all this happening, Thorazine, and then the other compounds began to appear on the scene. I got very caught up in them, because of my interest. One of the first grants I got from the National Institutes of Health from the psychopharmacology section was ten thousand dollars. Jonathan Cole gave me that grant. But I ran into a problem. If he gave me the grant, how was I going to administer it? I'd have to go through the whole state machinery and the bureaucracy. I said, "that is going to take too long and I'll never get started." So I set up a non-profit foundation called Friends of Psychiatric Research that was where the money was going to go.

LH: And it still exists, doesn't it?

AK: Still exists, and right now they've got a multimillion dollar program, and a lot of investigators. I started that. And then I got involved in doing more and more studies of one kind or another. They finally said to me one day, "look, we want to make it a little bit easier for you." I immediately became suspicious. "What are you going to do for me now?" "We're going to make you Director of Research here, because, after all, you know the impact of the drugs and what's going on in the literature and the excitement that's building up." Here I was, saying we should have research, and they say, "All right, you want research, we're going to let you do it. We're going to make you a director we're going to give you a department." So, I said, "Well, who's going to be in my department?" "It's going to be yourself; you're going to have a secretary and you're going to have a budget." I thought it was, maybe, my salary and, maybe something for a secretary. That was my budget. Well, anyway, you know about the early days. There's no point in going over ancient history. But I was vigorous. I was youthful and I began to attend the meetings in psychopharmacology. You know how it was at those meetings in those early days. Everybody was excited about things and you got into discussions. You forgot what time of night it was, and it was a very exciting time, at least for me. So, as I got all these things going, I began to realize I needed logistical support. So I went to the Superintendent at that time, who became later the commissioner on mental health in the State. It was a guy by the name of Isadore Tuerk. I said, "Look, things are happening, and I don't have a thing. Let's set up some kind of a research facility". He says, "What do you want to do?" "Let's set up a research facility where we'll have a number of resources available." He says, "Well, okay, maybe you could put something on paper." At that time, the NIMH began to solicit proposals for setting up research facilities. So, he says, "Well, see if you can do anything." So I said, "Sure, I'll try." I start writing and filling out these forms, and getting some ideas of what I would need, and, then I contacted Gene Brody who was head of the Department of Psychiatry at the University of Maryland. Remember, I'm doing this in a state hospital, without the University of Maryland, without Hopkins. I'm doing this from ground zero without their involvement.

LH: I remember the story of all the studies of chlorpromazine. They were all done in public hospitals.

AK: Right and, you know most of the work will continue to be done in public hospitals. I had a rather interesting and frustrating experience recently about this. I wanted to get involved with one of the newer atypical compounds, quetiapine or Seroquel, and I contacted the company, but I had to tell them, "Well, I won't have access to some of the state hospital patients because of the criteria in the protocol." They look over the protocol and they say, "Well we can't give it to you then." I say, "Why not?" "Well, we can't because if the patients are not competent enough to give you informed consent, we don't think we can go along with that." I began to remember the early days. Here's a state hospital with thousands of patients, including outpatients, I'm coming to them, knowing what I have to do and how to do it, and they get caught up in the nuances of a study which is complicated but which should be done. So I got shot down.

LH: Well, I hope at the time you started your research SK&F was eventually giving you the drug.

AK: Well, they eventually reached that stage. They reached that stage because they became aware that maybe I knew what I was talking about and I'd started to become productive, started to write papers. And what happened was that I went to Brody, who was the chief of psychiatry at the University of Maryland, and said, "Look, I want to write this grant. Are you guys going to support me on this?" He said, "Yes." Then, I went to Elkes at Johns Hopkins and I said, "Elkes, are you going to help me on this?" He said, "Yes."

LH: Was Elkes chairman of the department of psychiatry at Hopkins then?

AK: He was over at Hopkins at the time. So I put it all together, and then when I looked at the bottom line, I figured it was going to cost a couple of million dollars. I submitted my grant application, and in Washington, the NIMH says, "We shall give you some money, but we aren't going to give you all you're asking for." "So, how much am I going to be short?" "You're going to be short about a million dollars." I'm thinking to myself, where do I get a million dollars? As I was meditating about that, my wife got a ticket for going through a red light, so I had to speak to one of the local politicians about it. When I was talking to him I asked whether he could help in any way in getting some money to ameliorate my situation. So he referred me to somebody in the legislature to discuss it with them. As I discussed it with them, we got into other things, and they said, "Look, you need some money for that?" "Yeah, I need a million dollars." Now, remember, at the time the legislature was almost out of session. They've only got seven days left, but the guy thought maybe I was doing a meaningful thing, and he put himself to work and in seven days he got a bill put through. We got that million dollars, and we built the Maryland Psychiatric Research Center.

LH: Incredible, he must have been a wonderful legislator.

AK: He was. He was a judge at one time, and he became a legislator. So we have a friendship now that has existed over the years. At the same time, I built up the Friends of Psychiatric Research, and we began to get grants. We also had a lot of problems, because everybody was suspicious. They wanted to see whether the funds were being raked off into somebody else's pocket. You know how the public gets suspicious. Then, one day the Board of Directors said, "Look, you're entitled to some compensation for what you're doing, because you don't do it on hospital time." I said, "I never did anything on hospital time." So they went ahead and said, "We are going to give you a gratuity or something." And I said, "I think it's all right, the record is clear." Some enterprising newspaper character gets hold of this and it makes me look like I'm walking off with the state treasury. Of course, this was very shattering as far as my wife was concerned. Remember, I was only going to spend a year at the state hospital and here it is, fifteen years later, twelve years later, I don't know. I lost track of time. But in the meantime I was busy; I was working.

And, then, I got into another area of exploration. I mentioned that Charles Savage and Louis Cholden (who eventually was killed in an accident), had introduced me to LSD. About the same time, up in Canada, Humphry Osmond and Abram Hoffer had gotten interested in treating alcoholics with LSD. They thought that was a good idea. There was another outfit up in Canada headed by a man by the name of [J. Ross] MacLean, who had heard about the way some of the North American Indian cultures had treated their alcoholics with peyote and was doing research on that up there.

LH: And, a guy named Hubbard.

AK: Alfred Matthew Hubbard was working with MacLean up there. He was one of their research assistants.

LH: He was an engineer by profession.

AK: Well, anyway, he went to the Indians and observed it, and then he went back and persuaded MacLean to go ahead and try to incorporate what he observed in their treatment structure. Well, they did that and it seemed to be very helpful. Osmond and Hoffer heard about it, because they were working almost on a parallel track. They went and observed what MacLean was doing, then they brought Hubbard there to treat a couple of patients with LSD, and then a guy by the name of [Colin] Smith took over the project from Osmond and Hoffer and wrote the first extended series on it, indicating, "Hey, it's getting some good results."

LH: Now, wait a minute, you're getting way ahead.

AK: Yeah.

LH: When did you first publish your observations on chlorpromazine?

AK: It was around 1954, somewhere around that.

LH: So that was one of your first papers?

AK: Yes. Well, there was an earlier paper that related to what you had done with reserpine. We started off with reserpine, and then you had come out with a very important presentation summarizing it at that time and pointing out that it wasn't doing very much or words to that effect. I think that preceded the work with Thorazine. Because Nathan Kline was very much involved with the reserpine study. I had spoken to him and tried to see what I could do there. I was relatively unimpressed by it; but then when Thorazine came out, it was much less of a problem in terms of possible side effects, the depression and the apathy. So I got sidetracked and went off onto Thorazine, and then when the other compounds started coming along, we started looking at them, too. Tofranil (imipramine) came along and then the monoamine oxidase inhibitors (MAOIs). While Nathan Kline got involved with the MAOIs earlier, there was a guy by the name of George Crane, who had been working with Nathan Kline at that time, and maybe even preceded Nathan in terms of becoming aware that this was doing something to tuberculosis patients in terms of their moods. Anyway, George came down to Spring Grove and did a lot of that work on tardive dyskinesia. He went through thousands of records on patients, and began to provide some definitive evidence indicating that in some patients extended use produces this complication.

In the meantime, this chap from the NIMH, Sanford M. Unger, comes over and says, "Hey, there's all this work with LSD in alcoholics happening up in Canada," and asked "could we do this at Spring Grove?" I said, "Well, no, you've got the whole NIMH." He says, "I can't have any beds for alcoholics over there, but you've got a couple of wards filled with them." At that time, in about the early 1960s, the state hospitals were admitting alcoholics and treating them for a couple of weeks or longer, depending upon what they felt their needs were. That was the era that preceded managed "mangled" care. We could keep the patients there for as long as we wanted to, and I convinced the Superintendent that we ought to try to replicate this work. He was interested in alcoholism, and he said. "Sure, go ahead and do it." So we went ahead. We set up an experiment to replicate exactly what they were doing up in Hoffer's and Osmond's place and we began to see that there was something there that we couldn't discount. As you know, it's very, very difficult to quantitate in any way, but, on the other hand, the feeling was that we did see some dramatic changes in some of these patients. We became aware that there was something in their reactivity that seemed to be the critical factor, and we began to focus on what we called the Peak Experience.

At that time, my other difficulties began to pursue me, namely, in terms of getting the Research Center on stream. I built up a research unit, and was really looking at those possibilities very carefully, and I had good people working with me. There was a chap by the name of Stan Grof, who came over from Czechoslovakia, and had a fellowship with Hopkins. Elkes directed him to us because of his interest, and he worked with us. Savage came back. He had gone to the Institute for Advanced Studies or Training or something like that, and when he heard about what we were doing, he came and joined us. Then there was another chap by the name of Walter N. Pahnke, who was getting his PhD. He had an MD already. He was getting his PhD in theology and he got involved in what was identified at the time as the Good Friday Experiment. I don't know whether you remember that or not, where they took a group of seminarians and some of them got a hallucinogen and some of them didn't, and then they followed these people, some of them for twenty years. There was a recent review of those studies in one of the papers I get.

LH: You mentioned Charlie Savage; he came out to that Institute for Advanced Studies at Stanford, I guess, around 1963, wasn't it?

AK: Somewhere around that time.

LH: And, while he was there, I got him involved in a study we were doing on hallucinogens in psychotherapy. He'd give them four or five different treatments, three of which were hallucinogens, taped what happened, and then edited the tapes. It was a difficult job to listen to those damn tapes and evaluate the psychotherapy. But then he went back to Baltimore after that.

AK: Well, he heard about our work and I knew about his interest.

LH: Didn't you organize a fairly large control study with Thorazine in the early 1960s?

AK: Yes, we did a big controlled study. Everybody had some awareness of what the neuroleptics can do by themselves, but we became interested in what happened when you added an antidepressant or you added another type of compound to it. So we set up a big study, and we were trying to factor out whether the add-on drugs influenced the course of the activity. The bottom line in all that, in spite of the magnitude of the study, was that we didn't feel it did anything one way or another. It didn't influence the course of events. And then, we also got involved with the antidepressants and did a lot of stuff in that area. And then, another thing, which was very, very fortunate, was that the organization of the ACNP got started somewhere around that time.

LH: Around 1960.

AK: 1960. I learned about it from Frank Ayd. Frank Ayd was one of the original members who had been involved with some of the others and got the ACNP started. And when I heard about it, I said, "Hey, I want to come to your meetings." So he says, "You're welcome." I think I attended the second meeting, and then others began to join, too, because in those very heady days at the ACNP meetings, everybody was on the verge of a major discovery of one kind or another. But the interesting thing is, over the years that we carried on our research, and everything we were involved in – and we were involved in some very tenuous and sensitive areas – we never got in any trouble. Everything went along in a very carefully calculated way. And even with the LSD research, some of my associates wanted to be exposed to the LSD, and said, "well, maybe that will enhance our capacity for interacting." I said, "Before anybody gets involved, we're going to have some rules. The rules are, you have to go through a procedure just like the patient. You have to be interviewed by a number of psychiatrists; and, the other thing is, to keep the thing on a level playing field, we're never going to tell anybody who was treated and who wasn't." I wanted to make sure that the thing was balanced, so that the people who had been exposed and the people who weren't would be equal, so that we couldn't feel it was biased. And even as that got shot down, when they finally said, "You are not handling this so well administratively," I didn't feel very badly about it. I felt disappointed. I felt that, all right, maybe I could have done a lot of other things, but I said, "Well, maybe somebody can do a better job."

They put Will Carpenter in there (in charge of the Maryland Psychiatric Research Center) and Will Carpenter, you know, is focused on schizophrenia. But I see in the *American Journal of Psychiatry,* the 1995 issue, there was an article about him on clozapine in schizophrenia recently, and Meltzer took him to task. He wrote an editorial about it and, so, the ball started going back and forth. I read this, and then Carpenter sent a big letter to the editor of the *American Journal*, it came out twelve months later, but I read each of these documents very carefully, and while they accused each other of misinforming, misinterpreting, misconceiving certain concepts, I came to the bottom line: They were both right.

LH: Well, that whole issue of the specific action on negative symptoms has been somewhat iffy all along.

AK: It's iffy, because of the rating scales the criteria that they're using to identify and to grade them. The companies seized upon avidly to promote negative symptoms with Compound A vs. Compound B.

LH: Quicker action and negative symptoms were the gimmicks they all used.

AK: I don't fault them for that, because they've got to have some way of promoting their compounds, plus the money goes back into research, a lot of it, anyway. I've never gotten involved with the drug companies or given anybody a hard time about it. I've always been sympathetic to what they're doing. If they want to make a few extra dollars, that's their problem, not mine.

LH: Now, are Will Carpenter and Carol Tamminga and the people now working in the same unit that you started?

AK: They're using the facilities, but they've kept me hands off, never invited me to anything; never acknowledged, anything that we've done to bring this facility into existence. Sometimes I wonder about it, but, then, I figure, well maybe that's part of the cultural system.

LH: That's what the Eskimos do; when you get old, they put you on an ice floe and let you go to sea.

AK: Right. At one time I would go down to the university, because they gave me the title Research Professor of Psychiatry, never Professor of Psychiatry, but Research Professor of Psychiatry. I didn't check it. I don't care what they call me, as long as I could get in there and do something I felt was useful. What they asked me to do was to supervise the residents in terms of the psychopharmacology they were employing, and my feeling was, okay, I'll do it. I did that for a number of years, but then they started getting more and more administrative – you've got to sign off on all the charts and you've got to do this, and I don't even know when they follow through what they're doing – and I thought, I can't do that, because I can't assume responsibility that I really can't follow through on. They said, we have to do this. Well, I said, "I can't do it. Goodbye." So I quietly departed. I tried to get a number of drugs at Taylor Manor and I worked on a number of things with different drug companies. Then, finally, my last hurrah was trying to get established a specific research facility devoted to the exploration of the hallucinogenic drugs. I think there are phenomena going on in some individuals what I call a psychic healing influence. You have that in religious activities; and I've seen it enough times to realize that it reaches into an area which we know very little about. I think is going to be very important in the future as we move into the twenty-first century and we start learning more about how we really develop maturity within ourselves so we can deal with equanimity with a lot of the things we have to deal with. One of the elements in the psychedelic peak experience is this transcendental experience. It's something that's way out of the ordinary and has to be explored.

LH: The work with hallucinogens sort fell apart after about 1957.

AK: It fell apart.

LH: And, then, it's only been in the last four or five years that a chap named Rick Strassman, whom I don't know, but he's in Arizona, has been getting some grants and doing some publications on it.

AK: Rick Strassman, I'm familiar with his work. I'm familiar with what's going on in the past several years, because this institute that I'm talking about is called the Orenda Institute. They just got their foundation. They're tax-free. It was set up by a chap by the name of Rich Yensen and his wife Donna Dryer. She's a psychiatrist and he is a psychologist. He was involved years ago with us in our work with LSD, and they decided to pick it up and work with it, so they've gone through this laborious process. They've been to a lot of meetings on the West Coast and in Europe. Some of the Europeans are still interested in it. It has to be pursued because you know and I know that when we take a schizophrenic who has gotten better up to a certain point, there's a certain residue of symptomatology. Many times we find individuals who get to a certain point and then somehow there remains something that's unresolved. The only powerful element that I feel that might have some impact on it, at least from our observation, is in some way to create what we call a peak or transcendental experience. Now, the question is how to differentiate it from that which happens in a religious revival? What's the difference? Are the same things occurring? Many of these people have been through religious revivals or thereabouts, but that doesn't work. But, with this "transcendental experience," it seems to work. And then, in the cancer patient studies, there was no uncertainty that we were doing something that was important, because where we got these experiences, the amount of narcotics these patients were using decreased. The patients began to have a more wholesome relationship to the people around them. The conspiracy of silence seemed to be ameliorated, and in whatever time was left there was a much better relationship between the individual and the family, because the individual seemed to have a better way of communicating, and was more philosophical about things, There's much to be done, but I think it will be done in the future, because we know the limitations of the drugs we're using today. We treat a panic disorder, we treat alcoholism, we treat depression, and we ameliorate the symptoms, but what are we doing so far that is adding to the individual's capacity for development?

LH: Each person has a somewhat different experience with hallucinogens. I remember Jack Shelton, who used to be one of my collaborators, had extensive experience with LSD, and he always likened it to a near-death experience where he felt that he had been close to the edge, and then come back. My own experience was a feeling like I'd been terribly ill and now I'd recovered and felt so vibrant to be back with the living. So, you know, it's a different kind of reaction, I guess depending on our own personality, to so much of an extent that it's hard to quantitate it.

AK: It's hard. I went through a couple of years of analysis and I sometimes say to myself, well, what did it accomplish for me? I'm not so sure, maybe better insights, maybe a more humble attitude towards myself, my fellow man, maybe a capacity for tolerating the shortcomings of others.

The other thing that's very important, that nobody realizes, is that the organization of the ACNP, with the structure and the role it has played in getting drugs, getting people interested, and making it available for the younger generation, the people that are about to carry on the organization, was a tremendously important development. Carpenter presents his papers, Tamminga presents her papers at the ACNP, and we need that. We need those kinds of activities.

LH: Well, the remarkable thing about the ACNP is the ability to bring together so many different disciplines, so we can talk to one another. For instance, when I go to the ACNP meetings, I don't go for the things that I know about. I always go for the things that I don't know about; but, of course, every year there's more and more to learn, so I have trouble making my selection. And, of course, some people like Don Klein overreacted to it by saying, we're no longer interested in clinical psychopharmacology, and therefore he started a separate organization. Do you remember that?

AK: No.

LH: The American College of Clinical Pharmacology?

AK: I'm not a member of it, but I follow their proceedings, because I need to keep abreast for my work what is going on. I see a lot of patients and I use a lot of drugs. I don't just use drugs, because I have the advantage of having had a background and training in psychotherapy and analysis, so I can integrate these things.

LH: Have you retired from the state hospital system?

AK: I retired about fifteen years ago.

LH: And now you're doing private practice?

AK: I'm working for the Taylor Manor Hospital organization.

LH: Which?

AK: Taylor Manor.

LH: Oh, Taylor Manor, which is essentially a private hospital.

AK: A private hospital.

LH: Does Joe Taylor still live out in California now, Palm Springs?

AK: Yes, the old man and his wife live out in California. They moved out to some other place on the West Coast.

LH: The son has taken over?

AK: Bruce is very bright, very knowledgeable and he handles a very, very difficult situation with all this managed care and all the issues and things that are going today, which would drive me up the wall. They're providing a service. They're trying to deal with the demands. I'm studying and trying to constantly think of ways of dealing with new things, For example, at my age, would you think that I would be involved in the study of Attention Deficit Hyperactive Disorder (ADHD)? The stimulants are the only things that seem to do a pretty good job there, and the question is, why? So I get involved with comparisons, and then I get involved with bupropion, and I get mad at myself, because, "geez, I say, you're getting grandiose; you're getting caught up in all these things and nothing is going to be accomplished."

LH: You had too much analysis. Well, from your vantage point, what do you see in the future?

AK: The way I see the future is that this is just the beginning. It's like Churchill said a long time ago, "This is not the beginning of the end, but it may be the end of the beginning," because we're just getting oriented. We're getting some awareness of the techniques and the sciences and everything else. In neuroscience alone, we've got thousands of people working on different aspects of these problems, and if you're trying to keep abreast of all this, it's very difficult, but we need to have people in there who are knowledgeable and can tell us what is going on, and they need support. For example, somebody starts talking about dopamine receptors to me, and when he starts getting into the pharmacology, it's like Greek. They can say what they want. I can't criticize it one way or another, because I don't know when they're right, but I know that they're doing something that may ultimately be meaningful and it's important that they have an audience, that there's interaction. I think the needs are going to become even greater. They'll become greater because there are a lot of things in our society that we don't even have a handle on yet: for example, in learning difficulties, kids that develop all kinds of problems, and then they're mistreated and become psychopathic, because the parents and the people working with them don't understand. We've got to deal with the parents, because otherwise they become sociopathic in one way or another. And how do we affect our learning capabilities? How do we go about making what we're doing more effective? We've had neuroleptics for fifty years, and you know what, we still don't know how to regulate a dose in a really precise way. The other day I got a letter, written by a man by the name of Haase, saying get people just to write a simple verse and repeat it a number of times, and then look at the handwriting and the way it changes in structure and space, and you can tell very quickly whether your drugs are too much, too little or whatever. There are all kinds of crazy things we measured, prolactin, dopamine receptor assays, neuroleptic-plasma levels and try to correlate them. Nothing works, but the point is that one thing does work: looking at the patient. We make a judgment as to whether he is getting better or not, and we go along from that.

LH: All right. What you touched upon is a major point in all of medicine. The technology has become so powerful that people tend to rely on that rather than looking at the patient and deciding. I remember about three or four years ago, I came in to my urologist and said, "I have an atonic bladder." So what does he do? He does an urodynamic test to prove that I have an atonic bladder. It doesn't make sense to use some of this technology when you can make the diagnosis, clinically, but that's the story.

You mentioned Frank Ayd, who of course has been a neighbor of yours, although he worked out of a different hospital. Do you ever have much interaction with him?

AK: Yes I see him occasionally. Frank is very busy. He's put out this encyclopedia now with the different terms.

LH: Didn't Frank have some contact or consult with Taylor Manor, too?

AK: He's emeritus. He was the first Director of Research and Education. Incidentally, I have a title there, but I always keep forgetting about it. I'm supposed to be the Director of Research, but for me, it's just like being back in the state hospital. If you want to do something, you figure out how to do it, and if I get outside funds, I can go ahead and do it. But most of the times, I get shot down, because it's hard to do things without the proper logistical background.

LH: Do you know Fritz Freyhan very well?

AK: I met Fritz Freyhan when he was up at Delaware. Then he came down and took over, I think from Elkes when Elkes left the directorship of the research unit over at the St. Elizabeths.

LH: I'd forgotten that.

AK: He took over, and then he got divorced and subsequently remarried, and then he dropped dead.

LH: He died young, but he did a fairly large study of drugs over in the Delaware system.

AK: Yes, he was one of the first people that got involved on a large scale; he did careful work. He started that *Comprehensive Psychiatry* as well.

LH: He was an old fashioned clinician like you are.

AK: But, let me tell you something, clinicians, good clinicians never go out of style. They may get old, but if they know what they're doing, they don't go out of style.

LH: Well, whether you like it or not, you fade away. I was recently in the Far East sponsored by Pfizer and all these young employees, most of whom could have been my grandchildren, would come up to me and say, "What's your name?" And, I'd say, "Dr. Hollister." And, "What do you do?" Oh, god, fame is so fleeting, you know. My name meant nothing to them.

AK: Yeah, but you know what you did. Nobody can take that away from you.

LH: No. Maybe that's the consolation of old age.

AK: We're leaving things a lot better than we found them. Do you agree with that?

LH: Yes.

AK: Okay.

LH: Well, that's the only thing. Everyone I've talked to in these series has been so happy with their career and wouldn't have changed it a bit. Is that true with you?

AK: I'm not sure, and I'll tell you why. I've always had a passion for Space.

LH: You mean you would have liked to become an astronaut?

AK: Yes, I wanted to go out there and explore those planets, and one of my secret fantasies was that if I had unlimited wealth, what I would do is, I would make a deal with the world organizations, and I'd say, "Look, if you'll let me have a couple of hundred thousand square miles of land on the moon, I will go ahead and develop a transportation system that will get man from the earth to the moon, so he can communicate in a regular fashion." Now, is there a precedent for what I'm doing? Yes. In the nineteenth century, after the Civil War, when they were discussing whether they should build a railroad from the East Coast to the West Coast, there was a lot of commotion in Congress, because they said, "Well, why do you need the railroad out there? The only thing out there is Indians and buffalos. Why do you need it for them?" And the companies that were interested in promoting this said, "We'll make with you a deal. You give us land grants and we'll build that railroad." And, so, they said, "All right. The land didn't cost us anything, so take what you want." So, they did and they're still profiting and so is the rest of the country.

LH: You need another life. I tell you, if you'd invested in that SK&F stock, you probably would have had enough money to do that.

AK: All right. It wasn't my fate or my karma, whatever you want to call it.

LH: Well, we all missed opportunities in life but it's a lot of fun.

AK: It's a lot of fun, and that's the important thing. We can make it a lot of fun for a lot of people if we get to know more about what we're trying to do.

LH: Very nice talking to you, Al. Good to see you after all these years.

AK: All right. I'm glad to be here.

HEINZ E. LEHMANN

Interviewed by William E. Bunney, Jr.
San Juan, Puerto Rico, December 12, 1994

WB: I'm William Bunney, Professor of Psychiatry and Human Behavior, University of California, Irvine, and I will be interviewing Dr. Heinz Lehmann,* Professor Emeritus of Psychiatry, McGill University, Montreal, and Deputy Commissioner for Research for the Office of Mental Health in the State of New York. We're going to go through a series of question, about Dr. Lehmann's career and I wonder if you'd start by telling us a little bit about your training.

HL: My training was in Germany. I went to school there, the Gymnasium, and then to some various universities as it was the fashion then in Germany. You went to as many universities for your medical study as your father could afford to send you, so I studied in Freiburg; I studied in Marburg; I studied in Freiburg again, then in Vienna, and finally graduated from Berlin University. But it didn't go that easily, because when I was about twelve I felt what I can now diagnose as depression, which lasted for almost a year. In those days, children didn't have depression, so that wasn't diagnosed and nobody knew what to do about it, and my main symptom was that I couldn't work. I couldn't concentrate at all, and I couldn't do any homework. Now, when you're twelve years old and in the Gymnasium and you're supposed to learn Greek and Latin and mathematics, that didn't go very well. So my teachers told my parents that they had to take me out, that I just would never be able to get through high school, and I just wasn't made for it and I should learn a trade. Well, my mother didn't believe it and used her good judgment and got me a tutor. The tutor came every day. He was a student, and he did my homework with me, and much of the time for me, actually. He was interested in psychology and he saw that obviously I couldn't do it; I couldn't concentrate, so he would do the homework for me. That went on for about six months and I got out of my depression. And so, I did get through the Gymnasium. I got through the universities, and then I had to leave Germany in the late '30s, because of Hitler, and came to Montreal, Canada. I worked in a mental hospital there, the Douglas Hospital, then, called Verdun Protestant Hospital, and I didn't have the time to get any postgraduate training. I've always been interested in psychiatry. In fact, before I started medicine at the university I told my father, who was a surgeon that I would become a psychiatrist.

---

* Heinz Edgar Lehmann was born in Berlin, Germany in 1911 and received his MD from the University of Berlin in 1935. He took a post in 1937 at the Verdun Protestant Hospital in a suburb of Montreal, Canada, and stayed there for the rest of his career. In 1948 he joined the department of psychiatry of McGill University, and became professor emeritus in 1981. Lehmann died in 1999.

Now, back in the early 1930s, that was certainly something you didn't go into. There was practically no really good diagnosis, except Kraepelinian. The only therapy was psychoanalysis. But, anyway, I insisted on it, probably because I had gotten through the depression, and my tutor, who got me out of the depression and did my homework with me, was interested in psychology as a student, and he had given me all of Freud's works that had been written until then, all of which I read. By the time I was fourteen, I had read all of Freud's work. That got me interested in psychiatry before I started medicine, and I stuck with it. Everybody said, "you will change your mind about that," but I didn't. But then I didn't have any postgraduate training in psychiatry. There was no time for it. The War started when I started working in the hospital in Montreal, in the mental hospital, and there weren't many people left. I was one of the few, so I didn't have time and I didn't have the money for postgraduate training, so I never got any. I didn't get certified, and later when this came up I said, "Well, I certainly didn't have the time to go for the examinations now, and anyway, I wasn't so sure that the examiners would know more than I would, so I didn't bother." Eventually, they sent it to me by mail, the certification, I didn't even ask for it. So now, I'm a certified psychiatrist, without any postgraduate training. Well, what was the training? I learned it the right way, I think, by just working from 8:30 in the morning until about 12:30 at night. I had up to six hundred patients during the War, and there were only two or three doctors left in the hospital. We didn't have interns; we didn't have residents. I had one trained nurse. The others were untrained attendants, and up to six hundred patients. So I did learn a lot, because I spent my time with the patients.

WB: You taught yourself.

HL: I taught myself, and the patients taught me.

WB: Did you read during that time, too?

HL: Yes, I did read. That's what I did after 11:00 o'clock at night or 10:00 o'clock at night in the hospital library. I courted my wife, who was a nurse there, and word got around to her that I probably was a heroin addict, because nobody else would walk around the hospital library at 3:00 o'clock in the morning. So, I did read a lot, and I saw a lot of patients and I learned quite a bit, of course. I was convinced that there was quite a bit of difference between what we then called neuroses and psychoses, and I was convinced that psychoses, such as schizophrenia and the affective disorders, had some sort of a very strong physical component, and that wasn't necessarily so for the neuroses.

WB: How did the whole area of drugs come up? How did you get involved?

HL: Because I was convinced that there was a physical substrate for the psychoses, so I tried very large doses of caffeine. I came up with the notion that manic depressive swings may have something to do with acidity and alkalinity and pH, so I gave my patients very large doses of ammonium sulfate or sodium carbonate, in order to alter their pH. I was always hoping and dreaming about some drug that eventually would do something to psychosis. Well, then what happened is, that in 1953 – my wife is French Canadian, so we speak French at home – I read a French article by Delay and Deniker on chlorpromazine, on their first experience with chlorpromazine in 1952, and that intrigued me very much. I couldn't believe that psychotic symptoms such as hallucinations and delusions could be affected by a simple pill. But, anyway, I tried it. Of course by the late 1930s, early '40s, we already had shock treatments. I had been treating patients with insulin coma therapy, hypoglycemic coma, and with Metrazol (pentylenetetrazol) therapy before we had electroconvulsive therapy, and these treatments worked fine for a few weeks or a few months. But then, of course, the patients relapsed, as we know now, about seventy percent of them, and then we didn't know what to do. We applied the same shock treatments again, and the second time they usually didn't work as well.

WB: Didn't you have a role in the first use of chlorpromazine?

HL: In 1953, I read about this pill, and, so, we got samples from Rhône-Poulenc, who made the chlorpromazine. I read the articles one Sunday, I remember, and the next day, Monday, the first resident I met – by that time, in the '50s, we did have residents – I asked, "Do you want to try this fancy new drug? It seems to be incredible, what they claim for it." And he said yes, so we set up a clinical trial in, I think, seventy-two patients. We got it all arranged in about a week or two, because we didn't need any permission. I didn't even ask the director of the hospital. Certainly, there were no ....

WB: No Institutional Review Boards (IRBs).

HL: No IRBs, no informed consents, no Food and Drug Administration (FDA) regulations, nothing; also no money whatsoever. So we had to kind of fold these seventy-two patients into our regular routine. I didn't even have the heart to ask the hospital for a secretary. So I made my own cards out for each patient. Well, it worked remarkably well, because after two weeks, two or three of my acute schizophrenic patients were practically symptom-free, and that, I'd never seen or heard about before.

WB: That had to be an exciting week.

HL: Oh, yes. We started our study in May, and in August, we had finished, simultaneously, all seventy-two patients, and we had written the paper. I remember writing in the paper that these were the drug's 'unique effects,' and my boss, another psychiatrist, said in a short note in the manuscript, "don't ever say anything is unique," nothing is unique. But this one was and I insisted on keeping it. At the time, of course, there was no other way to describe it. At first, so, my co-worker and I thought that what we saw was a fluke, and perhaps some sort of mistake.

WB: Who else in the field was studying chlorpromazine at that point in time?

HL: Well, there was Nate Kline. He had started reserpine, which didn't last very long, but it also was an antipsychotic drug. And then I remember Frank Ayd, and I think, Douglas Goldman. I don't think anyone in Canada had worked on it.

WB: Did Fritz Freyhan study it, did he?

HL: Fritz Freyhan, of course. Now, Fritz Freyhan coined the term target symptoms, and that's fine. We did have target symptoms, typical psychotic symptoms like delusions, hallucinations, formal thought disorder. I think for awhile, he thought, like many others, that the drugs were anti-schizophrenic, but from the beginning that seemed to be very unlikely, almost impossible. But, we did find that it worked in psychotic manics, even in psychotic depressed patients, as well as in schizophrenics.

WB: You found that out fairly early.

HL: In our first seventy-two patients, we had about twelve different illnesses; a few manic patients where it worked miraculously well, of course, and a few depressed patients, and even a few organic psychoses, where it didn't work very well.

WB: So you had the whole story in those seventy-two patients, almost?

HL: Almost.

WB: In the first paper?

HL: Yes, and then in the next two or three months, before Christmas of that year, we tried it in a few anxious patients, and found out that definitely the drug wasn't an anxiolytic, so we really had the whole story.

WB: Now, in Europe, who was working with the drug at that point?

HL: In Europe, they worked with it primarily in France.

WB: The French, primarily?

HL: Delay, Deniker, and two or three others. Deniker came over to Montreal to visit us from Paris, and we had some jaundice cases, which the French hadn't seen. I haven't seen them since either. Possibly it was sub-clinical hepatitis. From then on, of course, there has been a never-ending chain of new drugs, such as Stelazine (trifluoperazine) ….

WB: What hospital were you in when you did the seventy-two cases?

HL: The same hospital I'm still teaching in. It was the Douglas Hospital that was called then the Verdun Protestant Hospital. I'm still teaching students there every Monday, so that's quite a long time. They have now a research center there. At the time, it was one of those big, well, snake pits, really. It's very nice to see what, over a lifetime, can happen with a snake pit becoming a good research center. Well, that is how I got into psychopharmacology, but really it was realizing a dream. I had hoped there would be a drug for those patients. I'd been looking for it, hoping to find it eventually. From then on, Tom Ban joined me. He had just come from Hungary and for the next ten or fifteen years, we did a lot of clinical trials. There's hardly any drug between 1952 and 1970 that we didn't do clinical trials with.

WB: Well, tell me some of the most interesting findings in those clinical trials.

HL: Of course, nothing can match the unbelievable thing that there was a drug, chlorpromazine, first time in history, that could in two weeks wipe out hallucinations and delusions. After we had really believed that was so, which took a year or so or more, nothing else could really....

WB: Anti-climactic.

HL: Everything else was anti-climactic, yes. But, then, I remember a funny story. I went in '57 to Zurich to the international psychiatric meeting, and there on the way back from Zurich to Montreal on the plane, I read Kuhn's first paper on imipramine, which he had given at the meeting in Zurich. I wasn't there; apparently he had about only twelve people in the audience. I read the paper he had written in German on the way back that there is possibly now a drug for depression. I immediately called Geigy when I arrived in Montreal, and their branch in Montreal hadn't heard of this; although their company had worked with it, obviously, for more than a year. Well, they felt a little embarrassed, but got me the drug from Europe, and, then we did one of the first trials with imipramine in Canada, and probably North America, and found that it worked, too. But that wasn't so surprising. I had told the various drug representatives, after we had anti-psychotics, it shouldn't be so difficult to find an antidepressant, because it's likely that there's a metabolic disturbance in affective disorder as in schizophrenia.

WB: Do you think we're going to find drugs for the twenty to thirty percent schizophrenics and twenty percent or fifteen percent depressed patients that don't respond to anything; do you think we're going to find a drug for them?

HL: I think so, not one drug, but probably a half dozen, and we'll learn how to make diagnoses based on the substrates involved in depression and schizophrenia, probably. That's where the new imaging technology will help us, probably. So far, we can't make any diagnosis with it, but we may be able to distinguish substrates. So far all our diagnoses are based on phenomenology, just the way Kraepelin did it, but we will probably be able to find certain traits with endocrinological measures, molecular research or functional imaging that will allow us to make distinctions between various depressives and various schizophrenics.

WB: Do you remember where your first paper on Thorazine was published?

HL: It was in the *Archives*, the *Archives of Neurology and Psychiatry*. It wasn't easy to get it published. We sent it in August and since I hadn't heard anything by December, it seemed that something was fishy. So I wrote them that I wanted the paper back, and "I'll get it to somewhere else." Then, they immediately published it. It came out in March of the next year. I think what happened is that we were in Canada, and the Americans that were working with it, I think Winkelman, wanted to be the first one out. His paper came a month later. He had worked with chlorpromazine in neurotic patients.

WB: The usual story.

HL: Yes.

WB: Who was the editor of the *Archives* then? Do you remember?

HL: No, that, I don't remember.

WB: Was it Grinker?

HL: No, it wasn't him.

WB: It was before him?

HL: It was before Grinker.

WB: Well, you've worked on a lot of different hypotheses and tested a lot of different drugs and had a lot of different theories. Are there any that particularly come to your mind?

HL: No, what I would like now is to find methods to determine sub-clinical minor stress. I'm thinking of that, particularly, because I have a notion that many aging people suffer from subclinical – to them probably unknown – chronic stress that actually kills their hippocampal cells. I think Ewing has shown, and several others have shown it too. In California, there's a group showing that corticosteroids produce atrophy of hippocampal cells, and a chronic stress condition would of course produce a chronic outflow of corticosteroids. I think a lot of elderly people suffer from chronic stress conditions without knowing it. Now, if we could, well, test, for instance, their saliva for corticosteroids, their electrolytes for corticosteroid receptors, we would possibly be capable of finding in a lot of people, who would never know about it, and the doctors don't know about it, that they are chronically stressed. If they are chronically stressed, then one would have to find out why, and probably with psychotherapy they could be helped to get over this change in their lifestyle or whatever it is. There's a lot of undiscovered chronic stress. Some people have suggested that post-traumatic stress might be due to an outflow of corticosteroids.

WB: Going back to your first major study with chlorpromazine, did you present it at a meeting before it was published? Do you remember?

HL: No, I didn't. I presented it a year later at the American Psychiatric annual meeting.

WB: After it was published?

HL: After it was published. And I was very much surprised when people clapped and applauded when I went up to the podium. I never expected it, and didn't know why and that was the first time....

WB: That was the first time you presented it?

HL: That I presented it.

WB: And, they, obviously, knew about it?

HL: They knew, because they read the paper.

WB: Right, right.

HL: But, I didn't realize that it had caused the impact.

WB: You didn't know the impact.

HL: I didn't know the impact.

WB: What do you think was the biggest contribution that you've made?

HL: To psychiatry?

WB: Psychiatry.

HL: Psychiatry needed a big contribution to show that the psychoanalysts were wrong. Up to the early 1950s, the teaching in most American universities was that it is simplistic to believe that there's any kind of organic substrate to schizophrenia; that most psychoses, except the organic ones, could only be treated with psychoanalysis and that any other treatment than psychoanalysis was anachronistic and just simplistic. We had to show that there was a physical cause, a physical substrate, physical pathophysiology for the major mental disorders. And the only way to show this, and therefore, to help patients to get the right kind of integrated treatment, was by proving that with a pill you could remove hallucinations. Having shown that, the analysts had to admit that there was a physical cause, and we could begin to use the biopsychosocial model that we have now. I think that was the main contribution I made.

WB: Just go to the various positions you've had.

HL: Well, as a refugee from Germany and untrained psychiatrist, I was a Junior Psychiatrist at the Verdun Protestant Hospital the hospital I'm still working at once a week, and then I became Senior Psychiatrist there, then Clinical Director, and I stayed there for thirty five years, full time. Incidentally, I don't know any other psychiatrists who stayed that long, full time, with a mental hospital, so I think I have credibility in knowing my schizophrenic patients. I became Director of Research and Education at that hospital, and then I became Chairman of Psychiatry at McGill

University. I didn't want to, because I didn't want to have anything to do with administration. I hated anything that had to do with administration. I thought it was just a waste of time; so when they asked me whether I would take the chairmanship, which was open, I still remember, I told the dean I needed it like a hole in my head. Well, he didn't like that, so he insisted then, and finally, eventually, I took it on. I took it on because the department was almost falling apart at that time. That was in 1970 at the time of the Quiet Revolution in Quebec. There was a lot of unrest and a lot of psychiatrists and university teachers were leaving, so I thought, well, I'd better take it over, because I was from there and I knew about holding things together, anyway. So I took on the chairmanship. Then later, after I had finally left the full time hospital job, I took on, originally for about a year, the job that I still have now, since 1980, as Deputy Commissioner for Research for the New York State Office of Mental Health. I have no license in the state, so obviously, I'm not practicing there. It's all adminis-tration, the one thing that I've hated all my life and kept away from, but I thought, well, at that age, then, after sixty-five, it was about time to learn a little about it, and, so, that's when I came on.

WB: What does that involve?

HL: Well, I have a budget of some thirty-six or thirty-seven million dollars a year on paper, but it actually involves being responsible for the adminis-tration of two major research institutes, one of which happens to be the Nathan Kline Institute, and actually for all the research that is going on in the state of New York, I have to sign off on all of the research protocols. I have to make sure that every IRB is working all right. I have to deal with all the political inside fighting about the various jobs in the various hospitals and research institutes. I have to fight about budgets and try to outwit people, get around and manipulate; you know, I do the things that administrators have to do. But, since I'm there only two days a week in Albany, and I live in Montreal, I live, really, in two worlds. The Canadian world is very different. I don't know what the Americans are going to do with their health care, but in Canada, of course, there's no problem. But it's interesting to have a position that all my life I never dreamt about, and in another country, in another political world, altogether.

WB: And it's a very responsible position.

HL: It's a very responsible position. Well, I had the experience, obviously. It's interesting, I think, that I know more researchers in the States than in Canada. Some of the Americans took quicker to developments, and I was more in communication with American researchers than with Canadian researchers.

WB: Let me ask you, since this is the ACNP, what was your involvement in the beginning with the ACNP? You were one of the founding members.

HL: Yes, again, against my wishes. I remember quite a few of the people that I knew quite well asked me to join them in founding the ACNP, the American College, and we had had meetings, and I said, "well, that's fine, but leave me out of it." I said, "I had no time, definitely no time, and I hate institutions, anyway, and I don't want to have anything to do with it." Then, I think it was Malitz who told me, "Well, we'll draft you," and I said, "I don't know what you mean." He said, "You don't know what drafting is?" So he explained to me what drafting is, and so anyway, they got me into it, and, I finally became one of the founders. Eventually, they drafted me again for being a president. I think it was in 1964. Again, I didn't want to, and I said, "I don't know anything about the procedures of running it." Anyway, I got into it, and as I was doing it, I was learning it. Now I'm very glad that we have an ACNP. In fact, it's very difficult to imagine that we didn't at any time.

WB: Looking back on your life, were there key turning points?

HL: No, really not, except that I had to leave Germany, which I didn't like at the time. I made one big decision within the first three weeks after arriving here, never to have a car. I kept this promise to myself. I think that helped me; otherwise I wouldn't be alive anymore. I was driving in Germany as a student. Otherwise, my life has become, really, remarkably the way I wanted it to go, step by step by step, no great crises, no great surprises. One of the surprises was chlorpromazine, but that wasn't such a surprise. My father, as a surgeon, told me "it's ridiculous to want to go into psychiatry," which was ridiculous at the time. I thought, well, perhaps I can do something about it if he knows so little about it. So, you know, that wasn't planned.

WB: Okay, well, maybe one last question: as you look to the future, now, of our field, what do you see as the challenges?

HL: After we had the serendipitous discovery of the drugs for the affective disorders and for the psychoses, we didn't know what they were, so we challenged the neuroscientists: "Now, you've got to find out why the antipsychotics work, why the antidepressants work." They found out first why the antidepressants work, and another five years later, why the antipsychotics work, and, from then on, neuroscience took off. Before that, we had a lot of anatomy but we did not learn very much more about what goes on in the brain. And now, neuroscientists are far ahead. We clinicians set them going, and they are very successful; they have left us behind. I don't think we have enough communication, and perhaps the focus isn't right. It's difficult for me to see the focus of the neuroscientists and molecular biologists. Well, there is a C-fos and N-RAS, and that works on a receptor on the cell wall, which then enables certain chemicals to get into the cell, which enables something else to help in the cell. You don't even have an aggregate of neurons anymore. It's all within one cell and, from the neurons to the brain and from the brain to the behavior and from the behavior to the human being, there's a gap.

WB: The gaps.

HL: Huge gaps, so we have to find a way to communicate and to get a general focus, which is the same for research and clinicians.

WB: Okay. I've been interviewing Heinz Lehmann, who has been and is one of the pioneers in the field of neuropsychopharmacology. He's past president of the American College of Neuropsychopharmacology, and clearly, one of the greatest neuropsychopharmacologists that ever lived. I enjoyed interviewing you.

HL: Thank you. I think you exaggerated a little.

WB: No, I'm not exaggerating. Are there any other things you'd like to add? We can always go back and dub it in if you want.

HL: No, I also want to make the point of having had this long-lasting depression which was so disabling at twelve years of age that the experts said that I would never make it. I got over it and have been doing fairly well for quite a long time without any drug therapy or any definite structured psychotherapy.

WB: Have you had subsequents?

HL: Subclinical ones.

WB: Subclinical ones?

HL: I had one or two, that's all. I never had to stop working. Once I took a drug, for a short time. For me that indicates that the prognosis is not as bad as recent follow up studies have shown.

WB: Right. There are many stories of educators who've told people they can't do it, and fortunately, a parent said, "but you can do it" and stuck with it.

HL: And the therapy of my tutor, doing the work for me, the homework, you know, which was considered to be horrible, his bibliotherapy of giving me all of Freud's stuff to read, when I was thirteen, apparently worked.

WILLIAM J. TURNER

Interviewed by Jo Ann Engelhardt
San Juan, Puerto Rico, December 13, 1994

JE: I am Jo Ann Engelhardt. My husband, David M. Engelhardt, has been the treasurer of the ACNP for many, many years. I have been asked to interview a colleague of my own from my home county of Suffolk in New York State. It is indeed a great pleasure to bring to your attention Dr. William J. Turner,* Professor Emeritus at Stony Brook University, State University of New York. I would like him to recollect his early years in the field of mental health research and treatment; to go back in time and trace his unique contributions as a researcher and geneticist as well as a well-known advocate on behalf of the mentally ill. Is that a big enough assignment, Bill?

WT: Jo Ann, I'll see what I can make of it. I got involved with psychiatry in 1937, I think it was. I went with the Veterans' Administration (VA) and they said, "You're a psychiatrist." Well, it took about thirteen years for me to feel comfortable with that designation, all those years with the VA. I was at Little Rock for a couple of years; I was a pathologist; I was a cysto-scopist; I was sometimes the pharmacist. I did all sorts of things. We had, in North Little Rock, an enormous range of medical and surgical and psychological problems with vitamin deficiencies of all sorts. There was a constant challenge! I started my scientific life as a chemist. I read everything that came under my eyes, and one day I read about the account of nicotinic acid being used in treatment for black tongue of dogs. Now, black tongue of dogs is the same as human pellagra.

JE: It is?

WT: Just the day before, I had admitted a man who was dying of pellagra and amebic dysentery. His amebic dysentery was being treated all right, but I had no treatment for pellagra until I saw this silly squib in a street newsletter. Well, I didn't go to the administrators of the hospital, I went to the business manager who was a foresighted man, and he called all over the United States and found 5 grams of nicotinic acid in a warehouse in St. Louis. He got an army airplane pilot to pick it up and bring it to me personally. We gave this dying man 100 mg of it on Saturday morning.

---

* William J. Turner was born in Wilkinsburg, Pennsylvania in 1907, and received his MD from Johns Hopkins Medical School in 1933. He trained in pathology at Baltimore City Hospital and took a course in psychiatry at the Veterans Administration Hospital in North Little Rock Hospital in Arkansas, where he came on staff in 1937. In 1941 he joined the VA hospital in Northport, NY. In 1950 he left the VA system and opened a private practice in Huntington, NY, serving also on the staff of the local hospital. In 1954 he accepted a courtesy appointment as research psychiatrist at the Central Islip State Hospital. In 1994 he moved to Albuquerque, New Mexico, and joined the department of psychiatry of the New Mexico State University. Turner died in 2006.

The following Thursday he walked firm and healthy into a staff conference room. This sort of thing is really hair-raising, and it's been my good fortune again and again to have equivalent kinds of experiences. The VA then sent me to West Los Angeles, and then in 1940, I was sent to the psychiatric unit in Northport, Long Island where the VA administration opened its very first research division.

JE: What year was that, Bill?

WT: 1941. Imagine a research division of one chief, one Indian, one psychologist, one secretary, one biochemist and one scrub woman – a research division, for heaven's sakes!

JE: Today, they would call that cutting back, wouldn't they? Bill, before you proceed any further, I would be interested where you received your medical training and from which medical school you graduated. Where you did your psychiatric residency? I think that should be recorded here.

WT: Well, first I started out as a chemist. Chemistry has always been something that I have loved and love to read about and know more about than anything else. I got out of Penn State in 1927, I believe. Then, I spent a couple of years moving around and went to Johns Hopkins University to get a PhD in biochemistry, but instead, the following year I found myself at Johns Hopkins Medical School. I graduated there in 1933, and had a couple of years wandering around as an intern. Then, I had a year of pathology at Baltimore City Hospital, and then a year of internal medicine, at The Billings in Chicago, and, almost a year working at the Tuberculosis Center. It was sort of a political job at the Tuberculosis Center because the man who was the head of it thought I was trying to get his job. He practically tried to frame me as if I had murdered one of his patients. I felt it would be just as good for me to get away from this political scene. That's why I went with the Civil Service and they sent me to Little Rock. So that's how I came into psychiatry, purely by chance, but I love it! I love it!

JE: What do you love about it, Bill?

WT: Well, like any doctor who loves his profession I love it because it's healing, because it should be compassionate, because it's ennobling to be given the privilege of taking care of the ill and the troubled and finding happy people at the end of a period of pain and turmoil.

JE: Although I would like to hear your regard for the profession, I am obliged to have you recount some of the important things that have happened in the development of the practice of the psychiatric profession and what role you played in it?

WT: When I first began, we had no medications. The only thing we could do was psychoanalysis. It was a dramatic year when Thorazine (chlorpromazine) was introduced. I had just finished four years of personal psychoanalysis and I was looking around for what to do. I wanted to do some research and I met Dr. Sidney Merlis, who had opened up a research division at Central Islip State Hospital. He and I hit it off immediately and for two years I worked there without salary. There are very funny stories that connect with that. However it was in that year the people in power, I don't remember now their names...

JE: In the State Hospital System?

WT: In the State Hospital System.

JE: Henry Brill?

WT: Yes, Henry Brill. Henry Brill ordered that all the patients in the State Hospital system should receive Thorazine. Maybe that was a too broad an order. But it was miraculous to see a woman who came in, in a terrible state, accompanied by a husband who was tormented and distraught, leave the hospital couple of weeks later, radiant, buoyant with life. Thorazine, in just a couple of weeks, transformed this woman from the drab terrified person to a happy mother.

JE: Bill, what was the patient population of those state hospitals? You were talking to me about that yesterday evening and described this "deinstitutionalization," or dramatic reversal from the warehousing of patients, that could be directly attributed to Henry Brill and Thorazine.

WT: At that time, the largest concentration of mental patients in the world was in Suffolk County, Long Island. We had Pilgrim State Hospital with something like 17,000 patients, 16,000 of them inpatients. There were at the Central Islip Hospital 11,000, and at Kings Park 5,700. Oh, the drabness, the terror, the horror of these hopeless people. I once drove my son around the hospital and he saw these men clinging to the bars on the windows and he blamed me for all these troubles. It was a frightful thing! Then, Thorazine came along. Within a year, well, at the end of that year, there were fewer patients in mental hospitals than at the beginning of the year. It was a dramatic change. People who say that the drop in state hospital populations was the result of changes in social conditions are absolutely wrong! There was a kind of effort to release patients and force them out of the hospital, but they came back. As a matter of fact, at the time this was going on in 1954 and 1955 people would go out of the hospital and wouldn't take their medication because there was no provision for taking it after hospitalization. So, within a year, they were coming back. It was like a revolving door, and something had to be done about it. And that began a whole series of state activities to find someplace for these patients to get their treatment without having to be re-hospitalized.

JE: I was very impressed when you mentioned to me the other evening that hospitals, particularly in New York State and in Suffolk and Nassau County in Long Island, which has the largest concentration in the country of state hospital populations, are again emptying out and putting patients back into the community. I had the pleasure and privilege of working with you as an advocate in this modern movement to care for the mentally ill in the community. So, speak to that now.

WT: Well, the major part is the education of the relatives. They're helpless and they're hopeless. They were condemned and humiliated, and then abused. Now, with the National Alliance on Mental Illness (NAMI) families are getting some education for the first time and there is hope beyond medication. The advances in humane treatment of the mentally ill, having provisions for care throughout their life, is largely due to the activities of the relatives. I don't know how to express my admiration for the guts of these men and women who have to establish a place for their loved ones to live.

JE: Thank you, Bill I know that is from your heart. Could I take you back to when you came to Stony Brook and worked with blood samples? I think that is a passageway leading toward the high point in your career. Would you do that?

WT: Well, sure. You see, having started out as a chemist, it just felt natural to me to look for something that I could do in genetics, since there seemed to be strong evidence that these mental illnesses have something to do with a genetic pattern of some sort, although we still don't know what it is. To pursue this line of research I was impelled to get blood samples. There is quite a story here. We had been advised that in England there was a movement afoot to search for the genetic basis of schizophrenias, whether there was an etiological one or not. So I went to England to investigate what was going on there and visited half a dozen hospitals. I also went up to Scotland. At one of the hospitals, Hammersmith Hospital, I was told that there was a woman by the name of Marrileena Fortino, who had been working at that hospital and doing some work on what was called HLA (Human Leukocyte Antigens). I was advised to go back and look at what she does. Well, it so happened that I had been working with the New York Blood Bank for about three or four years looking for something connected with treatment and drug reactions. When I went back to the Blood Bank I was told that they had just got a new service doing work on HLAs, and that they had Marrileena Fortino there. By golly, it was a hair-raising event! I went downstairs and we fell in love immediately!

JE: You mean clinically?

WT: Oh, clinically. I am not talking about sex, but I am talking about love.

JE: Tell me about it.

WT: I would go to the hospital, and some woman came in one day and wanted to talk with me. It turns out they had heard about my interest in genetics and had gone to Stanley Yolles, who was the head of the department of psychiatry at the time.

JE: That was Stanley Yolles who had been, if I recall, the director of the National Institute of Mental Health before and came to Long Island at Stony Brook to become chairman and director of the Department of Psychiatry.

WT: He had been the director and the Chief of Psychiatry. So, when these women heard that there was some doctor looking for genetic inheritance, they went to Stan. He said, "Well, I think Turner may have something there." So they came over and I can still see them, five of them, standing in front of me and talking in the lab.

JE: These women were mothers?

WT: Of mentally ill patients.

JE: People with schizophrenia?

WT: Schizophrenia. I saw the despair on their faces when I talked to them and listened to their hopes that something might be done, so we immediately formed a coalition. I got blood samples from them and all their relatives over a couple of years. It must have been more than 100 families that I worked with. And then, I took the blood into the New York Blood Center. They did, not just studies on HLA, but a lot of other proteins that were genetic markers. At the end of about three years, I was able to publish a paper saying that HLA was a good marker for mental illness. I identified chromosome 6 as the locus for schizophrenia. Well, only one group of people from Italy agreed with me. Elliot Gershon is claiming chromosome 18 is the locus of the gene for schizophrenia. But in doing this, my work went beyond the laboratory, because these ladies formed an alliance which is now associated with the National Alliance for the Mentally Ill. You know a lot more about that than I do, about the families forming organizations for promoting housing and better care, closer supervision, and all the things that parents have done by promoting the best and most humane treatment for our patients, my patients, your children.

JE: Yes, I have worked with those parents of mentally ill children. They were the very first in Suffolk County to join and promote the fledgling National Alliance for the Mentally Ill. These same parents, Mary Siegel, Audie French, Susan Etts and others, continue to work for NARSAD (National Alliance for Research on Schizophrenia and Depression), the other outstanding mental health organization. Now, if I may, I would like to lead you into your first involvement in the formation of the ACNP.

WT: Sure. The chief of the research division at Central Islip was Sidney Merlis, who had just opened his laboratory. We had done all sorts of studies and we had contracts with drug companies to use the new drugs.

JE: Were these all psychotropic drugs?

WT: Yes, we were probably the first ones to study Stelazine (trifluoperazine).

JE: Stelazine?

WT: Then, one day someone said to me that there was a group wanting to form a new organization in psychopharmacology and asked if I would like to go into New York and meet with them. Well, I was delighted. So I did, and we met in a hotel on three different occasions. At my age memory sort of fades and I'm hesitant to say....

JE: Go ahead

WT: Henry Brill and Max Fink were there.

JE: Max Fink, he is still with Stony Brook isn't he?

WT: Yes, he is one of the foremost investigators in the use of electroshock treatment. But we had, if you name some of these other people....

JE: Well at dinner last night we were talking about this, and I jotted down the name of Heinz Lehmann.

WT: Yes, indeed, I can confirm that, Heinz went to one of the three meetings.

JE: Was Nathan Kline there?

WT: Nate Kline was there and Leo Hollister, I think.

JE: Jon Cole?

WT: Jonathan Cole. We met and eventually decided to start a new organization that became known as the American College of Neuropsychopharmacology. I really had almost nothing to do with it. I was a passive observer and participant but was not an organizer; I was just going along. But it was a wonderful thing because the stimulus of Thorazine was keeping all of us just thrilled at the possibility we could find something better, something more lasting, and that we could really, really accomplish something. So the papers were drawn up and the arrangements were made for the college to be established, and we met in Washington for the first four or five years. It was just up the street from the hotel which was famous for being the rendezvous of Senators and their mistresses.

JE: Oh, Bill!

WT: It was astonishing; it was fun! Those early meetings were dramatic in ways that I can't really convey. Nowadays, there is a need for a format and things become stereotyped. At that time it was an explosion of devotion. I really don't know what words to use; it was transforming my world. The ability to continue outpatient treatment and to actually communicate with patients in ways you couldn't before, was transformative. In my previous work when I had no medications, I formed very close attachments with some of my male patients and female patients. I had wonderful relationships but that wasn't healing. Now with these new medications, there were so many more of them. Even now I get a letter or card from somebody that is living in Tuscaloosa or someplace else, whom I knew fifteen, twenty or thirty years ago, still thanking me. But I didn't do it! I was the messenger who carried this medication to them, a message of hope, a message of communication with the families. Boy, I tell you this has been a wonderful life!

JE: I'll, at the risk of being intrusive, studies say that the use of medication plus the involved, interested physician therapist is the best combination. You epitomize for me, as you do for thousands of people, this therapeutic partnership. You are a legend in Suffolk County and beyond because of the humanitarian feeling, empathy, and concern for your patients and their families, but also for your vast clinical knowledge. You are a pioneer here. I know and you know you are. And now, perhaps a lot of other people will recognize that. Do you feel that devotion and excitement still exists today in the research on biological psychiatry and psychopharmacology?

WT: I would like to think so. I would hate for the medication aspect to override the humane. Your actions transform simple medication into a miracle. It would be wonderful to find and get to a specific target, to a particular molecule and bring a person back to stable lifelong normality.

JE: Do you remember whether these four meetings in Washington, included an increasingly large number of people?

WT: The idea was that the organization would consist of one-third of government, one-third industry and one-third university people, and the membership would be kept small enough so we could interact actively instead of sitting passively to listen to lectures. And that has worked out very well, except now there is pressure to increase the size. Each time when I come to these meetings, there are fewer and fewer people I know. On the other hand, I am getting along in years and it's proper that there should be younger people coming in, and I hope that they will bear the torch. I don't know whether this is a satisfying response to what you have asked. At this meeting there is still that excited buzz; with heads nodding and chins bobbing and I think that the organization is doing what it set out to do.

JE: I think that is very well put. Since we are in San Juan, try to recall back around 1952 when you were staying at the fancy refurbished Normandy hotel. You mentioned to me that you were doing some research with hallucinogenics at the time?

WT: Oh, yes.

JE: Do you remember that?

WT: There were a lot of ideas going around in those years that hallucinogenic drugs mimic schizophrenia. Well, having worked with schizophrenics enough, I had a feeling that I would know if these ideas were true. So, I tried a whole bunch of different compounds. One of my experiences was quite accidental ....

JE: What was the compound?

WT: Well, that was adrenochrome.

JE: Adrenochrome?

WT: Adrenochrome; that it would cause schizophrenia. Well I had an ampoule of adrenaline in my pocket one day and accidentally broke it. And in breaking it I inhaled a whole lot of adrenaline. My nose ran blood red from the adrenochrome created by the reaction. It didn't have any effect on me! I tried to collect a lot of these drugs, and at one time I brought my younger son down here. We stayed at the Normandy Hotel and drove out to a little plot of land on the top of the hill on the western end of the island and I got some Piptadenia Peregrina seeds.

JE: Piptadenia Peregrina?

WT: Peregrina seeds, and I ground them up and I did what the natives are supposed to do in order to produce their magic trances. My wife refused to blow it into my nostrils the way they did, but my younger son did. All I got was a stuffy nose and wished the damn thing had never been found! It didn't produce any psychological effects on me. Then, I got from South America a jar full of Yajé.

JE: Yajé?

WT: Y-a-j-é. Richard Evans Schultes was the curator of the Herbarium at Harvard and he had taken some of this stuff which produces quite an active hallucinogenic effect. So I got some of it, put it in double boilers so I wouldn't contaminate myself with some parasite and I took a little sip every now and then. I was playing bridge with some friends and when I began to feel the effects we stopped playing and, as our guests left, I had an image in my mind of an enormous bowl of ice cream with a cherry on top. Well, it may seem indecent, but my feeling was that the cold dish was a woman who cherished her cherry.

JE: What about your experiments with hallucinogens at the Hotel Normandy in San Juan in 1952?

WT: After taking the stuff for the next eight to twelve hours I was studying my own translation of images into ideas and words. And of course it helped me a great deal in understanding many of the images my patients told me about, so that I could begin to put what they couldn't put into words and to help them find the words for it. It was quite an education.

JE: For understanding schizophrenic patients who have hallucinatory images?

WT: Not knowing and not trusting my memory, I took a tape recorder and taped everything that went on. And later, when I was on a TV program we played the tapes. There were images of me fading in and out and shimmering, things like that. It was very interesting. I'd already been through psychoanalysis but this was a new kind of education. I would not say these were hallucinogenic drugs that ought to be used, and certainly I don't approve of that. Cocaine was used on me as an anesthetic when I had an operation. Otherwise, these hallucinogenics and cocaine and drug abuse leave me absolutely uninterested and cold.

JE: Well, that's your personal reaction.

WT: Yes, it's my reaction and I think this may be genetic. There are some people like me that simply cannot and will not tolerate these things.

JE: This leads me to associate your work with blood enzymes and your keen interest regarding responders and non-responders from a genetic point of view to medication and drugs. I don't know if you are still doing work with the Dreyfus Foundation?

WT: Well, my Dreyfus connection is very interesting.

JE: Tell us about that.

WT: When Jack Dreyfus suffered, he was irritable, antagonistic and bitter. He saw his psychiatrist, I think, seven days a week for several years. One day he said that he felt as if he had too much electricity in his brain. And, he asked the doctor if there wasn't something that controlled too much electricity in the brain. The doctor said, "Well, yes there is, and it's used sometimes for people with epilepsy who have electrical abnormalities in the central nervous system." So Dreyfus said, "Well, why can't I try that?," and so he got some and he took it.

JE: Got some what?

WT: Dilantin (phenytoin) and he tried it that night. The next day he told the doctor that, "Oh, that's a wash out there's nothing to it." Well, they continued talking and the doctor said, "So let me see, you didn't bawl out anybody and didn't blow your stack." Dreyfus replied, "No, why should I? Everything is working smoothly; Oh, that's the first time in years!" So he continued to take the Dilantin. Then, he realized that there were a lot of other people that were short-tempered, intemperate, easily agitated, difficult and nervous in various ways. He began to hand out Dilantin to those people and was surprised to find a lot of changes in attitudes from dour to cheerful. So he went to see the people from Columbia, where Dilantin was first developed for epilepsy. And he gave them thousands of dollars to do a research study but in two years they couldn't find a suitable capsule to mimic the effects of Dilantin from Parke-Davis. He began looking around elsewhere, and finally he went to Downstate Medical Center where, after a series of circumstances, I was introduced to him. I said I don't know whether this would be helpful, but I have three patients who are not doing well in psychotherapy, I'll see what Dilantin will do. I am not going to tell the full details but one of them, a woman, had been starved as a child and saw her own baby as being starved. This woman, who is now a secretary in New York, was unable to eat in the presence of another person. She would take her lunch and eat in the women's lavatory. After she had been on Dilantin for a couple of weeks I heard that she had joined some people in the cafeteria and was sitting at the same table with them. Well, the other two patients were similarly affected. So I said to Dreyfus, "I think I will join you and let's see what happens." We set up a clinic in Huntington for about three years and we were in *Life* and *Reader s Digest*; something like 800 people came to us, who all had received various medications and psychotherapies. We didn't do any psychotherapy but we took their history and offered them Dilantin. More than half benefited and some of them very dramatically, so I continued to give Dilantin to almost anybody who asked for it after I was pretty well satisfied that it worked. Dreyfus was then given the opportunity to present a talk at the annual meeting of the ACNP.

JE: At the ACNP?

WT: At the ACNP, about ten or twelve years ago. It seems implausible a layman could introduce something to experts and yet after a little while people began to use carbamazepine and valproate. But you see no mention of Dilantin in any of these studies because I think there is still a suspicion that it is a fraud. But it is not.

JE: I could pick up on your statement of how a layman could influence scientific experts. I believe I attended, together with you, a plenary session, during this 1994 meeting and a standing ovation was given to a consumer, a layman with a diagnosis of schizophrenia, who at the invitation of the college, got up to do that very same thing. I thought that was exceptional. I don't know what you thought about it?

WT: Well you know the story of the man whose car got stuck in the sand just outside of the state hospital, and he was trying to get out when someone came up to him and said, "Why don't you let some of the air out of the tires so you can get better traction?" So, he did and after he got out he asked, "How did you happen to know that?" The man replied, "Well, I may be a patient in the hospital, but I'm not stupid."

JE: Bill, thank you for that bit of levity. I would like to wind down and I know you are a modest man, but you must do this for yourself, for the College and for me. What do you think was your biggest contribution, as a practicing MD, a chemist-scientist, as a geneticist- researcher? How do you think you will be best known?

WT: Well, it's a funny thing, and has very little to do with science and medication. It has to do with giving information to relatives of patients and sharing with them all I have learned and try to learn, so they can see their own sons and daughters in a different light, and can support further research.

JE: Well, that says a little bit about Bill Turner. How do you think you will stand in the annals of history?

WT: I will be forgotten. I am not anybody special. I am just a guy who happens to be passing by as the scene changes.

JE: All right, let me rephrase that; are you pleased with or are you happy with what is happening in psychiatric research and clinical practice of psychiatry and biomedical research?

WT: Yes, because what thirty years ago was just a molecule trying to find a place to land has grown into a substantial movement of vast, developing power and significance, which, in the next thirty years, will continue to transform the world we live in.

JE: Bill, I am so pleased that you and I were together at this meeting. I thank you so very much. It has been a great pleasure, as always, and I hope that I will continue to work with you.

WT: Yes, indeed. Thank you.

Pharmacologists

JOSEPH V. BRADY

Interviewed by Leo E. Hollister
San Juan, Puerto Rico, December 13, 1994

LH: Joe,* it's really an unusual pleasure to be assigned as your interviewer, for many reasons; first, for our long standing friendship and, particularly, all of your contributions. Of everyone I know in the field of neuropsychopharmacology, you represent a person who has contributions over a very wide range of areas and the work you've done with colleagues, has had an enormous impact over three to four decades. Now, I thought we'd chat a little bit, first of all, about your personal background, in terms of your schooling and let's start with college. I think you went to Fordham.

JB: Yes, I was trained by the Jesuits.

LH: Did anything happen during college, perhaps, that steered you in the direction in your career?

JB: Well, obviously, the main event was the war, you remember the period from 1942 to 1945?

LH: Yes, I was there.

JB: I had no choice but to take ROTC (Reserve Officers' Training Corps) and was inducted into the Army even before I finished my degree. That sort of launched me on a career in the infantry. I ended up in Germany at the end of the war, and for reasons that only the United States Army could fathom, I was picked up bodily and sent to the Neuropsychiatric Center of the European Command. That was in 1945 at the end of the war. I spent two and a half years as the Chief Clinical Psychologist of the European Command, with absolutely no training, whatsoever.

LH: That clearly got you oriented in this area.

JB: I began to learn a little bit about what went on. We did not have all the fancy and effective psychopharmacological approaches. People were plugged into the light circuit in those days. Along with your slippers and your bathrobe you received a set of electrodes and electroconvulsive shock, a major therapeutic intervention. And we also had the tubs. All those good things were in effect.

LH: In regard to your impact in neuropsychopharmacology, I know that you go way back, to Walter Reed. What people or events steered you in regard to your activities relevant to ACNP and neuropsychopharmacology?

JB: Well, I was picked up from Germany and sent to the University of Chicago in the late 1940s. I took my degree there with Howard Hunt. I capitalized

---

* Joseph V. Brady was born in New York City, New York in 1922; in 1951 he earned a PhD in Psychology from the University of Chicago. He worked for a number of years at Walter Reed Army Institute of Research, before joining the faculty of Johns Hopkins University in 1967 as director of the Behavioral Biology Research Center. Joseph V. Brady died in 2011.

a bit on what had gone on in Germany and I did an experiment with elec-troconvulsive shock. We had some methodologies that we developed, conditioned emotional responses in animals, and that was really the beginning of my interest in this area. After finding that the electroconvul-sive shock effects were clearly demonstrable experimentally, we began to look at what kinds of pharmacologic agents would produce these attenu-ating effects on conditioned emotional behavior. There wasn't a helluva lot available in those days.

LH: Why don't you talk about your paper on reserpine?

JB: That was just one paper, right?

LH: Yes.

JB: That was done after I had left Chicago for Walter Reed in Washington. Reserpine was the first of the tranquilizers. The major tranquilizers appeared on the market and we tried the effects of reserpine on the con-ditioned emotional response. Our paper was published in *Science* in the mid 1950s, and it provided the basis to develop screening for compounds, using behavioral procedures, to determine ones that had an effect on chronic psychiatric illness.

LH: So, you're saying that experience was pivotal in getting you in the field?

JB: Oh, no question about that.

LH: Were there any people, individuals that had a significant effect in regard to your career at that time?

JB: Well, obviously, Howard Hunt at the University of Chicago was a major influence in getting me into this sort of animal model type of research, but the people I interacted with at Walter Reed were also largely influ-ential. Also people from other disciplines had an influence: Dave Rioch, Murray Sidman from Columbia, Bob Galambos, a neurophysiologist, John Mason, an endocrinologist, and, of course, Walle Nauta, a neuro-anatomist. We did a lot of work together on lesions of the central nervous system and it was an easy transition to begin to look at the effects of drugs. Reserpine turned out not to be the panacea, needless to say, and we gave it to a lot of animals who never recovered.

LH: What were some of the problems you had to face at the time? What was going on in terms of drug interaction with behavior? What were the early concepts you had that may or may not have changed, regarding the interaction of drugs and behavior? What were the issues?

JB: I have written and spoken before about progress in this are. It's an inter-action between conceptual changes and methodological developments, essentially. It was the methodological developments which were the driv-ers at the beginning. We had a technique for measuring effects on emo-tional behavior; we looked at how lesions, electroconvulsive shock and drugs were acting upon the organism. That was the major conceptual thing. Needless to say, this has changed dramatically.

LH: In what way?

JB: The development of the tranquilizers, both minor and major, with the monoamine oxidase inhibitors opened up a whole new field with respect to areas we hadn't expected, that is, drug abuse and dependence. It was there the notion of an interactive effect between drugs and behavior became crystallized. When it was demonstrated animals would self-administer drugs through indwelling catheters, this had a dramatic effect upon looking at drugs having the same kind of stimulus functions all other events in the environment could have, both internal and external. Not only did they function as reinforcers, as consequences, which control behavior, but they functioned as signals and this was where the whole drug discrimination area has come from. So these are the results of a conceptual shift, which then produced methodological changes over the next 30 or 40 years.

LH: During your very successful career, in which you've had impact in so many areas, what were some of the problems that you faced in carrying on this very important research? Was it easy as pie? What did you have to do?

JB: I don't remember any great problems. I, obviously, was involved in a number of different areas, not only the neurobehavioral and psychopharmacological, but one of the great satisfactions of my life is that the domain I selected, or was driven into, was the study of behavior, every man's dependent variable. No matter what new fad comes along, whether it is microwaves, whether it is electroshock, whether it is drugs, whether it is space, everybody wants to know what the effect is upon behavior, so I've been sitting pretty for 50 years. No matter what anybody had, what they always wanted to know was about behavior.

LH: I would be remiss during this interview, if I didn't ask you how about the executive monkey?

JB: Quite a serendipitous finding, needless to say. We were, of course, interested in the physiological changes that occurred in animals who were doing avoidance performances, an extremely stable performance over extended periods of time. We were measuring hormones with John Mason at the time, 17-hydroxycortisol, steroids, all those sorts of things. We had a young pathologist working with us by the name of Bill Porter, who had done post-mortems on a number of the animals that had died, and he came in one morning with a handful of guts, essentially, showing me the stomach of one of the monkeys and saying it had a very serious duodenal ulcer. I said, "Well, that's too bad, we'll have to do something to see if we can prevent that." When he repeated this finding on several occasions, it became obvious maybe something we were doing actually produced it. So we launched a systematic series of experiments, and when we did control and experimental animals it was clear that there was a difference between them in this regard.

LH: I'm always impressed by the wide impact you have in so many significant events, even training a monkey for space.

JB: That's part of the business I'm telling you. Anything that comes along, everybody wants to know what the behavioral effects are. That was again a consequence of being in the right place at the right time. While we were doing the monkey experiments, which of course got a lot of wide exposure in the press and elsewhere, we had a visit at Walter Reed from Werner von Braun, who was working for the Army on the Ballistic Missiles Agency, even before NASA (National Aeronautics and Space Administration) came into existence. He wanted to know if I'd be interested in putting one of my livestock in the nosecone of one of his rockets. I had not much idea of what he was talking about at the time, but we ended up with very small rhesus monkeys, two of them in a plaster cast, because they got knocked around a lot in those cones, with one finger left out; my job was to train the finger so the animal would make some response during orbit. Well, the initial flights were ballistic. You went up 300 miles at 10,000 miles per hour and came back down. And there were no physiological or pharmacological measures at the time for the integrity of the organism. This is another reason why behavior is every man's dependent variable. It's the best indicator of the integrity of the organism, because with this behavior you know he's alive and well.

LH: Let me jump ahead. We'll come back to the continuation of your career. I personally find, as you probably do, a shift in regard to research attitudes, using gross-criteria behaviors as opposed to molecular biological approaches. I think there's been some moving away from research in the whole animal using these behavioral measures where people who are not behaviorists but are molecular biologists may have a different attitude than you or I in terms of its relevance to research. What thoughts do you have, in terms of the role of behavior in the future, how it's going to sustain itself, in view of all of these breakthroughs at the molecular biological level?

JB: Well, I also have an appointment in the Neuroscience Department at Johns Hopkins with Sol Snyder. I regard my job there as to keep these guys honest, and the way you keep them honest is to having them recognize that why they are interested in the nervous system is because it has something to do with the way organisms interact with their environment, and that's the major objective. Furthermore, the illusion that your mind accounts for that very complex interaction process, by identifying receptor sites seems to me to be a little farfetched.

LH: Do you think that we're going to continue to impress people about the importance of behavior?

JB: I don't think there's any question about this because that's where they end up eventually, anyway. As I've said to Sol on numerous occasions, understanding the nervous system is a piece of cake compared to the complexities of the way organisms interact with their environment.

LH: Let's go back again, now. You had a very heavy influence in regard to your consultantships with various drug houses, and they incorporated a number of test procedures you had worked out at Walter Reed.

JB: I think that influence was more on the direction of people that ultimately went to work for the pharmaceutical industry. And, to go back to where we left this earlier, it was that 1950s paper on reserpine that caught the attention of a number of people in the industry and flagged the notion that maybe every pharmaceutical company in the country had hundreds of compounds on the shelf that could potentially be useful without any good way of telling their behavioral effects. In other words, the behavioral effects were the ones they wanted. That's what caught the attention of people, and you know the pharmaceutical industry better than I do; once one company gets something that begins to look promising, everybody's got to have someone doing that. We had a reservoir of people at Walter Reed to meet that need.

LH: Who were they?

JB: Guys like Dick Herrnstein, Murray Sidman for example, and Tom Verhav, Larry Stein, and John Boren, and people who were provided to us by General Hershey, as a matter of fact. These were the days when the draft was widespread. So these people were assembled there, putting in their couple of years of service.

LH: What about Irv Geller during the 1950s and 1960s. Wasn't he at Reed?

JB: Absolutely, he was my first research assistant, as a matter of fact.

LH: So, we both saw that, during the 1950s and 1960s, the phenothiazines and benzodiazepines with the meprobamate series were primarily identified by behavioral tests.

JB: It was a behavioral endpoint that was of interest then.

LH: The behavioral endpoint was what decided companies to invest our 30 or 40 million dollars and develop a drug. As people go on in the future, they're not using as many of these criteria to identify drugs. How are drugs going to be discovered in the future?

JB: It could well be that molecular biologists will provide fertile leads in this regard; you know, receptor dynamics are clearly a most efficient way to proceed in some areas, but the ultimate test is going to have to be some changes in that interaction between organism and environment.

LH: You were a very good seer of the future. If someone said, okay, we've had the antipsychotics and we've had the anxiolytics and we've had the antidepressants and we're beginning to see drugs that may modulate cognitive processes....

JB: And, enhancers, clearly. Incidentally, that is not a new idea, as you know.

LH: So, we have these classes of drugs and I'm sure that we're both going to see, in the next decade, drugs appear that will be therapeutically effective in modulating neural processes.

JB: Yes, the memory area is clearly one.

LH: Where do you think psychopharmacology is going to go 20 to 30 years from now? Do you have any thoughts about that?

JB: Well, obviously, we're going to be creating drugs according to a model that is not even available to us now. But, in terms of the kinds of measures that we're taking, it seems to me the major methodological advances will have to come from the behavioral side of events. We've seen it in the drug abuse field, the notion of measuring a subjective response, that was a real breakthrough and was a behavioral measure we couldn't now ask animals to discriminate between contact measures. I think we'll see similar kinds of advances occurring.

LH: I know that, now, among the many things you're doing, drug abuse is something you're spending a lot of your time on. How does it fit into your continuing concept? What are some of the things you're doing in drug abuse?

JB: One of the things I've seen developing over the past 10 or 12 years is a broadening of the arena for behavioral pharmacology in this area. The dramatic effect and the thing everyone looks at is drug self-administration; then drug discrimination came along to tell us to use animals to tell us whether the drug made the animal discriminate. But there's a third area that has not received much attention and it's classical behavioral pharmacology, and what I think of as behavioral toxicology. That is the abuse liability of the drug, determined not only by whether it is self-administered and whether you can discriminate it, but the effect it has upon the organism and the price the organism and the community pays for that. This is a dimension of the whole drug abuse field we have started to develop pretty well now at Hopkins. We see this as a sort of three-pronged approach, the abuse liability being defined dependent upon self-administration and drug discrimination, but we now have a whole battery of auditory measure thresholds, that we can now measure very carefully with drugs in animals.

LH: Drug abuse continues to be a problem. If you had your druthers and you were kingpin, making decisions as to how to address drug abuse, how would you direct the national posture to the problem?

JB: There would have to be a substantial shift from the supply to the demand side. The notion that we can win the drug abuse problem by sealing the borders was crazy. On the other hand, we can do something about controlling the demand and there are some rather substantial contributions that have been made. In my view, there are some convincing experiments of nature, the Lee Robins work, for example, respecting returning veterans who had very heavy drug habits. Once they got here, they were all right. Being able to control drugs at the work place by setting up certain contingencies would be a major way we could use to control drug abuse.

LH: I have been asking you questions to give the audience some perspective and windows into Joe Brady. What are the things that I haven't touched upon that you feel have been very significant in your career?

JB: Well, one of the things about that early 1950s experiment that is frequently overlooked is the nature of the conditions under which that reserpine effect was demonstrated. Most of us look at drug effects in very acute way. We've got this animal trained and give him the drug; very few people paid attention to the details of that experiment, namely that the drug was given after the animal ran each day, not before. So, the animal ran for an hour or two and then we administered the drugs.

LH: So, you were testing the residual effect 24 hours later?

JB: Exactly, and nothing happened for a week. Only after two weeks of running with it, all of a sudden the condition appeared. At that time, who would have ever thought that's the way to do screening. But now we're looking at the antidepressant effect, that's exactly the kind of dimension that is critical.

LH: You just touched on something that I feel very strongly about and that's the residual effect of the drug behavior interaction.

JB: You can produce change in behavior very frequently but we also discovered early on, the organism changes too and, then, you can take away the drug and the effect.

LH: Plus, that the animal was different yesterday.

JB: Exactly. I think that's very important, but it's one that people don't look closely at.

LH: No, because they look at how did the drug affect behavior rather than what is the residual effect of the drug- behavior interaction.

JB: I guess the other point worth making is that all of the kinds of methodologies and conceptual changes we find of value in an area like behavioral pharmacology don't necessarily come from our intentions. The experiments, which we have done over the past couple of years in the programmed environment, where people live for periods of two to three weeks at a time, have measures that are not acute but continuous. That didn't come from our interest, in fact, that came from NASA. The necessity of developing methodologies that would make it possible for people who are going to be in NASA, talking about sending people off in little boxes for two years; under those circumstances, it was necessary to develop a behavioral technology that would maintain performance under isolation and confinement over extended periods of time, a technology that was at least as powerful as the engineering that made it possible. After we spent a few years working on this, we realized that's a great place to study the addiction cycle. I wanted to look at the effects of drugs and we did marijuana studies where it's been virtually impossible to demonstrate anything related to the long term "motivational" effects of marijuana. But in a setting like that, we had a fighting chance and we were able to demonstrate a lot of interesting changes that occur with repeated use when you're looking at everything as a process, not simply a given moment, like an X-ray.

LH: Over the forty years we've known each other and dealt with each other, I've always noticed that you always enjoyed what you were doing.

JB: Put in more technical language that I'm in a reinforcing field. Every time you do something and you got reinforced for it, this is career-enhancing.

LH: You've had fun though.

JB: Absolutely. Now, the latest things I'm involved in, of course, have been pretty heavy duty. I've been running a mobile drug abuse program on the streets of beautiful downtown Baltimore.

LH: Tell me about it.

JB: If you're interested in a research career in behavioral pharmacology, this is not the way to go. Once you get into a field of this sort, the notion that you have control of what's going on is the difficult part. So, it hasn't been a rich research area, but it has had the effect of opening the field up; we run a full service drug abuse program without a fixed site. By going out to various areas and making treatment accessible to people who would not normally have it, the most striking effect is retention.

LH: One of the aspects of the last forty years is that you, I and others like us started with a blank check, a blank piece of paper, as the field emerged and there was nothing for us to read to help us. There were no books.

JB: But we had a repertoire. I mean you were a pharmacologist. You still are a pharmacologist, so you knew that area and I was in the behavior analysis area. What we did was build upon that repertoire by expanding it, not with dramatic big changes, but little by little.

LH: Sequential steps.

JB: That's right. Let's see what would happen if we did experiments? That's the way progress is made.

LH: I want to follow that with a point. What we're doing right now with this videotape is we provide information for the generations that follow. Who is Joe Brady? What did he look like? What were his thoughts? Now, it's an opportunity for you and others to look at the next generation, or the one after that, in terms of any advice guidance principles you may want to relate. I don't mean for them to be the great seer, but there must be thoughts that you have projected for the future. Is there anything you would to like say, on a serious note, in regard to the research you see today and where the future is going? Any comments you would like to make to the young people that are going to see this video, perhaps, ten to twenty years from now?

JB: Well, my best advice is to keep making responses. The important thing is to, at least, make sure you have your field down cold and you know what you're doing. Another important thing is the idea of trying new things. I've always thought of myself as leading an experimental life, and if something doesn't work, you try something else, and essentially that's the way both you and I have progressed. Everything you do doesn't always work, but if you have enough foundation you can return to and you have some domain you care about, it seems to me that is the way to go. You can't be all things to all people, but if you have some area of confidence, some discipline, if you develop a high degree of confidence you can move from that. But you always have that to build on that foundation.

LH: We enjoyed something at that time, which was enormous freedom. We had the resources during the Golden Era to do almost anything we thought was worthwhile. Today, and I'm concerned about the future, the resources may not be there to allow a scientist to follow his nose. He doesn't know if he's going to be dictated to. His research is going to be highly programmed, overseen by different committees and that type of thing. What is your concern?

JB: I don't have that pessimistic view.

LH: You don't?

JB: No, and simply because having been around for the past forty or fifty years, I've seen us go through cycles like this before. I was at Walter Reed when there was no interest in basic research, and the Secretary of Defense felt it should not be funded. Well, "that too will pass" and I think that's the only way to look at it. The era we're in at the moment always seems to be the one that is unique. Either, "there's never been anything like this before" or "it's going to be a disaster".

LH: So, you're optimistic about research?

JB: Absolutely, no question about it. Just keep making responses and every-thing will turn out all right.

LH: What is it you'd like to say that we haven't touched on?

JB: Seems to me we've touched on just about everything. I wasn't sure I was delighted about doing this in the first place. Yeah, you'd take anybody! But, I'm quite content. I think we've done very well covering my life.

LH: Well, I could tell you, Joe, that I've always been your fan.

JB: The only thing we haven't touched on is that meeting in Rome we went to.

LH: Do you really want to talk about that?

JB: Maybe; what was the year of that?

LH: 1958.

JB: My Lord. About forty years ago.

LH: And, we enjoyed Rome.

JB: We enjoyed Rome and that was the beginning of the International College of Neuropsychopharmacology, as I recall.

LH: Right. That's when I gave my first paper on chlorpromazine. I don't know if you joined us when we went to visit the Pope.

JB: Of course, I had Rosary beads blessed.

LH: So did I; I gave them out to all my neighbors.

JB: Well, they told me "you've got to take them out of your pocket." I said, "well, what kind of blessing can it be if it doesn't go through my pants?"

LH: Joe, it's been an absolute pleasure to know you, in all sincerity, over these years and I just hope that the scientists of the future have the drive, the intelligence and the perspective of research you have.

JB: And have as much fun.

LH: Okay, thank you.

JB: Thank you.

CHARLES JELLEFF CARR

Interviewed by Thomas A. Ban
Nashville, Tennessee, July 19, 1999

TB: We are in Nashville, Tennessee. It is July 19, 1999, and this will be an interview with Charles Jelleff Carr* for the archives of the American College of Neuropsychopharmacology. I am Thomas Ban. Let us start from the beginning.

JC: I started my professional career in the Department of Pharmacology of the University of Maryland. After 20 years with the University of Maryland I moved to the Department of Pharmacology of Purdue University but stayed there only for about two years.

TB: Could you tell us something about your activities during those years?

JC: Well, John Krantz and I wrote a textbook in the late 1940s.

TB: What was the title?

JC: *The Pharmacological Principles of Medical Practice*.

TB: When was it first published?

JC: In 1949 and then revised in 1950, 1951, 1952, 1953, 1954, and 1958.

TB: Who was the publisher?

JC: Williams and Wilkins. It became a very popular textbook, and it sold very, very well, but had to be continuously brought up to date. And, I just got tired of it.

TB: So, the first edition was published in?

JC: 1949.

TB: And the last edition?

JC: In 1958.

TB: Whose idea was it to write a textbook?

JC: It was John Krantz's idea. John and I worked together and we coauthored the book.

TB: Was the book translated into any other language?

JC: Oh yes, it was. It went into several different translations in other countries.

TB: I know there were Spanish and Portuguese translations.

JC: I think that's right.

TB: So you had the first edition in 1949 and the last in 1958.

JC: It had to be revised almost every year, and I had to spend my whole time to keep the stuff going.

TB: Yes, indeed.

---

* Charles Jelleff Carr was born in Baltimore, Maryland in 1910. After earning a PhD in pharmacology at the University of Maryland in 1937, he held faculty positions at Maryland and at Purdue University, before joining the Psychopharmacology Service Center of the NIMH in 1957. He later edited the journal Regulatory Toxicology and Pharmacology. Carr died in 2005.

JC: Textbook writing is a very laborious task because the field is changing so rapidly all the time that one can't keep up with it.

TB: By the time of the last edition you moved from the Department of Pharmacology at the University of Maryland to the Psychopharmacology Service Center (PSC).

JC: Oh, yes.

TB: Why did you move from the University?

JC: I met Jonathan Cole at the National Institutes of Health (NIH), and I was attracted to this whole new field. I didn't know anything about it, but I learned pretty rapidly.

TB: What was your position at the Center?

JC: Senior Research Pharmacologist.

TB: What did you do at the Center?

JC: I was responsible for the Pharmacology Unit. We had to do a lot of things in those years because the whole subject of psychopharmacology was foreign to the thinking of physicians and people in general. It was a very unique moment in history, I think. You know that.

TB: Yes.

JC: It was believed for hundreds of years that when people got crazy that was the end of it. Now we were saying that one can give them a pill and they will get better. People did not believe us, and that was a problem.

TB: During the years you were with the Center a steadily increasing number of new psychotropic drugs were released for clinical use in the United States and all around the world.

JC: Yes. The pharmaceutical companies were first skeptical about these drugs, but later on they began to jump on the bandwagon and were trying to see what their beneficial effects might be.

TB: What did you think about these new drugs?

JC: Well, I was excited about them as a pharmacologist. They were drugs with potential benefit for psychiatric patients.

TB: Were you teaching pharmacology in those years?

JC: Well, yes, but while I was working at the Center I was not doing any outside teaching. And at the Center we did not do any research with the new drugs.

TB: Weren't you the one at the Center who was reviewing the pre-clinical aspects of grant applications?

JC: Oh, yes, I did that. People were expecting explanations about how these new substances were working, but we didn't know much about that in those years. It was also a challenge to me, because I did not know anything about psychiatry. We were also working with people who came from other countries. There was that wonderful man who came down from Canada.

TB: Heinz Lehmann?

JC: Yes, Heinz Lehmann. He was a genius and I will never forget him. Heinz came down one time, and I remember very, very well, we were both in a little group meeting, and he said, "You know I was walking across the campus of the University of Utah, and I saw some dandelions, and I wondered about those dandelions, they go to sleep and then they wake up and I wondered why. Why would a dandelion close up and open up again?"

TB: And, then he tried to see how dandelions respond to drugs.

JC: Oh, that was it? I remember a picture of him in a hotel with dandelions in a glass of water.

TB: He gave drugs to them.

JC: He did that. It was a novel approach, a very novel approach.

TB: For how long were you with the Center?

JC: Six years. During my stay I wrote a paper on psychoactive drugs with Jonathan Cole that was published in 1959 in a volume on *Research in Psychopharmacology in Children*, edited by Seymour Fisher. And then, I had a paper on psychopharmacology that was published in the *Encyclopedia Britannica* in 1959.

TB: You left the center in 1963?

JC: Yes, that was about right.

TB: Why did you leave?

JC: Well, I don't think I had a particular motive for leaving.

TB: You became the Chief of the Scientific Analysis Branch of the Life Science Division in the Army.

JC: Oh yes. I worked with Colonel Huber for several years.

TB: Then you moved to the Life Sciences Research Office of the Federated Societies for Experimental Biology?

JC: The movement from the Army to the Life Sciences Research Office was really an extension of the program in the Army. They financed that office, but we were not in the military.

TB: So, that was a continuation of your work in the Army. Weren't you director of the office?

JC: Yes.

TB: It was during those years that you became involved in food safety.

JC: That's right. There's always the opportunity to embrace something novel that hasn't been done before. In 1979, we had the opportunity to really develop a food safety council.

TB: And you also developed standards of safety for drugs.

JC: No, at the time it was primarily safety of food ingredients. The agricultural industry was very concerned about that, because there had been a lot of claims that food was not good and had bad things in it. So we had the opportunity then to establish a food safety council to investigate that kind of problem. And that was working very well. It was about ten people that constituted our original group. I had to get them together, make arrangements for meetings with them, and we had to come forward at the end, whether one or another foodstuff is safe, or no. It became a big job that went on and on for a long time and I was looking around for help. I needed a good competent secretary and I was very fortunate in being able to find one. It was through my secretary that I met Sallie Carr. We married and have been happily together for 19 years, and that's about my story.

TB: You have not mentioned the journal *Regulatory Toxicology and Pharmacology*. Weren't you the editor of the journal? How did that come about?

JC: My friends, who were always looking for jobs for me, came and said "Look, a new journal is going to be published by Academic Press in California and we need somebody to be the editor of that journal. I said I didn't want to do that; "I don't want to go to New York; I don't want to go to Washington, I don't want to go anywhere". And they said, "You can do it right out of your own home." I said, "How do you do that?" They said, "You can have an office in your home." Well, that's when I met Sallie. You met Sallie, my wife. And Sallie said, "I figure that's a good idea. Let's try it." So we did that and the darn thing took off. Now I get so many manuscripts coming in that I work from early morning till night. We work very, very hard. We have a beautiful office in our home. The journal was growing faster than we wanted. It's the price of success. I guess.

TB: And, you are the editor-in-chief of the journal, right?

JC: That's right. Well, I get the manuscripts that are submitted for possible publication and then I have a whole bunch of people that I use as peer reviewers. I look at the manuscript and I pick out two peer reviewers and the manuscript goes off to them. Very rarely they come back with, "That's a great thing; publish it; go ahead." It happens that one reviewer says, "it is great, publish it," and the other one says, "it's terrible, don't publish it." That's also rare, though. Usually they have some kind of objection or suggestion for doing such and such, and they lay it out for me. Our role is only as an intermediary. The manuscripts then go back to the authors and they have to decide whether they will do the suggested revisions.

TB: So, the journal keeps you very busy.

JC: If I had not had Sallie to help me out, I wouldn't have been able to do it.

TB: As editor-in chief you are working with a group of people.

JC: Well, out of the journal in 1984 grew an organization known as the International Society of Regulatory Toxicology and Pharmacology. It is composed of scientists who give their time and effort to evaluate for companies whether their products are safe and should be pursued for approval by the Food and Drug Administration. Products, especially in the medical field, have to be approved by the Food and Drug Administration. So, the companies come to our group and ask us to give them an opinion about the safety of their products. It may save them a lot of work. The companies have their own scientists who do reviews for them, but they like an outside person who is independent who can give them their opinion. We do a little bit of that. It's a lot of work, but, anyway, it's also a lot of fun. We don't make any money out of it, but it's nice to be able to do that.

TB: How many members do you have in the society?

JC: It's a small organization, has always been small with about 250 members from around the world. I would say that, at least 200 are domestic and from Canada and the rest come from elsewhere. We hold annual meetings; we usually try to hold at least one meeting and, if possible, we have a second or third. Now this year alone, we have already had two meetings and are anticipating a third. We have dealt with the Food Quality Protection Act in March that is going to be published in the journal.

TB: Who is organizing those meetings?

JC: Sallie, my wife. Some of those meetings are quite small. We had one on DNA (deoxyribonucleic acid) in 1995 in Florida with about 20 in attendance. The report was written up, and then published in our journal. So now, four years later, we've been contacted and asked if we would now hold another meeting on DNA.

TB: In most of your meetings you evaluate whether one or another product is safe.

JC: Yes, that's right.

TB: And you publish the reports of all those safety evaluations by your group in the journal.

JC: We don't publish all the reports. Some of the reports are confidential. The firm pays the money to bring the scientists together. We are sort of an intermediary.

TB: Intermediary?

JC: Our role is to organize the meeting and to give them a report on what transpired at the meeting.

TB: I understood from you that the society is international.

JC: Well, yes, but most of our members as I indicated before are from the United States.

TB: Who are the people involved?

JC: Most of them are well known scientists from the pharmaceutical or food industry. I don't think I can name them all. We have a lot of them.

TB: That's fine. What would you consider your most important contribution?

JC: Well, I got an award in the mid-1980s from the University of Edinburgh for my work on chemical anesthesia, the history of chemical anesthesia.

TB: So you had also been involved in chemical anesthesia.

JC: Long time ago John Krantz got me interested in the nature of anesthetic agents, and for my review I read all the literature related to the discovery of the anesthetics. At the time they were first discovered no one knew that if you put a person to sleep by the inhalation of an anesthetic, or suspected anesthetic, that they would ever wake up again.

TB: A last question: Are you still continuing with the journal?

JC: Yes.

TB: In concluding I would like to add that your work has had a major impact on toxicology.

JC: I like to think that.

TB: Thank you for sharing this information with us.

JC: Okay.

LEONARD COOK

Interviewed by Larry Stein
San Juan, Puerto Rico, December 14, 1994

LS: It's a very great pleasure to have the opportunity to interview, for this important series on the history of psychopharmacology, my close colleague and very dear friend, Dr. Leonard Cook.* Perhaps we could start by you telling us a little bit about your early history and educational history which you think stimulated your interest in becoming a scientific investigator.

LC: What the various critical factors were would be hard to recall, but I was always interested in science even when I was a kid as well as in college. What spurred me, in terms of graduate school, occurred at a picnic. My wife worked for a Dr. Mulinos, who happened to be a pharmacologist. After graduating college, I wasn't really sure what I wanted to do. Dr. Mulinos had a back yard picnic, to which my wife and I were invited. While I was eating my hamburger and potato salad under a tree in his back yard, he came over to me and we started chatting. I had just graduated college and he asked, "What are you going to do?" I said, "Well, I'm not sure. I'd like to go into science, but I'm not sure exactly what field of science would interest me." He said, "How about pharmacology?" I said, "Well, I didn't really want to work in a drug store and make ice cream sodas." He replied, "No, no, no. Let me explain to you what pharmacology is." And he did, sitting next to me under that tree. And that back yard potato salad conference determined my career. I was fascinated. He told me where to apply.

LS: So, you applied to graduate school. Which school did you apply to?

LC: Well, I was already accepted at Rutgers in endocrinology, but I must admit it didn't turn me on. He said, "Well, Yale is a great place where they train pharmacologists." The sequence of events was, I went up there and had my interview with the department chairman, Prof. William Salter. After the interview he said, "Fine, just walk down the street and see the dean of the graduate school." And I looked at him and said, "You mean I'm accepted?" He said, "Of course, you start in two weeks." So that was the turning point and the start of my career in pharmacology.

LS: This was when? What year are we talking about when you started graduate school?

---

* Leonard Cook was born in Newark, New Jersey in 1924. He received his PhD from Yale University in pharmacology in 1951 and began work for Smith Kline & French as the founder of their psychopharmacology division. In 1969 he became associate director of pharmacology at Hoffmann La Roche, and in 1975 director of CNS research at DuPont.

LC: 1948. I served in the Army, in the Air Force during the war as a navigator. The GI Bill of Rights took me through most of my college. After graduation I still had a year left under the GI Bill, and this enabled me to start my graduate training at Yale.

LS: And, you worked at Yale with whom?

LC: Well, they had at Yale, which was unique, not only a training program in pharmacology, but a program specifically designed to meet the growing need for pharmacologists in the pharmaceutical industry. It was a very special training in regard to the elements and skills that industrial pharmacologists would need: such as organic chemistry, statistics, pharmacology, and of course, test development, and drug screening procedures. It was an unusual program and did me a great deal of good. The primary teacher was Dr. Desmond Bonnycastle, who was also my mentor.

LS: At that early phase of entering graduate school, you already had an interest in a research career in industry. Can you tell me a little bit about that, because I think at that point in time, basic research was heavily academic? There was a distinction made – almost a class system – between academic and industrial pharmacologists. So what kinds of thoughts were going through your mind?

LC: Well, I'll give you this young student's mind, not only my thoughts, but critical things that happened.

LS: We're going to return to this theme, because you are a very interesting example of someone who has made significant research contributions from the drug industry. It's going to be interesting to hear your thoughts as you entered your training.

LC: Well, thank you. I took only one course in psychology in college. I think that was Psych 101 and that's all I had. I will never forget my first week at graduate school in pharmacology at Yale. That's when we were asked to select a journal for which we would be responsible in the Weekly Journal Club. I had browsed in the library and I saw a journal called *Clinical Psychology*. And when I was asked for my selection I said, "I would like to give my weekly journal club contribution on *Clinical Psychology*; Psychology, not pharmacology."

LS: Psychology, clinical psychology.

LC: Now, this was in 1948.

LS: Before the birth of modem psychopharmacology, or at the birth?

LC: No, before the birth. So the chairman, Dr. Salter, came up to me, looked at me seriously and said, "Young man, we're talking science, not spooky science." He said, "We're talking about legitimate pharmacology, not spooky pharmacology." So I took another journal, because I didn't want to cross the chairman of the department during my first week in graduate school. I did, however, focus on the central nervous system by doing my thesis on analgesics.

LS: So, early on, even at the start of your career, you had an interest in behavior, in psychopharmacology?

LC: Yes, but I was quickly dissuaded about getting into what he called spooky pharmacology. I was hurt, but interestingly enough, four years later I was deeply involved in drugs modulating behavior and the beginning of psychopharmacology. Then, you referred to the issues which were involved in industry vs. academia. I didn't, at the time, even think of industry, quite frankly. My focus was going into research and pharmacology. During the last six months before my degree, I started interviewing and I was offered four jobs in industry and one in academia. There was a great need for pharmacologists. That was the beginning of the rapid expansion of pharmacology in the pharmaceutical industry, in terms of their research capacity.

LS: Let me take you back to graduate school to establish one point, because we want for the record: your thesis and your thesis research. Did you do a behavioral or psychopharmacological thesis?

LC: I did a thesis on "The Effects of Analgesics on the Spinal Cord," so there was no behavior involved. It focused on certain spinal reflexes, and the effects of analgesics on the brain and spinal cord. My mentor, Dr. Desmond Bonnycastle, had a PhD and an MD, and was very well known in the field of analgesics. Regarding my going into industry, I had a number of people come to Yale from different drug companies to interview me; there was Merck; there was Smith, Kline & French (SK&F); there was Frank Berger at Carter's Little Liver Pills (that was before it became Wallace Labs), and Dr. R.K. Richards from Abbott. I had five job offers, four industrial and one from academia. I took the one at SK&F. I was so excited, especially after going through gruelling grad. school. When I received the official letter from SK&F stating the salary, I was overwhelmed by the amount. Excitedly, I showed it to my professor.

LS: Dr. Bonnycastle?

LC: Yes, Dr. Bonnycastle. In 1951 I was to be making $6,000 a year and he as full professor at Yale was making $5,000 a year.

LS: And, as a PhD and MD.

LC: This did not sit well with him. He looked at me and was speechless.

LS: You both knew the salary differential?

LC: That was the problem. Yes, we both were aware of the salary difference. When I saw him the next day he said, "I'd like to speak to you, Leonard." I felt I was in trouble. I went to his office where he said, "You know, I've been thinking about your letter. If I knew you were going to prostitute yourself and go to industry, if I knew I was going to spend all my time training you and you were going to exploit my training by going into industry, I never would have taken you as a grad. student. Thinking about it, Len, I think you should spend another year here and we can do more research and further exploit the research you have achieved." I replied, "Dr. Bonnycastle, I've not only done everything in my proposal, but more," which was rare in graduate school. We talked about it and I told him what I would do, if he insisted on this. I told him I would ask for a review of the situation by a board. He said, "Okay, if you want to go out and be a prostitute, I wash my hands of you."

LS: Now, what was going through your head as you were being lectured by this somewhat formal professor, who obviously was deeply concerned about his student?

LC: Well, fear. I didn't have my degree yet. I was married. My wife was expecting our first child, and the job was threatened.

LS: Now, one final item of this early personal history before we start exploring what took you into the field of behavioral pharmacology. You had five offers and, in particular, you had an academic offer, which you could compare against those industrial offers. What caused you to accept the SK&F offer? It's most interesting, because that stroke of fate, of course, opened up a very distinguished career.

LC: An interesting question. Well, there are many factors. For starters, it was the highest offer. And, after going through lots of years of struggle, making that amount of money at that time, for a kid who came out of the poorest ghetto of the town, was compelling. Also, and probably equally important, was the fact that SK&F was just beginning to evolve. It had a great interest in research expansion. They had previously done most of their research at Temple University Medical School. So I saw this as an opportunity to start with a company on the ground floor. They were very nice to me and it was appealing. I had a dilemma since I also had an offer from Abbott with R.K. Richards. He was a distinguished pharmacologist and that tempted me a great deal.

LS: Was Richards from the University of Pennsylvania?

LC: No, Richards was at Abbott Labs. Also Merck, with Hans Molitor, offered me a job, which I would have taken, but the letter of offer was lost in the mail and I didn't know that. Had it not been lost, I might have gone there. But, in any event, as you pointed out, that was the most fortuitous decision of my life. It opened up an opportunity for me to get in on the ground floor and play this very critical role in developing the field of neuropsychopharmacology.

LS: OK, you arrive now at SK&F and, as we all know, SK&F bought the rights to chlorpromazine, and you were their first trained pharmacologist. Tell me what your role was in the decision for the company, because chlorpromazine had been passed around to a number of companies that turned their noses up at it. So, that would be an interesting bit of history to find out, how did SK&F opt to buy chlorpromazine and what role did Leonard Cook have in that important decision?

LC: When I went to SK&F, my first project was gastrointestinal pharmacology and the only reason they put me on that is that I had told them I knew how to surgically prepare what was called a Thirty-Vella loop dog, for measuring intestinal activity. This program lasted only a short time. We were also interested in drugs that would be sedatives, but were not barbiturates. I realized that I would have to have certain tests to identify sedatives. I went over to see Charlie Winter at Merck. He had a test chamber box, originally designed by Peter Dews, which was about the size of a shoebox with light beams crisscrossing it, for measuring locomotor activity. In addition, one of the tests I developed was a rat pole climb, a conditioned avoidance response test. I used a doorbell for the conditional stimulus, a brass plate floor that could be electrified with 120 volts to provide a shock to the rats' feet, and 12 inches of a broom handle to provide a means of escape for the rats, i.e., the pole climb. I called the test the 'conditioned reflex test.'

LS: A conditioned shock avoidance?

LC: A conditioned shock avoidance is a more sophisticated description. What was really interesting and crucial is that one of the other tests that I employed was developed by, again, Charlie Winter at Merck. It was a measurement of the sedative properties of a compound by how it prolonged the sleeping time of a barbiturate. At that time it was very difficult to measure sedative effects in rodents, because most of them, under the sedatives available at that time, would thrash around in excitement and not show sedation. In any event, I used this sleeping time prolongation test, and we found SKF-525-A (ß-diethylaminoethyl diphenylpropylacetate hydrochloride) that way. This was undoubtedly critical in opening up the entire field of drug metabolism and it also helped start a drug potentiation program. SKF-525-A was considered a drug potentiator, and importantly, that led to our interest in chlorpromazine, as I will explain.

LS: But your work with Thorazine (chlorpromazine) was critical research too.

LC: That was critical for the entire field. As a matter of fact, SKF-525-A, which I discovered, made my early reputation as a pharmacologist. I published several papers on it and it drew a great deal of interest in the field. At that time, I heard about a compound from the drug company Rhône-Poulenc, in France, which reportedly was also a drug potentiator. I wrote for it and I received a two gram sample. I compared its potentiation properties to my compound (SKF-525-A). It did prolong the effects of certain CNS drugs, but it did it in a very different fashion, the animals showed heavy sedation.

LS: Was SKF-525-A a stimulant?

LC: SKF-525-A wasn't a stimulant. It was a "silent" pharmacological agent that other than inhibiting the metabolism of other drugs produced no overt symptoms. I noticed a very special sedation or quiescence and indifference to the environment in the mice and rats treated with the Rhône-Poulenc compound.

LS: Without being put to sleep.

LC: Well, it certainly worked in the hexabarbital potentiation test. But this very special sedation the French compound produced was a type I had never seen before. I made a decision which retrospectively, was crucial. I decided to test the Rhône-Poulenc compound in my conditioned avoidance test. I set it up, trained a group of rats and administered the compound. I noticed that they were indifferent to the environment and didn't respond to the warning signal, i.e., the conditional stimulus, they just stood there, even though they knew they were going to get shocked.

LS: These were well-trained animals, who hearing the conditional stimulus would immediately climb up the pole and avoid the shock.

LC: They were very well trained to avoid the foot shock.

LS: Under the drug, they did not respond to the warning signals.

LC: But when we gave them the shock, they responded by climbing the pole. And I said, "My God, they obviously do feel the shock." They were indifferent; it seemed that they didn't care. When we gave them a shock, they jumped. So what was this unusual modulation of the avoidance behavior?

Another important point, which was most telling to me, was that when we gave the French compound to mice, over a very wide range of doses, the animals became immobile but they still remained on all four feet. Nothing in the drug armamentarium at the time would do that. When we turned the mice over onto their backs they righted themselves; when you pinched their tail, they pulled it away. They had this unusual sedation.

LS: So, you recognized the unique properties. Now, what year is this?

LC: That was the end of 1951, and very early 1952.

LS: At that early point, you recognized that you might be dealing with a new drug class.

LC: Yes, we recognized that we had a drug that was very different than anything else we had ever seen. And when coupled with the specific modulation of the avoidance behavior, I knew that this was the beginning of a totally new area of pharmacology. We noticed another thing, its hypothermic effect. Of course, we knew then from Rhône-Poulenc that their pharmacologist, Madame Courvoisier had also seen this lowering of body temperature.

I was very excited when I brought these findings to our research committee and told them about it. I was told that they had just heard that in France, it was reported by two gentlemen, named Delay and Deniker that this compound modulated certain psychotic behavior clinically. I excitedly requested that we contact the group in Europe. In fact, we arranged that they send some representatives from Rhône-Poulenc. A few weeks later they arrived for a meeting in Philadelphia at our labs. I showed them my data and they showed us their data. They discussed the anecdotal reports from Delay and Deniker. Suddenly, in my mind, the relevancy of the conditioned avoidance began to loom. I wondered if what we were measuring in that test had any kind of correlation or relevance to the psychotherapeutic effect they reported. We worked out a financial deal, and of course, SK&F then became the consignees of this drug in America.

LS: Now, this drug had a certain antihistaminic activity. At what point did you realize that this interesting activity profile was really not the antihistaminic effect?

LC: Well, all of the phenothiazines, the whole class of drugs, were, in their own right, antihistamines. You mentioned, in your opening statement at the beginning, how chlorpromazine was offered to seven different drug companies, who turned it down as an antihistamine. They turned it down for the reason that it had this heavy sedative effect, which they didn't want. So the special CNS effect it produced was the reason they rejected it.

LS: And it wasn't as good an antihistamine as, say, promethazine.

LC: Exactly right. We knew, up front, it was an antihistamine. What we didn't know is that the CNS effect of these antihistamines, of that class, had potential as psychotherapeutic agents.

LS: So, chlorpromazine became Thorazine and the sales showed a very sharply increasing curve. A lot of that money was funneled back into the research operation with this early success, and the fact that your early experimental results stimulated the company's appetite for a drug that other companies had turned their nose up at.

LC: Yes. And that was lucky.

LS: This was a very important discovery.

LC: Yes, I was only two years out of grad school at the time.

L.S: So, what did that do to your research program at that point?

LC: I requested an appointment with the vice president of research, a very perceptive guy, and I talked to him and I said ....

LS: Who was this?

LC: Kapp Clark. We chatted about my findings and their potential relevance and he said, "Len, what do you think of this drug?" I said, "Well, I think that we're dealing with a whole new area of pharmacology and I feel that we should exploit this. We're in a great position in what may be a new field." So he said, "Would you come back tomorrow? Go home and think about what we should do from this point. Don't even go back to the lab. I want you to go home, and on one piece of paper tell me, if you were me, what you would do about this." So, I went home and scribbled some thoughts, and the next day, I told him, "Well, I believe that we are at the beginning of a new field. This compound is probably just the first of what could lead to an entirely new class of drugs." And, he said, "Well, what should we do about it? If I told you that I will give you a substantial amount of money to build a new research program, what would you do?" I said, "Well, I thought about that last night." I put my scrap of paper in front of me. I said, "I think there are three approaches we could follow." Now, this is, remember, 1952, maybe the end of 1952. I said, "We could do work that relates to that of Mary Brazier at MIT, in the field of EEG and neurophysiology. We could do work in the area of biochemistry of the brain" –which was just beginning to emerge at that time, but was not very advanced – "or we could do work using experimental psychological methods." I said, "I think we should do all of them. However, if I did work with a compound in neurophysiology, biochemistry and behavior, and came to you with the results from testing in all three areas, I would be more secure in recommending to you that the compound be advanced to the clinic, on the basis of behavioral effects, rather than on biochemistry or neurophysiology." At that time, it cost about thirty million dollars to develop a drug. I then said, "And I would be more confident in predicting the clinical pharmacological effects from the behavioral results, rather than from the other fields. Not that the other fields wouldn't be important, and I do think they should be part of our research approach." It seemed to me that if a compound modulates behavior in animals, then that's a better predictor for modulating behavior in humans than anything else we had. Well, what happened is that we started building my research group. I was lucky to be able to build one of the best and largest neuropsychopharmacology units in the country, in fact, the world.

LS: Now that logic is commonplace now, because of a number of successes of being able to predict from animal behavior to human behavior. But back in 1952, we did not have that demonstrated success. We had a presumption that human behavior and human thought was something very special. And there might have been a lot of people to tell you, what sounded like a good logical argument, that it's foolish to try to predict from animal to human behavior. Do you have any idea as to why you saw, at that early stage, some evolutionary continuity between animal behavior and human behavior?

LC: Well, as you know, Larry, you're touching upon a critical issue for the last thirty or forty years. Maybe not so much today, but you're touching on what is considered the concept of dualism. You are touching on the fact that the physiology of the body is one thing, but the mind is independent. And, even people in our research committee felt that it was not possible that a drug could affect your thoughts and your mind, as a drug could affect the pumping action of the heart or be a diuretic. This has been, really, a struggle in the field of psychopharmacology, neuropsychopharmacology for decades, where people felt that behavior was a free will thing and that drugs really didn't affect the mind as they did, for example, the heart. You are very well aware of this. It took a long struggle for people in the field to establish experimental behavior as a legitimate area of pharmacology.

LS: It's interesting. This was a crucial inflection point in the investigation of a chemical entity, because on the human psychiatric side, it was proposed that chlorpromazine was effective as an antipsychotic in schizophrenia and was able to straighten out the deranged thinking of the psychotic. It's most interesting now that the correlate of that therapeutic action in schizophrenics turns out to be the conditioned avoidance test in animals that you had been studying.

LC: It was.

LS: I think that was a turning point in our field and you were a very important contributor to the understanding that, in fact, we could generate some kind of crude animal model of human behavior as a testing device for such a new class of drugs.

LC: Well, there are a couple of aspects to your comments, Larry. We were able to make a correlation of the compound's potency in the clinic with the conditioned avoidance response, and we had a correlation coefficient of 0.9. In most areas of pharmacology that is beyond expectations. At the end of your comment, you said something that I think we ought to discuss. You said models of human behavior. In no way, then or today, would I conceive of the conditioned avoidance as reflecting, say, any aspect of schizophrenia, and I don't think it's a model, necessarily, of human behavior. I look upon it, like other behavioral tests we have both used over the years, as a test procedure, which identifies a type of pharmacological activity, which has effectiveness in certain symptomatology in humans.

LS: Isn't the same pharmacological activity reflected, in common, between the human disorder and the animal test?

LC: Yes, yes, but never did I think of these as models, for a very good reason. I remember giving a talk, here at the ACNP years ago. I was talking about this particular work, and I said, "The greatest barrier," and that must have been about 1970, early '70s, "in pre-clinical psychopharmacology is the lack of definition of the clinical syndrome, in terms that have relevance to the pre-clinical science. If I went to a cardiovascular clinician and said, 'I could give you a drug that would do anything you want it to do on the heart, could you describe what you want it to do, specifically?' they could say, 'Yes, I want it to relax the blood vessel, enhance the blood flow, increase the contraction of the heart.' They could describe in physiological detail what that drug should do." I then said, "Now, I turn to you (i.e., psychiatrists) in the audience, can you tell me, specifically, what do you want that drug to do in terms that I could go back to the laboratory and find it for you? If I had a magic wand and I could give you a drug with any pharmacological property you want, can you define to me exactly what that drug should do, other than tell me, 'Make the patient well.?'"

LS: Well, they could tell you, at the human level, we want the drug to cure schizophrenia, but they could not tell what schizophrenia is. What is schizophrenia in a rat?

LC: What is schizophrenia, in terms that I could do research using animals?

LS: Using animals.

LC: That's been a great barrier. I wonder if it's changing now.

LS: And that is your objection to the term, model. It conveys to you that ….

LC: It's a schizophrenic rat.

LS: A truly schizophrenic rat. Well, that's most interesting. Why don't we now proceed in chronology, and tell me what happened in terms of the program? I assume that the program was accepted by Kapp Clark and by the people controlling the resources, and then you expanded your research activities. And what then ensued in research, following that?

LC: Well, I was given, essentially, a blank check. That's what you and I call the "Golden Era." At that time I had a young technician working for me named Bob Schuster, and he and I started developing a number of test procedures that would be sensitive to chlorpromazine. Bob Schuster had a bachelor's degree at the time and he said, "I want to go back to school." And Bob was accepted as a graduate student with Joe Brady. I also hired a consultant named Charlie Ferster and told him, "I can add more people to my group. I'd like to hire another psychologist, because that seems to be where all our test procedures are coming from." He said, "There's a young guy working for me who's looking for a job." I asked, "Who's that?" And, he said, "A young kid named Roger Kelleher." So we invited him to come up from Florida and I offered him a job. And that was, of course, a very important decision. Roger Kelleher was fantastic. He taught me a great deal of psychology. And Charlie Ferster was also great, but a very hard teacher.

LS: Roger Kelleher? You taught him pharmacology, because I know Roger didn't know much pharmacology.

LC: I taught him pharmacology. Going back a little bit, even before a psychologist worked for me, I had read a paper by Abraham Wikler. His paper described something about rats working for food by pressing a lever. I thought, "Gee that sounds like another test we can play with." And, as I read his article, as best I could figure out from their description of the apparatus, I tried to duplicate it. I made a cardboard box and I fixed the pencil with a needle in it as a fulcrum. Part of the pencil came in the box and the other was outside the box. Every time the rat pushed the lever, I threw a piece of food into the box. Well, the rat had us well trained. After a while, he would press the lever eagerly and I threw the food in. The rat trained me to throw food in every time he pressed the lever. Then I started to become acquainted with the work of Skinner. When Kelleher joined me he started what he called schedules of reinforcement. I said, "I don't understand. What's the difference whether the rat presses ten times and gets a piece of food or he waits ten minutes to press and gets a piece of food? The drug is going to have the same effect." Well, those of us in the field now know that it's not the case. The schedule of reinforcement was more important than the reinforcement itself. I was very naive and skeptical about this approach initially.

LS: In terms of its pharmacological profile?

LC: Yes, in terms of sensitivity to pharmacological effects. And, as we know, I then became one of the strongest advocates in the world regarding the value of schedules of reinforcement as probably one of the most sensitive measures in identifying pharmacological actions.

LS: Now, I still want to stick a little bit more with the antipsychotic field. Here, you had identified, with a relatively crude conditioned avoidance test, the most interesting property of chlorpromazine, which emboldened the company to actually buy the rights to it. What other compounds came out of that program in the antipsychotic field? What was your role in detecting those compounds and encouraging the company to proceed with clinical testing?

LC: We began to expand our pharmacology strengths. We also worked closely with Rhône-Poulenc. My role was that I did much of the original pharmacology. I used to go to Paris a lot to look at some of their other compounds and compared them to our compounds. So out of this came a similar compound, Stelazine (trifluoperazine), with a stronger effect as an antiemetic. It had the same profile as chlorpromazine, but was some-what different and more potent. And that was the beginning of the phe-nothiazine story. Importantly, the company at that time felt we'd probably had enough of these compounds, and that we should stop testing any more compounds for clinical studies. I said, "No, we should continue." But they dropped the phenothiazines at that time.

LS: But out of hundreds of these compounds synthesized, what identified Compazine (prochlorperazine) and what identified Stelazine in terms of pharmacological effects?

LC: I would say the behavioral tests, as well as the antiemetic test.

LS: And, was there some clinical need, in your view, for these compounds? Did they represent improvements as therapeutic agents?

LC: I would say, it goes back to what we mentioned before. We had at that time an entire battery of test procedures, many, many test procedures, all of which were sensitive to these drugs. The decision to recommend a compound to the research committee to go to development was pri-marily based on conditioned avoidance. That test had such face validity and that was in the 1950s. Even today, I feel just as strongly that that test would be the go, no-go for drugs. Stelazine was tested as a more potent agent, and Compazine (prochlorperazine) as an antiemetic.

LS: So, that test was not only good to predict activity in humans, but a quan-titative predictor of potency. From the potency in the animal test, you could predict the daily dose. It ended up....

LC: Clinically.

LS: Yes, yes, this is a very good point.

LC: We made this correlation between potency in rats with their potency in the clinic. Bert Schiele published a paper in which he tested about ten different phenothiazines clinically. He reported their relative potencies. I published a paper showing that the correlation coefficient between the relative potency of these drugs in the clinic and their relative potency in conditioned avoidance was 0.9. We now know that it goes beyond this single chemical class of compounds, well beyond the phenothiazines. Every clinically effective antipsychotic, regardless of chemical class, works in the conditioned avoidance test, and predicts its clinical efficacy.

LS: This would include then, haloperidol (Haldol) and the class of butyroph-enones and the atypical antipsychotics?

LC: Clozapine.

LS: And, even clozapine, yes.

LC: So, it stood up

LS: It sounds like there's something deep within the schizophrenic syndrome in terms of its biochemistry and its brain mechanisms, that is parallel to some similar kind of brain mechanism that is important in regulating conditioned avoidance. We can't identify that yet at the behavioral level and that's a commonality that warrants further research.

LC: Yes. Again, all we really know is that whatever pharmacological action selectively inhibits the conditioned avoidance it's strongly correlated and probably reflective of the psychotherapeutic effect in schizophrenia and severe mental and emotional disorders.

LS: Okay. I think I will now make an observation, the interviewer's observation. Rather than you being someone preoccupied with theories or deep biochemistry or brain mechanisms, you are a practical person and you selected out predictability from animal models to human, the ability of whatever test battery, if it works – if it predicts – then you are going to use it and you are going to be interested in it and it's going to guide your research efforts. Do you feel that's a correct observation, that you don't have an ax to grind other than that it works.

LC: Yes.

LS: Now, let's see how that theme recurs again in your career later in the SK&F years. What was the next major research project, perhaps, the next major class of drugs that engaged your interest?

LC: While I was still at SK&F, I tested a compound that Frank Berger had come out with, called meprobamate, Miltown. It didn't work in the conditioned avoidance procedure. It did however disinhibit behavior that was either suppressed or extinguished, and it worked in the conflict test and in the fixed interval test. Behavior which has been suppressed, because of environmental contingencies, never comes back with chlorpromazine or the phenothiazines, but drugs like Miltown, and of course subsequently chlordiazepoxide, anxiolytics, will disinhibit that suppressed behavior and bring back the behavior.

LS: It's most interesting, that behavior can either be suppressed by punishment or by an absence of reward. In either case, behavior becomes suppressed and this new class of drugs, the meprobamate class, produces a disinhibition of that suppression. And you saw that clearly in the conflict and fixed interval tests. It might be worth taking a couple of sentences to explain how inhibition is measured in a conflict test or the fixed interval procedure and how you used it to predict activity in meprobamate type drugs.

LC: Just to finish up, there were two major tests we were getting to. One is the test that identifies anxiolytics and a test that identifies the so-called antipsychotics. Conditioned avoidance will select the antipsychotics. The anxiolytics don't work in the avoidance test but they do work in the conflict and fixed interval test. Now both groups of tests, the conflict and the avoidance, both involve foot-shock. People used to say, "Well, these drugs work in conditioned avoidance by affecting fear." That's not sustainable. If fear was involved with foot-shock, then chlorpromazine type of drugs should work in both tests, and the anxiolytics should work in both tests. In the fixed interval test only the last response was reinforced. So, initially the animal works all the time, but soon begins to realize, I suppose, that all of the responses before the five-minute period were not reinforced. It doesn't pay off, so the first three or four minutes are flat, that is no responses, and the animal says, "I guess it's about time, one of those presses is going to be rewarded." So, it starts pressing, pressing, and pressing. As it nears the end of the five-minute period, it responds faster and faster and gets rewarded.

LS: When the five-minute period time is up, the next press ....

LC: The next press, yes, thank you. But, the thing is that in the beginning, that period of time was full of responses.

LS: Early in training.

LC: Early in training. The fact that it was no longer reinforced extinguished the early responses. Now even though that behavior was gone because it was not reinforced, with meprobamate, it was brought back. In the conflict test, if the rat used to be rewarded by pressing a lever, it would get a pellet of food. Then we add the additional contingency that it can still press a lever and get food, but it is also going to get a foot-shock if it does respond. Therefore they suppress the pressing of the lever, because they don't want to be punished. The anxiolytic drugs like meprobamate and Librium (chlordiazepoxide), later on, turned out to be very different classes of drugs. They disinhibited the electric shock induced suppression of behavior.

LS: And this is also recognized on the clinical side. Early on, both groups of drugs were labeled tranquilizers, one major and one minor, and it emerged, on the clinical side, that the meprobamate types are not effective in schizophrenia, but the phenothiazine types are; whereas, in anxiety or certain anxiety conditions, the chlorpromazine type drug is not effective, but the meprobamate type drug is. So, now the logic is, going back into the animal laboratory, to identify different behavioral strategies that will distinguish between these two groups of drugs. And you were successful in doing this. On the one hand, the conditioned avoidance test predicted antipsychotic activity, and the conflict and fixed interval test predicted anti-anxiety activity. But that's a long story. In addition, there was an interest in trying to understand some of the underlying biochemistry that was involved and you had a hand in that. In the case of the antipsychotics, catecholamines and in particular dopamine was relevant;

in the case of the anti-anxiety drugs, you were interested in other transmitters. Can you tell us a little bit about some of that research and some of the ideas?

LC: That's when you became a big part of my life, Larry. Remember, we've often talked about the fact that you had published this study and I said, "Larry, it can't be right." And, I went back and it was exactly right. I think when we got to the anxiolytics, even though dopamine began to emerge with the phenothiazines, the role of biochemical mechanisms really became exciting and prominent with the anxiolytics. I remember some of the papers on parachlorophenylalanine, and your work on the relative role of serotonin and epinephrine in anxiolytic effects. I remember one paper you had published with Margolis, where you had identified the relative role of these biochemicals in terms of their sedative and anxiolytic effects, and I was skeptical about it. We did the work and replicated it to a T, and I called you up and said, "Larry, I'm sorry, you are right." But it was in the era of the anxiolytics that the significant role of biochemistry began, and we began to make correlations in which a chemical in the brain may have particular relevance for different behavioral aspects.

LS: And that stood us in good stead as you entered still another therapeutic area. Now, you correct me if I'm wrong; you, then, became interested in learning and memory. Was this during your time at SK&F, just to get the chronology right? I know at some point Hoffmann-LaRoche was very keen to recruit you because of your important work on the benzodiazepines, and you made a move. So you continued your work on benzodiazepines at Hoffmann-LaRoche, but also started a program in learning and memory. Is that chronology correct?

LC: You're essentially correct. I left SK&F in 1969 to become director of research at Hoffmann-LaRoche when Lowell Randall was going to retire. But while I was still at SK&F, I kept thinking of the possibility that we could find drugs which selectively enhance certain behavioral processes. Early one day, I had a call from my director who said that the president of our company had just read a paper, I think by Cameron in Canada, who was giving RNA (ribonucleic acid) to people who had deficits of memory in aging. My boss said, "Gee, Len, can you take some of this yeast RNA and give it to rats, show that it doesn't work, and we can get the president of the company – who was a friend of Cameron – off my back?" I said, "I will test the compound." I took some of my conditioned avoidance rats we were training and said to my technician "Give half of these rats this RNA and half of them saline and see if the treated ones will learn faster with the RNA." The next day he came to me and said, "I did it Len." I said, "Good, give me the negative results and we'll go and submit it. Our boss will be very happy." He said, "They weren't negative. It worked," and I said, "You better do that over again." And, he did and it continued to work. Well, I don't know what was going on with the RNA. We also found that it prolonged extinction. I remember, in London, at a meeting where I gave a paper on these results you had asked me the question, "Why shouldn't it hasten the extinction?" We won't get into that. But that was the time we also did some work with nicotine, and I began to realize that it is possible that drugs could facilitate the processes of learning and memory, cognition. We may not have had a drug in mind at that time, but I was convinced of the feasibility of identifying pharmacological agents that would enhance memory and learning.

LS: Perhaps even in normals?

LC: Let me get to that, yes. One of the drugs we tested was strychnine. Now, we used doses 1/10th the convulsive doses, and strychnine has an enormous enhancing effect of certain discrimination tests, particularly in a "delay match" test in normal monkeys. Now, what was your last point?

LS: Perhaps even in normals? Back at that time, people were divided and some thought that in those subjects with normal function you're unlikely to get pharmacological enhancement, and most of the activity should be aimed at correcting deficits. I'd be interested in your opinion on that.

LC: I have my thoughts about that. Number 1: Is the normal animal the right model to test drugs that may enhance memory? I mean, normal people are doing pretty well. How much room is there to enhance? Number 2: If we're to look for drugs for Alzheimer's or senile dementia, should we use a normal animal or an animal with deficit? I've used animals with lesions causing all kinds of anoxic damage and micronecrosis, but my private thoughts are that the normal animal is a fine subject to look for drugs to enhance memory. Think about this. Let's take an Alzheimer patient. A drug which enhances the learning and memory processes of an Alzheimer patient is not going to work on the dead cells. It's going to work on whatever residual function that brain has. It's not going to bring back a cell that's dead. Well, the normal animal, we do know already, can do better with certain pharmacological effects, according to our test criteria. So there's room for the normal brain to do better. We can pharmacologically enhance the performance, the behavioral measures in animals that reflect cognition, learning, memory, discrimination, etc. So in all of the drug screening and testing that I did at SK&F, DuPont Merck and even at Hoffmann-LaRoche, I used normal animals. The drug is going to be working on those cell brain mechanisms that are still viable. I still have that strong feeling now, although I have used animals where we have burned out the nucleus basalis, which caused deficiency in cholinergic projections. But even there, the drugs I worked on affected the normal cells that were still left. They didn't work on the cells that were burned out. So I'm not saying that one approach is better than the other, but I really believe that the normal brain in test animals is a perfectly viable substrate to look for drugs to enhance memory and learning in people who have cognitive problems, or someday even in normals.

LS: And, again, Cook's law is: don't get too tied up in trying to create an animal model of Alzheimer's, but rather, try some tests and see whether you can predict a relationship in drug potency between animal and in humans.

LC: Yes, absolutely. I have always had research going on in my lab groups that reflect the best of our science, but I don't get hung up on it. I'm looking for tests that will predict those pharmacological actions in animals that will have therapeutic effect in humans. I have always worked in the drug industry where the motto is: we want drugs now.

LS: I'd like to turn to the subject of how does one make an impact in fundamental research working out of industry, as you have through your whole career, and what views do you have on industry versus academic or institute research in psychopharmacology?

LC: Well, first of all, I firmly believe that industrial research should incorporate every known breakthrough that exists, and I've always done that. But as I just mentioned, if your job is to discover drugs, it is important to get the clinicians to evaluate the drugs. You have to use expedient, meaningful and relevant methods. You have to act in concert with good basic research, too, and I've always tried to do that. I've been lucky to have some of the best scientists working for me, the best people in the field. But, you shouldn't lose sight of the fact that you're responsible for a group of up to maybe fifty, seventy, or eighty people, looking for agents, drugs in the area of CNS and psychopharmacology. Your job is to identify those drugs, set up mechanisms that are relevant, and find drugs for the market. I suppose relevancy of the approach has been the keynote in the operations that I've had at SK&F, Hoffmann-LaRoche and at DuPont Merck. Most of all, your group must be productive for the company.

LS: Do you have any observations as to why drug discovery has, with only a few exceptions, occurred within the industry and why not in government labs? Do you have some views on that?

LC: I have some thoughts on that. In universities, frequently they are interested in the mechanisms of why drugs work and certain research aspects. Basically, I have a personal thought, after having spent forty-four years of my life in drug industry, doing research, building a career in drug discovery, and it's this: I've learned that the strategy of drug discovery is different than the strategy of doing basic research. Not that, in drug discovery, you don't try to incorporate every element that you can of what is learned in research. The drug discovery process should incorporate and reflect every known useful finding. The strategy of drug discovery is different than the strategy of basic research, and what has happened is that in most cases when drug companies have tried to incorporate the strategy of basic research to discover drugs, it hasn't really been as profitable as when the individual scientist sets out with his own strategy and says, "This is how we're going to find the drugs. These are going to be our criteria. This is the kind of pharmacological spectrum we want." I feel strongly that the two research approaches are different.

LS: Now, just to explore this maybe a little further. Science is science, so to some extent, the science is the same. And I think what you're pointing out is that the mission is different and that the objective is different; therefore, there is something in the strategy of the science that is different which enhances the probability of success in the approaches taken in industry: one possible reason for the difference between a drug discovery strategy vs. an absence of strategy is that in academia and in government laboratories, the science centers on the PI, whereas in industry there may be more of a team approach. But you may have some expanded views on strategic approaches. I know that you are one of our philosophers in spelling out strategies for drug discovery. I'd be interested in hearing.

LC: It's difficult to talk about this. As a matter of fact, even within industry things have changed enormously. You and I both have worked in industry. Before you went to California, you were in industry. And we often mentioned the fact that we had the Golden Era of pharmacology and psychopharmacology and we came out with many, many useful drugs. We had a purpose. We knew what we were going after. The research you and I did in the laboratories and the drug discovery process was planned and generated at the bench by the individual scientist. You were not told what to do or how to do it. You had a purpose as I did, in deciding what we would like to get into, such as have a drug for anxiety or whatever. We decided what we would do and how we would do it. So the strategy was determined at the bench and we were pretty successful. Well, after about twenty or twenty-five years, our companies began to grow and got very worried about their resources, and they started what they called strategic planning groups. They had people come in from Wall Street and Harvard Business School. And, what happened was that concerns about resources, specific goals and "bang for the buck" were the issue. Management bought this, as their security blanket, to justify the money spent.

LS: Well, the time and dollars to bring the drug out changed a lot from 1954 to 1994.

LC: So, whatever good reasons there may be, things, as you pointed out, have changed. Now, what the individual scientist does and how he does it, his time frame of when he's going to do it, and how long he's going to do it, is determined by upper management.

LS: Who are not, necessarily, scientific people?

LC: Right. So what you have lost in this program of research discovery is the ingenuity of the individual scientists to follow their nose, and how long they should continue on something, because it's pretty hard to put a timetable on discovery. In many cases, management will say, "you now have twenty-two months to prove that the research program is going to work." After that, that's it. Well, we may find it in one month; we may find it in five years, so I think their logic is a total fallacy. So things have changed, in the industry. What we decided then was what we did, even as young scientists, to a large part. Today planning committees tell the scientists in industry exactly what they're going to do, when they're going to do it, and even though there's a little latitude for individual contribution, it's not what it really should be or was at the time.

LS: They're not going to be able to attract the same kind of individual, it sounds to me, into industry; that is, the creative entrepreneurial type individual.

LC: Well, they may recruit them, but that's not the way they're going to function. And I think that is a major, major change in the pharmaceutical industry, let alone their philosophy. I think, in a way, it's very good to analyze resources and the costs carefully, but you may be throwing out an awful lot. The history of drug discovery is not the result of planned working groups or strategic planning. When you think back on all drug discoveries we've had over the last forty years, they've come mostly through an individual who has championed some sort of research.

LS: He was an intellectual investment.

LC: He's the champion, an intellectual investment, most of the time fighting authority, putting himself on the line, and frequently, against the company. Without going into individual names, I can think of several instances where the person who made the drug discovery is no longer with the company, because his persistence to get that job done made many enemies. And when their drug came out, they were not there anymore.

LS: I think, in a way, you're explaining a new development in the pharmaceutical industry, and that's the emergence of small drug discovery companies that function the way we used to function twenty years ago.

LC: That's interesting.

LS: With, again, individual investigators, who have an intellectual investment as well as, perhaps, a personal financial investment.

LC: And a little freedom

LS: More freedom. A lot is at stake. We operated with financial security.

LC: Right.

LS: But what you're saying is that the board planning approach, in your opinion, is not going to produce the new drugs of the future.

LC: Well, it may, but it's going to be a very different world. I'd like to see it work, because that's the way things are now, but the individual scientist, even no matter what they're told and what the companies say, the individual scientists don't have the luxury we had of following our noses. We could tell the market researchers, the market analysis people that we knew what was coming up in the future and where the field was going. I remember a personal experience where I said, "I am looking for drugs that will enhance learning and memory." And at this one meeting, one of the market people said, "Len, why are you doing that?" I said, "I think it's a great need." He said, "No, there's no market for it." I said, "Yeah, that's true. There is no market because there is no drug yet." "Oh, no, no," he said. Market analysis has always been retrospective. It's not prospective. The prospective aspect of the market is usually done by the scientists.

LS: Before chlorpromazine, there wasn't a big market for antipsychotics.

LC: That's right, and before Miltown (meprobamate) and Librium (chlordiazepoxide), there was no market for anxiolytics. But I had to fight this. They said there's no market for drugs in learning and memory.

LS: So you had three industrial careers. You had a career at SK&F. You had a career at Hoffmann-LaRoche. You had a career at DuPont-Merck. What does Len Cook do these days? Are you still in drug discovery?

LC: Well, I loved it, absolutely loved it, and I'm very fortunate, probably as you feel yourself. I mean, I've done exactly what I wanted to do and I got paid for it. And that's been an exciting thing. I could never wait to get into work every day, that is, until the special new research committees took over. They did tell us what we were doing wrong and things like that. But I'm now partially retired and doing consulting work. I'm very fortunate to be involved with NIDA, the National Institute on Drug Abuse, in advising them on their cocaine and opioid program. I am an adjunct professor at Temple in pharmacology. And I am doing consulting work for several drug companies. I'm having fun. So I'm still keeping involved. I believe that we have an exciting period of time in drug discovery in our area. I think we're beginning to identify those processes that are most relevant to learning and memory and it's going to be very interesting to see how these particular substrate systems will be useful to identify drugs in the future. I think this whole area of drugs to enhance performance, to enhance our intellectual capacity will come. There's no question that there are already people in the field who have demonstrated, clearly, that it is feasible to expect pharmacological enhancement of these processes. What we have to find are drugs that will be safe enough and effective enough to produce. I think it's an exciting future. I just hope that the resources that everybody needs to do that will be there, and the freedom of the individual scientist to do it. It's not only in industry where the individual science work now is heavily monitored, but also in academia by the research study groups and the grants, places where support comes from. The problem is, of course, the limited resource availability for funds, but, somehow or other, we've got to make sure that we don't lose what we know has worked in the past, even though people say, "Well, all the drugs up to now were discovered by chance." Chance was involved, but it took the special people, the special skills and attitude and the fact that they were allowed to work in this area where chance could happen. You know, the old saying, "chance favors the prepared mind." And if you have the freedom to work in a wide area, that goes beyond the approved research of the company or grant people, we're going to have a greater chance to discover the drugs. I would like, very much, to see that the highly structured research programs are going to pay off. And they have in some cases. But, historically, in our field, that has not been true. Maybe if we go back in time to my talk, in which I told the audience at ACNP, if I had the magic wand and I could give you a drug that will do anything you want, then you just find it. And maybe if some day, they could say, "we want a drug to work in this cell or on this particular group of biochemistry to this extent," then we could duplicate the process in an animal. We then could set up the correct procedures in a highly programmed research project to do that. But we've got to have a little elbow-room as we go along. I feel strongly about that.

LS: As, perhaps, a final topic, what I would like to do is mention a few names to you and ask you how these people have impacted your career. I'd like to start with Dr. Goodman at Yale.

LC: Well, Lou Goodman, the co-author with Goodman and Gilman, was my surrogate father. I remember presenting the first pharmacology program proposal to the SK&F research board and Lou Goodman was a consultant. He was in the audience. He was spectacularly supportive to my research program and I remember he told them that of all the work he'd seen supported by Washington, of all the investment Washington has made in our entire grant program in this field, nothing compared to what I had done. It was a great, great moment for me. So, Lou Goodman was critical to the support that SK&F gave me to build up the great research effort we had there.

LS: And Lou offered you a job at the University of Utah, at some later point.

LC: Lou said he had a vision of having, at Utah, the greatest center for psychopharmacology in the world and asked if I would come and be its director. I decided to stay at SK&F because everything was rolling for me and I decided not to. I don't know if that was a wise decision or not, but Lou was a very important person in my life and still is.

LS: I know another important colleague was Joe Brady. That goes back a long way. Are there any other figures that had a special relevance to your career? Of course, there were your colleagues. You mentioned Roger Kelleher. You had other important colleagues. Perhaps, those could be mentioned.

LC: Yes, Bob Schuster and Roger. Bob went on to get his degree and did pretty well for himself, he became director of NIDA. Roger worked with me for five years and went to work with Peter Dews at Harvard. Then, I hired a young man named Charlie Catania, and Charlie taught me all about concurrent schedules of reinforcement, he was very useful. Then there was Bill Holtz who was timely in bringing in punished response behavior so we could look at anxiolytics. Of course there was Arnie Davidson. I hope I didn't leave anybody out. I went to Hoffmann-LaRoche and, Arnie Davidson joined me there. He was crucial as my associate at SK&F and as well at Hoffmann-LaRoche. Jerry Sepinwall also worked with me at Roche. Then at DuPont Merck, I had a number of good colleagues there. Overall, I guess that whatever success I had was really dependent upon these people. I couldn't have done it without them, obviously.

LS: But I think there's an interesting thread here, again, that indicates something about your scientific style. All of these colleagues, whom you worked very closely with, were meticulous investigators. Tell me about your style and your views about data and how one gets it right and how much care is involved, in terms of the way you like to do it.

LC: I was a reasonably hard taskmaster with them, but I was familiar with every bit of the data because I couldn't talk about it and go to research committee or go to scientific meetings without being intimately involved. Even though I couldn't personally program any of these behavioral tests, I told them exactly what I wanted and we talked about that. So I was always very involved in how the experiment should be done and how to interpret the data with, of course, the help of these great, great colleagues.

LS: Well, I think it's most interesting what you have accomplished when we consider you at the starting point of your career and the professor expressing displeasure with your choice of a first job. Leonard Cook, the president of this society, you've won research awards; you have been an exemplar of a researcher who has spent an entire career in industry, having a major impact in the creation of a new field, behavioral pharmacology. Thank you, on behalf of the field.

LC: Larry, thank you. I just have to say, of course, that talking about people who were critical in my career, you know you're on top of the list.

PETER B. DEWS

Interviewed by John A. Harvey
San Juan, Puerto Rico, December.12, 1995

JH: This is John Harvey. I'm at the Medical College of Pennsylvania at Hahnemann University, and I'm interviewing Peter B. Dews* tonight, from Harvard University. I think it's going to be an interesting interview, Peter. I thought we'd start out by you telling me something about how you got from, what I gather, was medical school, somewhere in Britain, and ended up at Harvard.

PD: Well, after I got out of medical school, I wanted to go into either physiology or pharmacology and it turned out to be pharmacology. I did a hospital job and I went straight back into pharmacology. It so happened, that one of the principal interests in the department at the time was marijuana. There had been a lot of interest in the late thirties in the active constituents of marijuana. There were synthetic compounds, with marijuana-like activity, and there were also extracts of the plant. And the mystery was that we knew that in the extracts of the plant there was a large amount of inert material, cannabinoidol and things of that kind, but yet milligram for milligram, it was as potent as the best of the synthetic compound. So we knew there was some good stuff in the right oil. They were working on it, and so I got involved in studying it. It was a very intractable problem. The methods were not available for doing anything quantitative with it, to do a decent assay. In fact, the most accurate assay that we had was for people to take a little of it, compare thirty milligrams of this with thirty milligrams of that. There was a rapid corneal anesthesia assay, which did not work. There was also, a dog ataxia assay, which also did not work, so it really was difficult from the point of view of guiding the development of drugs from the marijuana series or anything of that kind. They're basically useless. But my curiosity was aroused by the problems of dealing with an agent which doesn't do anything except affect behavior. Tetrahydrocannabinol, the active ingredient of marijuana, is the extreme example of a drug that does nothing else. It has no toxicity. It's less toxic than sodium chloride put into the mouse. So that's how I got started in pharmacology and that's why, from the very beginning, I had an interest in behavioral effects of drugs.

JH: Well, you went from that straight to Harvard, then?

---

* Peter B. Dews was born in Ossett, England in 1922, and earned his medical degree at the University of Leeds, England, in 1944. This was followed by a PhD in physiology from the University of Minnesota in 1951. After serving as a research associate at the Mayo Clinic in Rochester, Minnesota, in 1952, he became a member of the pharmacology department of Harvard Medical School and remained at Harvard for the rest of his career, becoming emerited in 1993.

PD: Oh, no. After I'd been in Leeds, where I'd been in medical school, and in pharmacology for about a year or year and a half, I was offered a position as a Wellcome Research Fellow, in the Wellcome Research Laboratories, in Tuckahoe, New York. It was a two-year Fellowship. I was young and single and two years in New York sounded like the thing to do. In fact, it was. I had a good experience there. There was a very fine Director of Pharmacology, called E. J. De Beer. I got along very well with him and I got to know people like George H. Hitchings and Trudy Elion. They were in sort of the next room. I had good colleagues and I had a good experience. While I was there, I had been looking at antihistamines. Before I came over, I'd been to see Bernard Halpern and Daniel Bovet in Paris. They were the people that developed the first clinically useful antihistamines, and I'd been working on antihistamines in Leeds.

After I'd been in Tuckahoe for about a year, I got a letter from Halpern saying he was coming to the United States. He was going to land at Idlewild, and he was terrified of the journey from Idlewild to Manhattan because he'd heard there were cowboys and Indians, and fights going on among the buses on the roads, and things of that kind. "Would I come to Idlewild," he asked, "and convey him safely to Manhattan?" and I did. It turned out that one of his reasons for coming to the United States was to give a Mayo Foundation lecture. There was a meeting of the American Physiological Society, half in Minneapolis and half down in Rochester, Minnesota, at the Mayo Clinic. And it ended up with Halpern and I driving to this meeting for him to give his Mayo Foundation lecture. His host at the meeting in Minnesota was a man called Cole, Charlie Cole, who was an important figure at the Mayo Foundation. Just in the first evening I met him, he said, rather casually, "Would you like to come out here for awhile?" And I said, "Yeah." I thought it might be very interesting, so I went back to Tuckahoe and said, "Well, instead of staying two years, I'll stay one year and go out to Mayo." And they were outraged. They said, "You said you'd come for two years; you're going to stay for two years." So I talked to Cole and said, "Can I come out a year later?" He said, "Sure." "But I want to come just for a year." And he said, "No, you'd better come for three years". And, we went backwards and forwards, and in the end they said, "Okay, you can come for a year." I stayed three years, and I was recruited from there by Otto Krayer, who was Head of Pharmacology at Harvard. He knew Will Wood, who was at the Mayo in Rochester, and he gave him my name. Wood had worked in Krayer's lab. Krayer was looking for a pharmacologist who was interested in CNS, and I had really done very little work on CNS. I'd done a little at Boswell Chemicals on motor activity in mice, but it had not really been my main activity. But he recruited me anyway, and I went to Harvard in 1952 as an instructor and found the environment and colleagues and support just better than I could imagine. I never had any inclination to leave, and still don't.

JH: Well, there was only about three years' time, then, between the time you arrived at Harvard in '52, and you published what's considered to be the seminal paper in the field, "Studies on Behavior" in 1955.

PD: Yes, actually, I got started even sooner than that, because when I arrived at Harvard in January 1953, Krayer said, "There's a man over in the department of psychology called Skinner who's been in contact with me, and he says he's developed techniques that he thinks will be useful in pharmacology. There's another man in the department, a Rockefeller Fellow for a year, who is interested in seeing effects of drugs, called Peter Witt." He became quite famous from his work on spiders and quantitative work on a variety of agents, in fact, in the web building of spiders. He went back home, and then he came back to this country and ended up in North Carolina. But, anyway, Krayer had this letter from Skinner, and he said, "What are they doing? See what the man is talking about." So Peter Witt and I went over to Cambridge, and I'm ashamed to say that I was not aware of Skinner or his work. I'd never had any contact with psychology. B.F. Skinner was very cordial and chatted for a few minutes, as was his way, then he turned me over to a man called Charles Ferster, and said, "Charlie will show you around the lab." Charlie was an enthusiast and he showed me around the lab, and it was very apparent to me, from the moment I stepped into the lab, that the techniques were of great interest and the main reason was that they were familiar. When people have talked about looking for the effects of marijuana, looking for behavioral effects of drugs, people would talk about a whole variety of things that generated information which was of an unfamiliar kind. Let me explain. In those days, a great deal of the classical pharmacology of the cardiovascular, respiratory, you name it, systems involved, the recording of events as for example, contraction of smooth muscles, usually on a smoke drum. The smoke drum would revolve and there would be levers and strings attaching and a tracing would be made on the drum. I was very familiar with dealing with information which came in the form of automatically made graphs in real time. And, in fact, I'd worked with droplet calls, for example, where you used to profuse rabbit ears and count the drops coming out.

Now, the lab that Charlie Ferster was showing me around was just full of recorders, recording in fact the pecking of pigeons. It was exactly along the lines that I was familiar with in physiology and pharmacology. It was immediately appealing as a method of studying behavioral effects of drugs. It was in the context of the pharmacology I was familiar with and it was love at first sight. Charlie was very enthusiastic. He was a very generous sort of person and he'd dug up some operators, so, for a week or two I used to go over there every day and we'd give a few drugs to the pigeons to see what they did, and then it was very apparent, from the very beginning, that things were happening. Now we could see them in the record. He managed to get some spare operators, which I took over to the medical school, a distance of about four or five miles. He gave me a lesson in real electricity and he gave me a whole lot of operators for pigeons. I didn't really want to work with pigeons, as they were quite unfamiliar, but that was what I got and that was all I had and, so, it was certainly a way of getting started. And he was a constant source of strength and help on the other end of the telephone. We used to have weekly Friday afternoon meetings, in which everybody took their part and I became part of the group very quickly. It was apparent from the very beginning that I was getting interesting results by injecting a variety of drugs. I started with phenobarbital. It's a nice short acting drug. You can give it every day without there being any tolerance or any change in its effect, and that made it possible to generate a dose-effect curve, and in fact, as early as that fall, I gave a paper at the meeting of the American Society of Pharmacology and Experimental Therapeutics, but it took me a little while to get around to actually writing a paper. The *Journal of Pharmacology and Experimental Therapeutics* was very particular about their papers.

JH: We still are. Did you have a hypothesis behind this, or some sort of guesses that led you to this distinction between the effects of schedules and drug interaction with that?

PD: No, I've never generated hypotheses. I followed Isaac Newton to not make hypotheses. I've been associated with and watched closely some of the most distinguished physiologists and pharmacologists of the generation, at work. I was in Gaddum's lab, and Feldberg was at Harvard for a time. I've known John Vane, closely, since he was a graduate student. I was across the corridor from Hubel and Wiesel when they were doing their classical work. I worked with Wiesel. None of these people were hypothesis-driven. It was always much more of, I wonder what will happen if we do this, if we introduce, if we manipulate this situation. Get a situation under a bit of control, so you will know what will happen if you don't do anything and you've got a good baseline, then intervene. I wonder what will happen. I wonder what will happen if you close the eye of a kitten, or I wonder what will happen if you perfuse these tissues with blood and stimulate nerves in another part of the body, as John Vane did. I think that in this field of science you find that most people are not hypothesis driven. I think that it's also true that statistics has very limited use in this sort of work. If you look at the classical papers of Dale, of Gaddum, of Feldberg, of Vane, of Hubel, of Wiesel you find a great paucity of statistics. I think, in this type of work, the best that statistics can do for you is to prevent you from thinking you've got something real, when it really is well within the limits of standard variation. I don't think you can prove that anything is there, no matter what your level of significance. All a high level of significance tells you is that it's not a random process, not to say that it's got anything to do with what you're doing. It could be something entirely different. So I think that hypothesis work and statistics played a relatively small part. I spent a year and a half of my life, in Rochester as a statistician. I'm not making a blanket condemnation of statistics. I think that there are important statistical problems, but they tend to be statistical problems and epidemiological problems, problems of that kind, very rarely experimental problems. I can really think of only one and that was Bernard Katz and his miniature end phytoderm series, and that was an application of statistics that was crucial and entirely appropriate and essential for the case, but it's the exception that proves the rule, I think.

JH: So, your feeling was more that if you could establish experimental control, then, you had, essentially, bypassed any use for statistics?

PD: You've got to be able to make a convincing case, I think, without statistics and, then, you may have to do some statistics to show that your convincing case is not fooling you.

JH: Right.

PD: But, the case has got to remain on the development of the experimental results themselves.

JH: Okay, so given that answer to the question of what were your hypotheses, I think you have a goal that you were striving at, too. Was there something that you were hoping to uncover, some general rules of drug action or certain classes of drugs, whether they were therapeutic drugs or something like that?

PD: It's very difficult to say anything more specific than that we were looking for things that made sense. The drugs that we used for psychotherapeutic purposes, I expected to have something in common in their pharmacology in pigeons and, later, in monkeys. But with the phenothiazines, for example, when they started to use them in psychotic disorders, I expected there would be similarities in their effects in a variety of species and, indeed, there were. I looked for generalizations about what one could say about the pharmacological effects of amphetamines. Amphetamine was a drug that was very reliable in its effects and very similar in a variety of species, and it gave one confidence that one was dealing with results of generality, and I was trying to make sense of it. I had to look at it for a coherent picture, rather than any particular theory at that stage of the game, and I still do to some extent, not necessarily having any neurological basis for what the effects were. I think that the situation has changed enormously in thirty years, enormously for the better. I think that most of the neurologizing in the fifties and before was largely gratuitous and just fooled people into thinking they were studying something which they really weren't. And, you know, I'm hopeful that we must keep going along these lines. I'm not happy with the state of affairs at the moment.

JH: Would you like to expand on that?

PD: Well, I feel as though it's very common in any branch of science that you have a period of tremendous revolution, the development of methods, a lot of people working in the field, and the field transforms itself in the space of a dozen years. And, then, somehow it sort of plateaus for awhile and people go on trying. You can't expect to keep that feverish pace of discovery forever and ever. Physics has had its periods; science has had its periods. I think that behavioral pharmacology has had a couple of spurts of extreme productivity and extreme change. I have a feeling that, at the moment, it's a little plateaued. I suspect that we need a discovery, in an unrelated branch, maybe, coming out of the neurochemistry or something of that kind that will start it off again on a new golden age, but I don't know what that's going to be.

JH: Well, in looking back, could you summarize what you might think of as your important contributions, at least as far as they affected you, that you feel were important for yourself or for the field?

PD: I think, without a doubt, the recognition that there was something that Skinner and Ferster called schedules that could control long sequences of behavior for long periods of time. And, even though this was a purely psychological behavioral device, if you will, it had the biological power to affect a purely biological, biochemical intervention such as giving a drug. I mean, even though it was not, primarily, a biological intervention, it had biological implications as was shown by the schedules being able to differentiate the effects of drugs. I still think this is an extremely important concept.

The appreciation of the power of schedules is still far from generally recognized as I think it should be. I think that a great number of daily human activities are basically schedule controlled, and they take place in the sequence they do and at the time they do and the intensity they do, because they are scheduled for the day. And I think that if we had some notion of how that was working, that might produce another golden age, not only in pharmacology, but also in behavioral science. These things go on over very long periods of time, you see. I worked with monkeys on twenty-four hour fixed intervals, for example. The whole twenty-four hour period is controlled by a single schedule. We've not any notion, whatsoever, of what the sort of new physiological process is that's involved in these extended time effects of schedules, no notion. We've no more notions, I think, than we had twenty-five years ago, and that's disappointing. It's learning, in a way, of course. It's learning, in the sense that it's through the operation of the schedule. The subject has got to go, quote, "I've been learning constantly where they are in the sequence"; otherwise, it's controlling the sequence of behavior, so, they've got to learn where they are. I think a lot of people think of learning as being something that most of the time you are not doing. Occasionally, you sit down and learn something. I don't see it that way at all. I think it's much more like writing continuously on a magnetic tape, and, then having some sort of process whereby the recording fades but is not obliterated, and if you record on the tape according to a schedule, regularly, over a period of time, then it becomes very firmly entrenched. I've got to believe that's molecular. I don't think it's primarily synapses. You've got to be writing something on a polymount and whether it's a protein or a nutrient, I don't know, but I think when somebody gets a notion of how the information is recorded, it could be a discovery that will have the same sort of effects as discoveries we've already had.

JH: You think, then, that the scheduled reinforcement is actually affecting the molecular biochemistry of the brain?

PD: Oh, absolutely. I think it's putting blips on the molecular coding of information, absolutely. And, I think it's also read back in a timely fashion so as to allow the schedule to control right or wrong sequences of behavior. This is purely speculation. Call that a hypothesis, if you will.

JH: I think I caught you on that one.

PD: I just can't conceive of it not being a polymount...

JH: The other sort of area that came out of your interest in the various schedules was the rate dependency hypothesis. Would you like to talk about it and how you feel which way it's going?

PD: I think that was simply a way of saying something about how schedules could control the effects of drugs. It started at a very modest sort of way. There were people who were studying behaviors in an animal that were clearly of different strengths, in the sense, that if we'd been doing it with a pigeon or a monkey, we would have said they had different rates. So you'd have an animal that would have this high rate under one set of circumstances, and then you'd introduce some variable, something to do with an electric shock, for example, that would change that rate. Everything else is the same. The subject is the same and the response is the same, but, now, you have two different rates. People would say, we'll put a drug in and they got a differential effect on these two components of behavior and they'd say, "Ah, ha, the drug is affecting the shock or it's affecting what the shock is doing to the animal". And I started by saying, "The simple fact that the subject is looking at different rates is, in itself, enough to occasion the difference in the effect of the drug". You must not jump to the conclusion that it's what you thought you were interested in. You've got to do a control for the rate, for the dependence of the effect of the drug on the rate of response itself. And that was a negative sort of thing at the time. It was an objection to people jumping to conclusions that I felt would have affected it. But, the more we looked around, the more instances we saw where over large ranges of different rates, one saw orderly relations in the effects of drugs. A lot of workers don't know amphetamine; amphetamine was a particularly good example, and it seemed to have great generality across species, across different types of response, and it was the first sort of generalization that we had. I don't think one ever thought that the rate itself was an independent variable that was doing this, but it was something that whatever it was that was controlling the rate, it was affected by the drug, and we never got very far in identifying what was back of it. But it was useful. You got such nice graphs.

The other thing that I think was, not my own contribution, but it came out of the lab during those years, was the manipulation of the electric shock, the use of it in such a way that it was a reinforcer, that you could maintain indefinite amounts of response and the only constraint was the occasional administration of a shock that we know was noxious because it would knock other behavior clear out. I think this is the importance of this line of work, which was developed, primarily, by Moss and Callahan. I think the importance of this is still not being recognized. There's a very strong tendency in the field to think that a positive reinforcer must have an effect on a positive reinforcement in a particular part of the brain. The fact is that you can get exactly the same sort of schedule control with a sharp wallop to the tail as you can from an electrode in the "rewarding" part of the brain and I don't think the full indication of that has really been appreciated in the field as yet. Sooner or later, it's got to be recognized, and people have got to reconcile their findings and their ideas with it. It is not a little gimmick; it's not a little trick. It's been seen in too many species by too many people under too many circumstances, and I think, again, it's something that we should be learning about, not trying to brush under the table.

JH: Do you think, Peter, that these kinds of approaches would lead you to try to look and see what kinds of schedules are controlling individuals who are depressed or psychotic? I mean, is it possible to take these kinds of conditions and try to see how they might be used to understand the therapeutic actions of drugs? Or do you think you're in a different domain?

PD: I do not think I'm in a different domain, and I think that the systematic application of schedules in therapy could be an extremely important contribution to therapy in the future, or certainly, combined with drugs, there's nothing incompatible about it, either. It's a very difficult area. The really good people who ventured into this field have had enough success to make me quite comfortable that if there was a widespread systematic effort by a lot of able people that there would be contributions, that it would help a great deal in the handling of psychotic people, as well as non-psychotic people with behavioral disorders. I'm thinking, particularly, of Charlie Ferster and his work with autistic children. It really was amazing what he was able to get autistic children to do, purely by using schedule controlling methods. These children who did nothing except damage themselves would engage in activities that were entirely normal, entirely appropriate to the contingencies that he was imposing. I think one could do that in mental hospitals on a very extensive scale. I'm not sure what Travis Thompson is doing at the present time, but Travis is a very ingenuous sort of person. I think he might very well be making a contribution. But, I think, really, you need hundreds of people.

JH: The recyclability, especially, of the approach that you began, in terms of drug actions on behavior and analyzing them, do you see yourself – as most of do – as the father of the field?

PD: Well, no, there were other people interested.

JH: One thing about it, how did they influence you or you influence them, then?

PD: Well, what has had the most influence on me was my long collaboration with Moss down the years. We've talked backwards and forwards about everything under the sun. We worked, surprisingly little together in the sense of doing the same experiment and publishing jointly, almost none. But, the reciprocal influence has been just immeasurably valuable. I've been influenced by Travis Thompson, I would say, in later years and a lot of the things that he's been doing. I've had good relations with Joe Brady, but I don't think we've influenced one another very much. I mean, I think Joe's got his own way and we've gone our own way. Those are the main people down the years.

I think, also, one way in which I may have influenced the field was sort of advantageous. At a federation meeting in the late fifties, I was approached by Howard Hunt and Lloyd Roth, both of whom I knew; they got me in a corner sort of at the back of a room and they said, "Lou Goodman says there should be more programs in behavioral pharmacology like that one at Harvard, and how about you coming to Chicago and starting one up?" And, I said, "Well, you know, I've got a program at Harvard and things are going well. If I move to Chicago, it'll still be only one program. You've got resources at Chicago; you've got a pharmacologist, Lloyd Roth there. He's interested. You've got Howard Hunt. He's interested in the program. Get your staff to collaborate together and put on a program and see whether you can find good students." And they went back, and the rest is history. From the very beginning, the very first students they got, fortunately, were very good students and they've had extremely profitable careers. So I feel as though I made a real contribution.

JH: Well, you made it into my life.

PD: I think I made a real contribution to double the number programs at that time. Lou Goodman was, also, a beneficial influence. Lou Goodman was a consultant to Smith, Kline & French (SK&F), as they were then called. There was a man called Len Cook at SK&F, who had the good fortune to apply the right test to chlorpromazine, one that showed it was an interesting drug. When Rhône-Poulenc tried to sell it, they tried to find an American company to take over the North American rights, and Merck Sharp & Dohme, and Lilly, all the major drug companies were approached, SK&F amongst them. Len Cook just did the right sort of test. It was, in fact, an opportune test, and he found that it was partly good luck involved, because he'd been studying SKF 525-A (ß-diethyl-aminoethyl diphenylpropylacetate hydrochloride), which was a drug that prolonged and intensified the effects of a variety of other agents by its metabolic effects. And, lo and behold, chlorpromazine did some of the same things as SKF 525-A, so he said, "This is interesting. Let's look at it." SK&F took the ride on chlorpromazine, and it was a very profitable move. They decided that they would go after other drugs of that kind. They gave Cook another position, essentially, and he recruited people for the next twenty years, maybe longer than that.

JH: There were large numbers of people that came through....

PD: And, they came through and did very good work and published. That was when Lou Goodman was very influential. Charlie Ferster was, also, a consultant for SK&F and he said that Lou Goodman used to beat on the table and say, "You came in kind of spoiled." There's a pharmacologist called Jack Strominger, who is known as Mr. Biochemical Pharmacology. He is the man that discovered the mechanism of action of penicillin. He was a medical student at Yale when Lou Goodman was at Yale. And, then, there's a paper in the literature on behavioral experiments done by Jack Strominger under Goodman's direction.

JH: I didn't know that.

PD: That must have been in the early fifties. He had an important influence.

JH: So, Peter, why don't we just start closing, unless you have some other things you want to say. I am just curious about what you are doing now and what your future plans are.

PD: I'm doing the most difficult thing I've ever done in my life. I knew when I started it that it would be a most difficult thing, and it's something I wouldn't have attempted in years gone by. It's been known that there are psychiatric problems amongst people with AIDS. At first, people were skeptical. They said, you know, you'd expect someone with a diagnosis like that to have psychiatric problems. At first, it was sort of dismissed, and then the pendulum swung, people started to find encephalopathies, and then they could see histological changes. The pendulum swung all the way; a very large proportion of people having behavioral deficits, even when they have no other symptoms. So everybody got very concerned about it, because all these airline pilots and policemen, and all these people who didn't know they had AIDS may have behavioral deficits. Well, where the matter rests now, as far as I'm concerned, is that people with no immunosuppressive symptoms don't show any behavioral deficits, but amongst the people in the later stages, usually with immunodeficiencies, there are substantial proportions that have a devastating psychiatric illness. I believe it's a relatively specific ailment; it's a psychosis, really, and it's got nothing to do with the psychological impact of the diagnosis. It's a genuine psychosis. And in the simian immunodeficiency virus which is so much like the human immunodeficiency virus, you can certainly get the same sort of neurological lesions in rhesus monkeys that you get in humans, and it seems to me that there's a good possibility that one could get psychotic monkeys as they develop their simian AIDS. So I've been following monkeys, in fact, with simian immunodeficiency virus, looking for behavioral changes. Now the importance of this is that HIV psychosis is a terrible thing and it makes the handling of the patients very difficult and it's an important problem in its own right. But another reason that I think it's an important line to pursue is that if it were possible to find a strain of virus that produces, say, psychosis in fifty percent, then one would have an experimental psychosis in a monkey to work with. You can't study schizophrenia in a rhesus monkey, because even if it has the same incidence in monkeys that it does in humans, it's a five percent lifetime incidence, something of that kind. You couldn't study that number if you wanted to, but if you get a psychosis that occurred in fifty percent of monkeys and study it, study some of the psychotic phenomena, then, you may have the very beginning of a way of studying psychoses in primates other than humans.

JH: Sounds like a good wise question.

PD: Now, because of the protracted nature of the disease, it's clearly a project that you could tell ahead of time, you're going to put years and years of work in your publication. And that's something that only somebody sort of at the end of his career can do these days. Indeed, I've studied it for about five years now, and I'm optimistic. I'll say no more. I'm optimistic that it's going to pay off, but it's been a hard job to keep everything under control from week after week, month after month.

JH: Sounds like a really fascinating project, Peter. It really does. It would be wonderful to have a psychotic monkey.

PD: Wouldn't it?

JH: On that terrible note, I guess we should end.

PD: Better than a psychotic monkey, a psychotic person.

JH: That was very nice, Peter.

EDWARD F. DOMINO

Interviewed by Christian J. Gillin
San Juan, Puerto Rico, December 11, 1995

CG: Hello. My name is Chris Gillin. I have the honor of interviewing Dr. Edward F. Domino,* Professor of Pharmacology at the University of Michigan. This is part of the ACNP Task Force on History. Dr. Domino has been one of the leading figures in American neuropharmacology, going back, Ed, I guess about thirty years now, isn't it?

ED: It's been a long time. I did my first work in clinical pharmacology in 1951.

CG: 1951.

ED: After I graduated from the University of Illinois as an MD, I really didn't know what to specialize in. I decided to take a rotating internship. Then I was offered a good deal when I was invited to be a part-time instructor in the pharmacology department at the University of Illinois Medical School. It was during my internship that I really got involved in clinical pharmacology. Prior to that, I worked on chlorpromazine in animals when it was not known as yet as chlorpromazine.

CG: Chlorpromazine wasn't even released at that time.

ED: It was a Rhône-Poulenc compound. My old professor, Klaus Unna, suggested I study it because Smith, Kline & French (SK&F) was considering it as an antiemetic. I had the job of working it up in animals, especially in dogs. I'd give them apomorphine alone and then with chlorpromazine. It had some obvious antiemetic effects.

CG: So, what was it that got you interested in neuropsychopharmacology?

ED: Believe it or not, it was nalorphine.

CG: Nalorphine.

ED: Nalorphine, that's right. Nalorphine was just being clinically developed at Lexington as a narcotic antagonist. Klaus Unna did all of the basic animal pharmacology on nalorphine, but never took it to man. Merck decided, for some reason, that they should temporarily stop further studies. It was decided a lot later to study it in humans. During my internship, I was on a cancer service where we had dozens of patients in great pain with inoperable cancer. We would usually give them morphine for their pain. We were working up a new experimental narcotic, called Dromoran, the l-isomer of which is now levorphanol. Dromoran is the racemic mixture. I ordered Dromoran for a woman who had disseminated breast cancer. Dr. Trout,

---

* Edward F. Domino was born in Chicago, Illinois in 1920, and graduated in medicine from the University of Illinois in 1951; he also gained a master's degree in pharmacology, becoming in 1952 an instructor in the Department of Pharmacology. In 1953 he moved to Ann Arbor, and was appointed instructor in pharmacology at the University of Michigan, serving as director of the neuropsychopharmacology research laboratory from 1966. He remained at Michigan for the rest of his career.

an internist, was the attending physician but it was my job to treat her. She needed a lot of narcotic medication because she was in severe pain. After a few days of therapy with Dromoran, I got an emergency call from the nurses that the patient was only breathing a few times per minute.

CG: That must have been scary.

ED: It was absolutely scary. I ran to see her. Sure enough, she had pinpoint pupils and was breathing very slowly. She was comatose so I had to ventilate her. It occurred to me that there was plenty of nalorphine in the dog lab at the University of Illinois Department of Pharmacology. I called my attending and said "I think I overdosed your patient with Dromoran. There is a treatment. It's just been published. As far as I know, the only source of the narcotic antagonist in the Chicago area is in the dog lab at the University of Illinois. The patient is terminal and has no relatives from whom to get permission." He said, "Well, if it works in dogs, it ought to work in people." I had a nurse call one of my colleagues in the Pharmacology Department and he came over with some nalorphine. The nurse gave me a syringe and I broke the vial of the sterile nalorphine and put it into the syringe. I then injected it into this comatose patient.

CG: Did that do the trick?

ED: Oh, did that do the trick! I tell you, it was remarkable! I'll never forget it. The woman was totally comatose. After I gave her the nalorphine, she started to breathe like this, "Ah, Hah, Ah, Hah." Shortly thereafter, she woke up. Then she started screaming in pain. Unbelievable! The nurses thought I was God. My attending thought I was God. I was obviously the Professor. That became my nickname. That did it!

CG: So, that was the event that really determined your new career?

ED: That was the event.

CG: I can see that it still has a lot of effect on you. That was an incredibly potent experience for you.

ED: It still is.

CG: To save a patient's life like that.

ED: Well, of course, I'm the one who almost did her in because of my stupidity. I didn't know drug metabolism. That's when I said, "Boy, I'd better learn some real pharmacology." What I didn't know at that time is that the liver is involved in the metabolism of narcotics through the P450 enzymes and glucuronide mechanisms. There's a complex story there. The bottom line is that my patient had disseminated carcinomatosis. She had a liver that was loaded with a breast cancer tumor and was in bad shape. Even though we were giving her therapeutic doses of the drug, they were just adding on accumulatively. I poisoned her but; in addition, I saved her life.

CG: So, where did you go after that? Did you go on with more clinical training?

ED: It was time to make a decision about what I was going to do with my life. I thought clinical pharmacology was a pretty great field. I also thought maybe anesthesiology was the field to work in. I had decided that although I liked OB/GYN, it involved too heavy a time commitment. All of my peers in clinical work, including my attendings at that time, were on a schedule every other night. The deal that I had at the time was as a part time intern at Presbyterian Hospital and part time instructor in pharmacology at the University of Illinois. Then I was offered a full time job as a pharmacology instructor. I was married. My wife and I had a couple of kids. Because of my family situation, I had to find a better job. In those days, the old Chicago Medical Center was in a very poor area. I'll never forget that when I came home one day my wife was crying. When I asked her what was the matter she said she wanted to leave immediately because there were mice in the building. My daughter was playing on the floor when a mouse ran by her. So I started looking for a job and I thought, "Well, I can't make any money as a resident. It's got to be in a field where I can make some money." In those days, as an intern I got zero dollars a month, and as a resident, the pay was twenty-five dollars a month. I figured to heck with that. So I decided to go into pharmacology. I looked for a job and that's when I came to the University of Michigan.

CG: And, you've been there ever since?

ED: Amazingly, I've stayed there ever since, even though it was originally only a one year job. When I was first interviewed, my old Chairman, Dr. Seevers, said, "Ed, if you're good and you can make it here I'll promote you to assistant professor. If you're no damn good, then in six or nine months I'll let you know and you're out here on the street at the end of the year." Fortunately, I made it.

CG: I think you did. How did things go after that? How did you get into neuropharmacology, as time went on?

ED: Dr. Seevers hired me particularly because I had electronic ability.

CG: You had been in the Navy before you went to medical school?

ED: Yes, I had been in the Navy during World War II and knew a lot about electronics. Because of my training in electronics, I got really good at handling such equipment. When I got out of the Navy, the reason I was hired in pharmacology at the University of Illinois was that I could put together an EEG machine. As a matter of interest, Bill Martin was also a graduate student with me as well as Eva Killam, then known as Eva King, and Keith Killam. The first day I started working at the University of Michigan in pharmacology, Dr. Seevers said to me that we ought to plan some things. I asked, "Well, what do you want me to do? What are my duties?" He said, "Well, number one, keep those darn medical students off my back." Of course he used other words. It turns out that the year before Mark Nickerson, who was a famous pharmacologist, had actually flunked about half the medical students in sophomore pharmacology. Dr. Seevers was upset because all those medical students had to take pharmacology over again. So that was my number one job, keeping those darn medical students off his back. Dr. Seevers said, "You don't have to be a good teacher, just good enough so that you don't get any complaints. I don't want to hear any bad things, okay." And then he said, "Your second job is to make me happy." I said, "Well, what does that mean?" He said, "Well, I'm your boss. As long as you don't have any money, I want you to do some of my research. What do you want to do research on?" I said "What do you want me to do?" He said, "I want you to work with the monkey colony." That's how I got started working with narcotics and monkey brain waves. My first introduction to research and neuropharmacology was with Klaus Unna and Carl Pfeiffer, then later with Dr. Seevers, working with drug dependant monkeys.

CG: Did you ever have a formal training program in research?

ED: The only research program I had was when I got a Master's Degree in pharmacology. That was a wonderful program.

CG: When you were at Michigan?

ED: No, at the University of Illinois. Carl Pfeiffer, again one of our ACNP members, liked to bring medical students into pharmacology. He used them as a means of teaching in the laboratories. We had a lot of student lab teaching. I was one of those students. Therefore, I got a Master's degree at the same time I got my MD degree at the University of Illinois.

CG: Today, we put a lot of emphasis on training, research fellowships, research training programs and so forth, but it sounds like you didn't really have the kind of intensive two or three year fellowship that most young people are encouraged to get now.

ED: The reason is that we were told to go in the laboratory and do something. Basically, it was learning from the more senior graduate students. My first job was to put together an EEG machine, and once it was working, to try to do something with it. Subsequently, I got involved with other graduate students. So I learned by hands on. We were told to go in the lab and do it, and if you can't make it in the lab, tough for you, out you go.

CG: Did you ever take a sabbatical or go away for any extended period of time?

ED: For many years I was unable to take a sabbatical because Dr. Seevers wanted me to be available to teach and to keep the medical students off his back. Eventually, I did take several sabbaticals. They were crucial to my career.

CG: Where did you go?

ED: For two of my sabbaticals, I went to the Lafayette Clinic, which was associated with Wayne State University in Detroit. It was the best research facility in the State of Michigan, competing with the University of Michigan Mental Health Institute in Ann Arbor. Dr. Jacques Gottlieb, who was then the head of the Lafayette Clinic, called Dr. Seevers and asked for suggestions for someone to help regarding drugs. As a result of a consultantship that was set up through Dr. Gottlieb and Dr. Seevers, I went to the Lafayette Clinic one day a week. Later on, it was two days a week. This association lasted for 25 years. I had a third sabbatical in Ann Arbor, working with geriatric patients. I was also working with phencyclidine, PCP, as an anesthetic agent in connection with Dr. Seevers, who was a consultant for the old Parke-Davis Company.

CG: What years are we talking about right now?

ED: The late 1950s, early 1960s.

CG: PCP came back a long time before in your own career, I guess.

ED: That agent had a big effect on me and my career. That's how I got involved with psychiatry during my association with the Lafayette Clinic. During my three sabbaticals, I accumulated quite a bit of clinical time. I also had some training in anesthesiology. So I ended up with a mixture of psychiatry, anesthesiology, and a little bit of geriatrics. However, I never worked in one discipline or specialty enough that I could get board certified except in Clinical Pharmacology. It was clear that I was deeply rooted in pharmacology and neuropharmacology and that's where I've stayed ever since.

CG: When you look back, who were the people who had the most influence in your own professional career?

ED: There's no question that first person to get me into research was Carl Pfeiffer at the University of Illinois when he hired me while I was still in medical school. Dr. Pfeiffer had a lot of wild theories that would motivate you to go into the lab and test them. Usually you'd prove them wrong, but maybe you'd come up with a new finding that was perhaps even more important than his original theory. The second person was Klaus Unna who gave me a tough time but was really my scientific mentor at the University of Illinois. He thought very scientifically. And then there was Dr. Seevers who was absolutely critical for me at the University of Michigan. Through him, I got to know Dr. Gottlieb of the Lafayette Clinic. I ended up with two laboratories. I was able to stay at Michigan and commute twice a week to the Lafayette Clinic. It was great. Although I had a rather low salary as a basic scientist in pharmacology at Michigan, I had a pretty good income from the work at the Lafayette Clinic. Because of the two salaries, when I was later offered chairmanships and other positions, I decided I was making more money in Ann Arbor and Detroit than what I could get anywhere else. So, over the years, that's where we stayed.

CG: Were there any other scientists, in particular, whose work you admired or emulated?

ED: Well, I would say a lot of the people in ACNP. One of them was Jonathan Cole and another was Frank Berger. There were a number of other people who were important, for example, Ralph Gerard.

CG: Also, from Michigan, right?

ED: Yes. He was originally at the University of Chicago. He came to Michigan to build up research at the Mental Health Research Institute (MHRI), which, incidentally, has grown into something beautiful. After Bernie Agranoff stepped down, Huda Akil and Sam Watson became co-directors.

CG: Again, ACNP members.

ED: You bet.

CG: When did you first get involved with the ACNP?

ED: Very early. I wasn't one of the charter members but I think it was about the second year that I was put on the list, probably because of recommendations from people like Carl Pfeiffer and Klaus Unna. So very quickly I was asked to become a member of this society.

CG: What was the first year you attended, do you recall?

ED: Oh, I attended the old Washington DC meetings.

CG: Was that early 1960, '61, '62, something like that?

ED: I think it was within a year after the society was formed when the meetings were held in Washington DC. I always get colds in December and whenever we'd have a meeting in Washington, I'd be sick; when we finally started having the meetings in San Juan that solved that problem.

CG: That made a lot of difference?

ED: A big difference, indeed. So over the years, my life has been very interesting. I've maintained my professorship at Michigan where I've been always given a rather free hand. The name of the game is, go find your own research money and then pay yourself. If you can pay yourself enough, you can do research rather than have an excessive teaching load.

CG: When you look back, what have your main contributions been? What are your main interests?

ED: My interests have always been in the field of neuropharmacology. I had a big problem selecting a research topic. I asked "What's important in the brain? If you get rid of it, what will happen to you?" I knew that if you overdose on agents like atropine you develop organic psychosis. On the other hand, if you take an overdose of a cholinesterase inhibitor, you can die. If you get botulinum poisoning, it will inhibit the release of acetylcholine and you may die. I decided that I should work on the cholinergic system because it is important to life and also to mental processes. That's how I got involved with acetylcholine and, eventually, with nicotine. That led me to the role of cholinergic mechanisms in arousal and sleep. I first studied cholinergic mechanisms in the cat, particularly rapid eye movement (REM) sleep. I always had an interest in doing something with humans and had an opportunity to do that at the Lafayette Clinic. Dr. Gottlieb said, "I don't want you to work with rats and monkeys unless there's a good reason. Mainly, you ought to be doing something with our schizophrenic patients." And that's how I got involved in doing a lot of sleep research with Don Caldwell studying schizophrenic patients.

CG: What other contributions are you proud of?

ED: I'm also proud of the work that I did with minor tranquilizers. I was involved a lot with those early developments.

CG: In the medical controversy?

ED: Yes. I really got beat up by Frank Berger. I was a young guy and he a real acknowledged leader in the field. I had a big argument with him over the advantages or disadvantages of meprobamate. Nevertheless, I was involved in the area of sedatives and did a lot of work. Over the years, I have been a survivor by working with my chairman and with my mentors. Very early I got involved in tetrahydrocannabinol (THC) research. During the Korean War, Dr. Seevers got a big Army contract. None of us knew what the compounds we were studying were until a graduate student friend of mine, Harry Hardman, got the empirical formula of the red looking oil which had no nitrogens. He went to our chemistry library to look it up. We thought it was a great tranquilizer. It was a great agent for treatment of war casualties because it produced a hibernation-like state. What we were studying turned out to be a synthetic red oil congener of THC, a marijuana derivative.

CG: THC wasn't recognized at that time, was it?

ED: No.

CG: That came about fifteen years later, I think.

ED: You're right. As a matter of fact, the derivatives that we were working with were the Roger Adams compounds from the University of Illinois in Urbana. I was an undergraduate student in Urbana majoring in chemical engineering. In the same department, they were working with these analogs of the active ingredient of marijuana. Later on, THC was isolated and chemically described by Mechoulam to be the active agent in marijuana. I ultimately did a lot of THC research. Over the years, I've been involved with a lot of compounds related to drug abuse. I don't view myself as an expert in drug abuse. It is a field that I stumbled into out of a more basic interest in cholinergic mechanisms. I ended up using nicotine and I'm still doing work on nicotine now. I'd say my contributions over the years have maybe not been as important as they should have. On the other hand, they've given me one heck of a lot of fun. I've worked in many areas and been involved with all kinds of clinical projects. I'm kind of proud of the ketamine story too. After PCP was rejected as a useful anesthetic compound, I did the first clinical pharmacology on prisoner volunteers at Jackson Prison using early review board protocols. That got me further interested in the field of clinical pharmacology and anesthesiology. I ended up over 10 years doing a lot of work in anesthesiology, as well.

CG: When the PCP epidemic came in in the mid to late 1970s, you got back into that?

ED: Yes, I got back into it. Who would have believed that a goofy compound like PCP would be abused? Obviously, it was and continued to be, although not that much these days. In any event, I got back into the PCP field with ketamine derivatives and from there into ς agonists and antagonist compounds. Basically, I have to survive and at the University of Michigan the name of the game was then and still is either you bring in grants or get out. Over the years, I've been able to bring in grants, but in a number of different areas. I guess if you can't be employed as a singer then maybe as a dancer, or as a comedian, or as an actor. I've moved from field to field but this has usually been necessitated by grant availability.

CG: Have you spent a lot of your time in the lab actually using either analytic techniques or animal models? It sounds like you've done a lot of work that would interface with a lot of human work.

ED: The animal work is a very important part of my activities. I am in a basic science biochemical pharmacology department but the animal facilities are very important. In fact, for years I had a very nice colony of monkeys with Parkinson's disease.

CG: You mean at this time?

ED: Yes. We're actually doing nicotine research this morning. It's a crazy idea, but we're looking at nicotine as a supplemental agent in treatment of Parkinson's disease. I called this morning to see how some of our monkeys are doing. They're doing great but the nicotine didn't work at all so maybe I'll up the dose. I also do some chemical work. At one time, you and I were actually going to the same GC-MS (gas chromatography – mass spectrometry) course. I got very much involved with chemical analytic work and did a lot with GC-MS of acetylcholine. That work was supported by NIMH for a long time. We did a lot with precursor substances. Most of them didn't work in our hands. So, I've been involved in chemical analytic and some animal work, usually rats, cats, dogs, or monkeys, and then human volunteers or, occasionally, patients.

CG: What about your students? How have they done?

ED: I'm proud of my students and post-docs. I've had something like twelve PhD students most of whom are associated with either pharmaceutical companies or with academic institutions. They're in a variety of fields and are doing very well. Michael Lasko, for example, is a professor and chairman of pharmacology, mainly interested in substance P and other agents involved in pain mechanisms. Lindsey Hough is another professor of pharmacology mainly interested in histamine. There was also Dick Rech, who is one of the best. I have had a large number of post-docs, mostly Japanese. One of the reasons I enjoy going to Japan often is that my former post docs are now the "big shots." Now I'm just a little professor here at Michigan and I go over to Japan and these guys are big professors. One of them, Dr. Shigeaki Matsuoka, was head of neurosurgery at UOEH in Kitakyushu, Japan. He once said to me, "Ed, I'm not number one neurosurgeon, I'm number two." I do go to Japan once or twice a year and interact with a lot of my post-docs over there. In fact, that's where we're now involved in a study with nicotine and tobacco smoking and PET. I just finished a study with tobacco smoking in PET on cerebral blood flow which was done in Akita, Japan at one of the major PET centers. Hopefully, we'll be continuing that area of research there.

CG: Have you done functional MRI studies?

ED: Functional MRI at Michigan is starting to take off. We've got all of the equipment, as we heard at the symposium last night. The University of Michigan is competing with your institution, by the way. All the equipment is there but you need about a half a million to really get the appropriate software. I've been talking with the people in the MRI facilities about moving ahead in that area. Right now, my interests are primarily with PET experiments. As I said, I also have a very nice colony of MPTP (1-methyl-4-phenyl-1, 2, 3, 6-tetrahydropyridine) monkeys, where we're looking at new dopamine agonists. I have a reputation in the pharmaceutical industry where they say, don't give Domino that compound because what I usually tell them is "Hey, this thing is as good as carbidopa-levodopa, but not any better." For about eight years now that we've been looking at many different anti-Parkinsonian drugs which are usually selective so-called D_1 vs selective D_2 types. So far, we haven't found anything better than the carbidopa-levodopa, I'm still active in that area.

CG: Where do you see that you're going now?

ED: I think it's more of the same. I have a number of grants both at the animal and the human level. I'm concentrating on two areas. One is clearly nicotinic mechanisms in brain function. The other is with new anti-Parkinsonian agents. With the monkey colony, we're looking at different selective

D_1, D_2, D_3, D_4, D_5 agonists. We need medicinal chemists in industry to develop more such agonists. I interact with a lot of drug companies but most of them are on tight budgets and not too many are developing such agents. We've got a very interesting story with D_1 plus D_2 additive or potentiating effects. In humans, we've found some very interesting gender differences.

CG: What was found?

ED: With an equal blood level of nicotine, our female tobacco smokers get a bigger "bang for the buck." They're getting EEG changes that are more dramatic at a lower plasma level than the males. On the other hand, the end effect is pretty much the same. From the point of view of plasma concentration, there appears to be a difference. I want to pursue gender differences not just from an EEG point of view. It is a very limited tool because it is only measuring the noise of the brain. Hence, I'm interesting in pursuing PET or other techniques.

CG: Ed, I'd like to turn to a little bit more of a personal level. I know your family has always been very important to you. How have you been able to balance your family with your very busy professional life?

ED: Well, it's been quite a life! I have a superb wife, Toni, and she's maintained me. I've got a lot of energy. I'm not sure where I get it but I guess my dad was the same way. Our family started to grow and we now have a total of five kids and ten grandchildren. The bottom line is that my wife always saw to it that I was a dad first and that I was around whenever I needed to be. So even with out of town meeting such as this, if there was something important going on with the kids, I had to be there. Otherwise, my wife would really raise heck with me. Basically, the kids are doing great.

CG: I know one of your sons is a psychiatrist.

ED: That's Larry who's the oldest. He's getting a very good reputation in the State of Michigan as a forensic psychiatrist. He has an interest in psychopharmacology but more in clinical psychiatry. My two daughters are in anesthesiology. My older daughter, Karen, is an associate professor of anesthesiology at the University of Washington in Seattle. My younger daughter, Debra, is an assistant professor of anesthesiology at Washington University in St. Louis. My youngest son, Steve is an MD/PhD and has finished his residency in OB/GYN. He is learning how to knock out genes so that he can get a position as an assistant professor in OB/GYN at the University of Michigan. My middle son, Ken, is a computer expert. He may be the cleverest of all of them. While the rest of the children are killing themselves with heavy clinical work loads, he's able to maintain his own schedule and do some very sophisticated computer work.

CG: Do you have any strong interests outside of your work and family?

ED: I do a lot of photography. I enjoy travel, which I usually do with my wife. Basically, we're just enjoying life. It's been a lot of fun.

CG: Did you come from an academic background?

ED: Not at all.

CG: Where did you get your interest and drive in science, learning and education?

ED: From my mother and father. They were both from Poland. My dad was a barber. When they came to this country, my mother could barely speak English, my dad only very broken English. While I was growing up, I could only speak Polish because that's all we spoke at home. When I went to grammar school, I could only speak Polish. I told my mother, "You know, I can't speak good English. I'm a little kid and I'm having trouble at school. They call me Dum Dum." That day my mother said, "From now on, we speak only English at home." And, that's how I got good in English. Both of them felt very strongly that I had to go to college. They told me, "In America, you've got to go to school." And, that's what I did.

CG: Did you have brothers and sisters?

ED: I have one brother. He's working for United Airlines. He's one of the senior experts on jet engines. In fact, if you fly on United, he's responsible for the 747's. He does a good job.

CG: I hope so.

ED: I have a great sister, who is taking care of her family at home in Chicago.

CG: And, finally, where do you see the field of neuropharmacology going? Where do you think we'll be 5, 10, 15, 20 years from now?

ED: First of all, pharmacology comes from "pharmacon," that's drug, and "ology," the science. So to be a pharmacologist, you better keep the drug in mind. I'm very concerned that over the years too many of our younger people haven't been keeping the drug in mind. This is the key thing. And neuro, of course, refers to the nervous system. I believe that neuropharmacology is going to blossom even more. But, we have to take techniques from all of the scientific disciplines. Right now, we're taking all we can from molecular biology. That's the beauty of pharmacology. You can study the drug molecule and its molecular interactions. You go all the way from animals to patients. Questions that come up as a result of patient data require more data from animals, etc., then to the molecular events. It really takes in the whole circle of activity. Most importantly, it gives you the perspective that, ultimately, your interest is in humans. I feel that right now we're going through a phase in which we all have to learn a lot more molecular biologic techniques and use them. Ultimately, our field is going to become even bigger and better. We need to train more generalists and specialists in their own areas. You've got to go deep in your area but, at the same time, you've got to have the big picture of where this all fits. You've got to have interactions in the clinic. I feel very strongly that those who are strictly in a basic science area have to relate to what's happening in patients and, then, back again into the basic science laboratory. I see the field as really improving. Would I be doing what I am now if I were starting all over again? I think I would but I'd do things a little bit differently. I'd probably start by doing a combined MD/PhD program and I certainly would want to be board certified in a clinical specialty such as neurology or anesthesiology. I'd probably end up doing what I'm doing right now, except that I'd have a clinical appointment as well as a basic science appointment.

CG: If you were starting right now, what kind of training would you get?

ED: I would get all the chemistry I could. I'm convinced that you should start with high school chemistry and continue to get as much training as possible. Then go to a good medical school.

CG: What would your PhD degree be in?

ED: Oh, no question; pharmacology.

CG: Would it be molecular or genetic pharmacology, neuropharmacology?

ED: I don't know but I would end up in pharmacology regarding the brain, heart, or whatever. It's interesting that most of my kids are interested in these different areas and I am still too. You can get me just as excited talking about what's going on in the field of OB/GYN as in internal medicine, or anything else. I could also end up in psychiatry, but it would not be the psychiatry of the kind I knew, which was psychoanalytic. It would certainly be more biologically oriented. I would also be a darn good clinician. I am convinced that if you're going to get your MD, you'd better be a good clinician. Equally, you'd better be good in one basic science field and try to combine them. Whether one would be a specialist in only one or in combined disciplines would be up to the individual.

CG: Well, thank you very much, Ed. Any further things you'd like to add before we close?

ED: Well, I'm having a heck of a good time enjoying the meetings and learning all I can.

CG: One of the things that have always impressed me about you is your enormous enthusiasm and great eloquence at times. You always show great excitement in whatever you're doing and bring great joy to everyone you come into contact with. Ed, thank you so much.

ED: Thanks a lot.

LOUIS C. LASAGNA

Interviewed by Donald F. Klein
San Juan, Puerto Rico, December 10, 1996

DK: I am Donald Klein and I'm interviewing Dr. Louis Lasagna,* and if you will start by telling us something about you, your background and what training you have had?

LL: Well, I originally trained as an internist, and then went for a post-doctoral, a couple of years, to Johns Hopkins, where I for the most part did animal pharmacology. Then I was deeded over by the Public Health Service, in which I had a commission to work on an army project for Harry Beecher, who was head of anesthesia at the Massachusetts General Hospital. I was there for two years, and that's when I first started doing clinical pharmacological research. After that I went back to Johns Hopkins and started a division of clinical pharmacology.

DK: If you could tell us a bit more about your experience with Beecher, because that sounds very crucial.

LL: Yeah, that's how I really got into the whole psychopharmacologic area. I was fascinated by the work his group was doing on pain, because it seemed to me to be opening up the whole area of subjective responses, which had been deemed in the past to be beyond the ken of most people. How could you possibly know whether anybody had pain or not? He showed that if you used proper controls you could, in fact, quantify pain by relying on subjective responses, and I think that ultimately led to where we are today, where we had no qualms about trying to measure anxiety or depression, things that are not, quote, objective, unquote. So his interest in subjective responses, plus his interest in controlled trials and placebos, really got me started.

DK: That was pretty moving, wasn't it, the whole bit about controlled trials, placebos?

LL: Yes, actually, controlled trials had come into view, in modern times, at least, with the trials in the United Kingdom in the 1940s, I remember, on streptomycin and tuberculosis. It was after that that people began to realize that perhaps one needed controls of one sort or another, and one needed randomization, and things that we now accept as routine, which were not at all routine then.

---

* Louis Lasagna was born in New York City, New York in 1923 and received his MD from Columbia University in 1947. After training at Maimonides Hospital in internal medicine, he accepted a staff appointment in pharmacology at Johns Hopkins University in 1950, founding the clinical pharmacology program there several years later. In 1970 he became chairman of the pharmacology department at the University of Rochester, and in 1984 Dean of the Sackler School of Graduate Biomedical Sciences at Tufts University, serving simultaneously as professor of psychiatry and of pharmacology. Lasagna died in 2003.

DK: This was about when?

LL: In the 1940s is when it started, and I began in the early 1950s.

DK: So that was less than half a century ago, and things have really changed enormously.

LL: Yes, indeed.

DK: So, after you left Beecher and Mass General, you went back to Hopkins?

LL: I went there and started the division of clinical pharmacology and really spent sixteen years there doing research and training people for careers in clinical pharmacology. From there, I went to the University of Rochester, where I was Chairman of pharmacology and toxicology, but also had a sort of division of clinical pharmacology during the entire fourteen years that I was there.

DK: When you say clinical pharmacology, that in itself was a whole new development, wasn't it?

LL: Yes, indeed. That description, I think, harks back to probably Harry Gold and the people at Cornell Medical College, who began publishing what they called their Conferences on Therapy. It was there where one began to read about such things as placebos.

DK: So, when you say you were head of the division of clinical pharmacology, were there any other divisions of clinical pharmacology?

LL: When I started, there weren't, but within the next decade, groups sprang up in Kansas, in Nashville, in San Francisco, and following those, the discipline really got rolling in Europe where the Swedes and the Brits actually have done the best, in my view, in supporting the discipline by having chairs of clinical pharmacology, an infrastructure to support them, which we've never really had in this country, which I think is not a credit to us.

DK: Do you have any guesses why they were more successful in doing that than we were?

LL: I think they became convinced that clinical pharmacology was essential. In this country, I would submit that to this day, academia doesn't consider it essential. Where clinical pharmacology is considered essential, in my view, is within the pharmaceutical industry and the Food and Drug Administration, where it's the life blood of everything they do; but in academia, for instance, if a charismatic leader in clinical pharmacology retires or goes to another institution, the institution doesn't act the way it would if their head hematologist left or their head oncologist left. Then they would say, "We must replace this person," but that isn't necessarily the attitude in clinical pharmacology.

DK: A throw down to clinical pharmacology. So anyways, you were at Hopkins before you went to Rochester. What was the area of your involvement then?

LL: Well, I started doing research on pain in the early 1950s and I continued to do research on pain through, I would say, 1984, when I left Rochester to become a Dean at Tufts Medical School in Boston. But I also got interested in hypnotic studies, research with the newer psychotherapeutics agents that were coming along, like the major tranquilizers, the major antidepressants. I began to do work on Attention Deficit Disorder and the Hyperkinetic Syndrome in children, studying stimulants in that area. What I'm saying is that I began to broaden out as I became interested in applying the principles of controlled trials in almost any area where they were required.

DK: And, the move to Rochester, was that an amicable move?

LL: Well, when I moved to Rochester, I acquired new responsibilities, because prior to that time I'd never had the responsibility of teaching medical students all of their pharmacology. So that was in a sense a distraction, but on the other hand, an opportunity to bring to the teaching of second year pharmacology what often didn't happen, which was emphasizing the relevance of animal data, for example, to human experience.

DK: Was that sort of the first time that somebody who was really a clinical pharmacologist became the head of a department of pharmacology?

LL: That's a good question. It may well have been. I'm trying to think of other situations where that had occurred and I don't believe it had happened before that, nor has it happened very much since, I might say.

DK: I remember that when I went to Columbia in 1976, that bringing in a Director of a department of clinical pharmacology was scotched by the pharmacology department.

LL: Yeah, and things haven't gotten any better with the accent these days on molecular biology and cellular biology, so that these days, as you know, it's hard to tell what basic science department you're in any more. It's as if all one needs is an institute of cellular or molecular biology, which makes it even harder to sell the notion that a clinical pharmacologist ought to be head of a department of basic science.

DK: And, at Rochester, you said you got new responsibilities about teaching. What else did you do there?

LL: Well, I continued to train people for careers in clinical pharmacology. It's been my great pleasure over the years to have had recruits to this discipline from, I don't know, maybe twenty-five countries around the world. I think we had one of the best groups in the world with regard to training people as generalist clinical pharmacologists. I always thought that it was important for them to be generalists, rather than to be only cardiovascular clinical pharmacologists or only infectious disease clinical pharmacologists, because I thought that any academic medical center really needed

generalist clinical pharmacologists, on the one hand, to be the therapeutic conscience in the institution, and, then on the other hand, to give
advice about the economics of drug utilization.

DK: That's something that you considerably got interested in, the economics
and the institutionalization of it.

LL: Yes.

DK: Didn't you start a group at Rochester on that?

LL: Twenty years ago this year, we celebrated the twentieth anniversary of
the founding of the Center for the Study of Drug Development, which
began with the hope that by acquiring information on drug development
and drug regulation, the quality of the national and international debate
about drug development and drug regulation would rise from the rather
low level of which it existed in the past; wherein the various characters in
the drama, sort of most of the time, threw harpoons at one another and
criticized one another without really having any factual basis on which to
base those criticisms. I would say that over the years we have contributed to raising that debate. We have gotten good data on how much it
costs to bring a new chemical entity to the market. We've got information
on delays in moving from one country to another, and while, Lord knows,
we haven't solved all the problems, I think we have called to the public's
attention the need for doing a better job at bringing new chemical entities
to market.

DK: But that put you in something of a critical role in regard to both industry
and FDA, though?

LL: Yes, as a matter of fact, Walter Modell, the first editor of *Clinical
Pharmacology and Therapeutics*, and I were the witnesses back in the
early 1960s that were really responsible for the ultimate language, some
of the ultimate language of the Kefauver-Harris amendments to the Food
and Drug Act, specifically that part that talked about the need for adequate and well controlled trials, because prior to that time, we felt that
the regulatory system and the drug development system had not really
appreciated the progress that had been made in what constituted persuasive evidence with regard to drug efficacy.

DK: So, with that Act, it really changed the whole practice of the pharmaceutical industry. and maybe, in many ways, gave us a lot of contrasts that we
wouldn't have otherwise.

LL: Yes, because prior to that time, legally, the government could only require
evidence on safety. In fact, of course, the companies did have some
evidence on efficacy, because, otherwise, how could they promote a
compound without having some idea about what it was good for? But
after 1962, one suddenly had to provide the regulatory agency with really

persuasive reproducible data on both safety and efficacy and it revolutionized the whole scene.

DK: Actually, there's been sort of a swing against that idea recently, hasn't there? Some more conservative forces have argued that we should just go back to safety.

LL: Yes, I've testified before Congress and had the subcommittee chairman ask me, couldn't we go back to the old days? Couldn't we really demand data on safety and let the marketplace decide about the rest? I'm not persuaded that the people either want or need that, so I don't believe we're going to go back to that point. On the other hand, I must say I spend a lot of my time these days trying to persuade people that controlled trials are the only way to get information that's reliable about drugs. For example, the naturalistic study of medicines, a term that I have used for some years now, I think is very important as a complement to the clinical trial data, because, as you know, the clinical trial situation is really a hothouse atmosphere, because you have relatively skilled physicians dealing with rather circumscribed populations that don't have multiple diseases, aren't taking multiple drugs and, then, the drug is marketed and everything changes. You have physicians of varying degrees of experience treating patients with multiple diseases and multiple drugs and the situation might well be expected to be quite different after registration and before registration. For instance, only by doing pharmacoepidemiologic studies do you find out, for example, that a drug that looked terrific in the controlled trial arena in fact isn't terrific, because patients won't take the medication.

One of the fathers of the controlled trial was A. Bradford Hill, who was the statistician in Britain and was involved in those first streptomycin studies, and, he, thirty years ago, in the Heberden oration given in Britain, pointed out that we still don't tell the doctor what the doctor wants to know about a drug. That is, who is it good for? Is it better for Mr. Jones to have this drug or the one that's already been on the market, or how do you pick the best drug for Ms. Smith in advance of trial and error? We're spending very little energy today, as he was criticizing us for doing back thirty years ago, on what one might call the fine tuning of drug prescribing, where you don't treat people as if they're average people, because nobody is an average person, but you individualize a treatment. I would say that that represents one of the great challenges still remaining before us.

DK: So Bradford Hill had a big impact on you?

LL: Oh yes, he and Harry Beecher were the two people that, I think, had the greatest impact on me, because Bradford Hill was a statistician who talked in a way that non-statisticians could understand.

DK: What an angel!

LL: Yes.

DK: In terms of your own contributions to the field, do you have any favorites?

LL: Well, I'd say the work we did, reminding people of the importance of the placebo phenomenon is something that I'm pleased with, and I'm pleased with our contribution to analgesic methodology because that required some doing after Beecher had started the field. I'm proud of the fact that we, like others, contributed to a destruction of the old concept that the morphine molecule was sacrosanct and you couldn't diddle with it, because you'd lose all activity; and by controlled trials, just plain experience, it was demonstrated that that theory wasn't correct. You could chew away at the molecule and, not only not lose activity, but actually sometimes have more potent chemicals. I guess that, plus two other things I would add: one is, selling the notion of controlled trials, and then, setting up a unique center to study drug development and drug regulation.

DK: That really is unique. I mean, has anyone else?

LL: Well, there's a Centre for Medicines Research in Britain, a man named Stuart Walker had started after we did, and that's quite successful. And, then, there's very recently been a new group started by Dr. Peck, who used to be at the Food and Drug Administration, at Washington University, but that's it.

DK: In terms of your own professional career, after Rochester, I think you wanted to become, I think, a Dean?

LL: Well, I found myself, after ten years of being a department chairman, being more or less persuaded that I had done about as much good or as much harm as I could do to that department, and I was getting bored with it and thought, well, what else could I do? I also had resigned my Chair after ten years but stayed on in the department, and I realized after awhile that that was big mistake, because the department was torn apart by loyalties to me, and loyalties to the new man, and I realized that having been a Chair, being retired, you really should get off the premises and Rochester wasn't clever enough to figure out something for me to do outside of the department. So I began to look for other things to do and also was attracted to the New England area, because most of my children lived in one of the states of New England; and I thought, well, somebody's got to do the Deaning in this world, and maybe it's what we do to pay back to science and society all the wonderful things we were able to do before we became a Dean.

DK: The Dean's job sounds worse than a Chairman's job nowadays.

LL: Well, I, fortunately, am not the real Dean, who is the Dean of the Medical School. I'm the Dean for Academic Affairs and the Dean for Scientific Affairs, which more or less makes me a minister without portfolio, and then, I'm the Dean of the Graduate School and all of those jobs are really a piece of cake compared to the Dean of the Medical School, who has unbelievable pressures on him. When I first went to Hopkins in the early 1950s, the Dean was also the Chairman of Physiology, because the Dean in those days had little to do besides recruit a new set of students who were entering class in September and deal with the curriculum. One year they would take a little free time from them and the next year they'd give them back the free time and there was none of this outreach to the community and dealing with affiliated hospitals and so forth. Today, I would say that the medical school deans in this country are probably the most underpaid professionals going.

DK: So, basically, you're pretty happy with the way things turned out for you?

LL: Yes, I've had a wonderful time. Sometimes students would come up to me and ask, would you do it all over again, and I say, in a minute, except that, of course, one couldn't do what I did over again today, because the scenario is so different. So many things have changed. I still believe that clinical pharmacology, in general, can be a very satisfying way of conducting a medical life, so I don't discourage people from entering the field. It's just that they have to face up to the fact that, in contrast to my early years when money was almost too easy to come by, now it's getting increasingly difficult to come by and the world is just tougher and harder in many ways.

DK: Do you have any feelings, given the tremendous advances in terms of molecular and sub-synaptic in pharmacology, that it's not what you were doing, in terms of clinical pharmacology?

LL: Well, I find myself very ambivalent about this cellular and molecular biology revolution. I continue to feel that we're more clever at identifying receptors, or at least sites where drugs attach, than we are in translating that into something that's clinically relevant. I hope we're not seduced away from empirical clinical evaluation of drugs, because as I said before, the theories about the morphine molecule turned out to be wrong in practice, and I believe that our notions, for example, about needing clean drugs that only attach to one receptor may not be valid at all. I don't want us to discourage cellular and molecular biological research, but I do believe that whatever we put into perspective and people ought to be, at least, more humble about it for the moment until we find out that combinatorial chemistry and all the other goodies that should be very helpful are shown to be helpful in practice. Thus far, I would say that the promise has not been met by the achievements.

DK: Do you have any ideas about the next five or ten years, what's likely to happen?

LL: Well, I think it's going to be a tough decade. As far as the pharmaceutical industry is concerned, they're faced with the need to come up with new drugs that are, if not breakthrough drugs, at least advances in some way over what's already available or the Health Maintenance Organizations (HMOs) and hospital pharmacology committees will not pay for them. The process of drug development continues to be excessively lengthy, ten to twelve years from discovery to marketing. It's getting more and more expensive to bring a new chemical onto the market, because you have all these dry holes that you dig, as well as the occasional gusher, and then you have what they call the cost of money, that is, what you could have been earning with your money if you'd invested in something giving you eight or nine percent interest. So, here, we have a lot of unmet challenges in medicine among the sick and a prospect of a lot of hostile factors that are going to make it hard to come up with drugs to meet those challenges. I don't think that means we should give up, but I think we do have to take a hard look at some of the axioms that one hears these days, like fourteen percent of our GNP is all that we can give to health. Well, I don't know that it's all that we can give to health, or that the drug bill is too high, for example. I'm not sure that those experiments that have been tried in other countries that try to cut down on drug costs have necessarily cut down on health care costs. So I see a difficult and tricky decade ahead, which I hope we'll continue to see the survival of the pharmaceutical industry and the survival of the research enterprise of America, which is one of the glories of the planet.

DK: I'm not sure of that one. Thank you very much, Lou

LL: Thank you.

LARRY STEIN

Interviewed by Arvid Carlsson
San Juan, Puerto Rico, December 13, 1995

AC: I am Arvid Carlsson from the University of Gothenburg, Sweden and I have the great pleasure to interview my old friend, Doctor Larry Stein.* Doctor Stein is professor and chairman of the Department of Pharmacology, University of California at Irvine. The question I would like to start with Larry, is how you got into the area of CNS pharmacology, and which area has been most important for you?

LS: That is a frequent question, because my formal training was in psychology and behavior. the pharmacology was more informally acquired after I had been out in the field and had a job. My first contact with drugs and finding out how wonderfully drugs can be used to analyze behavior was when I was drafted into the Army after my doctoral work at Iowa was completed. I had the good fortune to be assigned to the Walter Reed Army Institute of Research in Washington, DC, and my mentor there was Joe Brady. They were doing some very new things at Walter Reed, two of which particularly stimulated my interest, both then and throughout the entirety of my career. The first was that Joe and others at the institute were working with the then-exciting new drugs, reserpine and chlorpromazine, and were starting to describe their behavioral effects. And secondly, Joe's laboratory was the first to confirm the very important discovery of James Olds and Peter Milner that one could electrically stimulate the brain to produce reward effects. Specifically, Olds found that animals would work very hard to self-stimulate certain points in their own brains. Incidentally, it was Joe Brady who coined the term "self-stimulation" at that time.

AC: Yes, this concept of reward was new, entirely new at the time, wasn't it? The whole idea that there is in the brain a system that operates to give us reward for what we are doing, wasn't that entirely new?

LS: Yes, although it seems perfectly obvious now, since anything we can experience or feel is currently thought to be a result of brain activity. So it must be the case that if we can feel the reward, then the brain must be responsible for producing it. But the theories of positive reinforcement popular at that time were based in part on Freudian theory. Freud held the Victorian idea that reward is not so much excited by hedonically positive or pleasurable stimulation, but rather that it consists mainly in

* Larry Stein was born in New York City, New York in 1931 and received his PhD in psychology at the University of Iowa in 1955. After a stint at Walter Reed Army Institute for Research and the VA system in the late 1950s, he joined Wyeth Laboratories in 1959 as a research scientist, staying there until 1979, when he became professor of pharmacology and head of the department at the University of California, Irvine.

the reduction of pain, or satisfaction of drives such as hunger. Thus, most psychologists at that time favored drive-reduction theories of reward with the implication that reward was mediated by decreases in brain activity. According to these theories, it should have been impossible to electrically excite the brain and produce reward until James Olds' discovery.

AC: One thing I would like to ask here. Olds, of course, discovered this, but did he really go into the enormous potential of this in terms of pharmacology?

LS: Yes, Olds did many of the early pharmacology studies, and discovered, for example, that chlorpromazine had quite selective reward-diminishing effects at doses that did not significantly impair motor behavior. But he left a little segment of work for me. I will always appreciate Professor Olds for always using a little bit too high a dose when he studied amphetamine. He found that high doses of amphetamine, like all effective doses of chlorpromazine, will diminish reward effects. I was able to discover, by coming down in dose, that amphetamine's very large reward-augmenting effects can readily be displayed. This finding opened up this little career of mine.

AC: That is an understatement. And also, I would guess that you must have been more or less the pioneer of the area of drug development using these techniques, or what do you say? I mean, that you are the one that really pioneered this, isn't that true?

LS: I was one of the early workers, and I think that it is fair to say that I was there at the time that we investigators were making up the field as we went along. But it would be taking too much credit to make me the pioneer of behavioral pharmacology. I would think that it was such people as Joe Brady and Peter Dews and a number of other investigators who first understood how nicely behavior and drugs go together. In contrast, electrophysiology and drugs didn't quite seem to go as nicely together. It's almost as though drugs cut along the analytical lines of behavior in a very deep way. The chemical theory of neurotransmission was not so old at this time. But now, and in large part from your own efforts, Dr. Carlsson, we understand that messages are communicated in the brain by means of chemical transmitters. Thus, if one manipulates the brain's chemical messaging system with drugs, it just makes very plausible sense that one can readily manipulate behavior.

AC: Yes, and this is how I understand your contributions in this area that you bring in the concept of chemical transmission into your thinking at the very, very early stages.

LS: Yes. I guess both of us were influenced by the early powerfully simplifying ideas of Bernard Brodie.

AC: Yes.

LS: Who dared to think that with as complicated an organ as the brain, the functions can be analyzed in terms of the actions and interactions of a small handful of neurotransmitters? This was just a wonderful and simplifying idea to be pushed as far as it would go. It is astonishing, I think, how far that simplifying idea can be pursued. Obviously in a complicated system such as the brain, everybody understands that it is a gross simplification. But how do you make progress unless you start with a simple alphabet and build from that, rather than start by being overwhelmed by the complexity?

AC: What you have brought up here I think is extremely interesting. Brodie was, of course, a very, very bright person, but he was really not at all burdened by too much knowledge about the brain. And he was so courageous to go right into it and to make this fantastic discovery that we have profited from so much; that was in a way, career. . . .

LS: Career openers?

AC: Career openers. That was very generous, in many ways, I must say. Not to digress, he was a very generous person.

LS: Yes, I think so. Just to return to this reward subject for a second (and to get just slightly historical and a little bit personal), when I left the Walter Reed I went to the VA Research Laboratories in Pittsburgh that were directed by a pharmacologist by the name of Amadeo Marrazzi. Another simplifier, Marrazzi had a simplΔe electrophysiological transcallosal system, and liked to analyze it, "Brodie-like," in terms of the interplay of a couple of important transmitters. And I developed with the secretary of the ACNP, Oakley Ray, who was my first post-doctoral student a sensitive self-stimulation technique where an animal traced out continuously its threshold for brain reinforcement. The rat operated two levers; one lever gave brain stimulations but the current came down in small steps with successive responses. When the current no longer was reinforcing, the animal would hit a second lever to reset the current back up to the original top reinforcing level. When plotted, the jagged edge of the reset curve (reflecting the sequence of reset currents) traced the approximate reward threshold. And, lo and behold, moderate doses of amphetamines lowered the threshold of reward, and chlorpromazine, the opposite partner, elevated the threshold for reward. Other CNS drugs, such as the anticholinergic agent scopolamine or the anesthetic pentobarbital, had negligible effects on reward thresholds. Because amphetamine was known to release catecholamines and chlorpromazine to block catecholamine receptors, these results opened up my catecholamine theory of brain stimulation reinforcement. And if one assumes that brain self-stimulation is not just an artifact, but, in fact, that the map of reward sites reveals the brain substrate for natural reinforcement, then these findings support a catecholamine theory of both natural and drug-induced reinforcement. This theory has been a theme in my research for a long period of time. And, although I have closely followed your work, I probably could have been more attentive and saved myself some time if I had featured your important advances in dopamine pharmacology at an earlier point than I am doing now.

AC: Tell me a little bit about how you got into this area of catecholamines, and a little bit more in detail what you have in mind when you mention dopamine here? Also, how you felt about the catecholamines when you started to focus on them?

LS: This is very much the Swedish connection. At the time that Oakley Ray and I were doing our studies with amphetamines and self-stimulation and trying to analyze the biochemical action of amphetamine, amphetamine's action was not connected so robustly to dopamine as it is now. And, indeed, there is a Nobel Prize winner, who will remain unnamed, who felt that amphetamine's behavioral actions were mediated in fact by serotonin. But this was in the early 1960s, and our best brain stimulation electrodes were located laterally in the hypothalamus in a structure called the medial forebrain bundle. Animals would work very hard to stimulate their lateral hypothalamus, and we also knew that they would work even harder for small currents if they had a little amphetamine. And then, lo and behold, in 1964, papers by Fuxe, Hökfelt and others appeared out of the Karolinska Institute showing these wonderful dopamine and norepinephrine fiber bundles running through the lateral hypothalamus on their way upstream to the limbic system and the neocortex. These fiber bundles were the obvious places where reward electrodes might be stimulating, and a light went on. It just seemed very possible that those electrical stimulations that were so highly rewarding for the rat were activating catecholamine fibers and splashing catecholamines onto their cellular targets in the brain. So, that was the catecholamine theory of reward, formulated in the early days before there were good pharmacological tools for differentiating noradrenaline effects from dopamine effects. So, as a young man, I sadly emphasized only noradrenaline and could have taken a cue from you, Arvid, and given dopamine its rightful place.

AC: Well, I must say in this context that that you were not the only one to put emphasis on norepinephrine to start with; as you remember, dopamine has been, how is it called in English?

LS: The precursor?

AC: No, no, well, it will come a little later. At any event, it took a long time for dopamine to come into glory. I mean, it was maybe ten years after the discovery of dopamine before people started to think that maybe there is something important about dopamine. So, what you had in mind was really quite in line with what people felt at that time.

LS: I had the advantage of doing an experiment in the early 1970s. I had moved from the VA to the drug industry, into a basic research job at Wyeth Laboratories. Curiously, Wyeth Laboratories did not make an explicit decision to hire a basic research psychopharmacologist to work in pure science. But this is what I wanted to do, and they were willing to support this activity, and indeed, they did so generously and I never had to worry about the funding of research for the many years I was there.

I had several collaborators at Wyeth, one of whom was Bruce Baxter, who did self-administration. In this type of experiment, the reinforcement is an injection of a drug (typically an intravenous injection) in place of the electrical brain stimulus. I realized that perhaps one way to settle the nasty little dopamine versus norepinephrine issue in the catecholamine reward theory was to offer a rat the dopamine receptor stimulant, apomorphine. You see, I knew that apomorphine treatments in dogs and in people can make them very sick and they throw up. Of course, the rats should not like apomorphine and should not self-administer this powerful dopamine receptor stimulant. So, one possible way to dispose of dopamine as a reward transmitter candidate was to test apomorphine in the self-administration experiment. I was so sure of the probable negative outcome of this experiment that, rather than troubling to set up the self-administration procedure in my own laboratory, we went downstairs into Bruce Baxter's lab.

By God, I can still remember vividly Bruce Baxter coming up to me one day very excited with the tracings, showing me that the rats loved to self-administer apomorphine! That was a very big, early hint that dopamine should get more prominence in the reward theory. And if we have a chance to discuss my more recent cellular work, dopamine comes to full glory in these cellular reinforcement experiments.

AC: So, let's do that for sure. Now, the name that I couldn't remember a little while ago, of course, was "Cinderella." Dopamine is the Cinderella of neuropharmacology.

.LS: But we know how Cinderella ended up.

AC: Well?

LS: She married the Prince.

AC: Yes. One thing that I think is kind of common in our work, yours and mine, is that we have focused on catecholamines, but then all of a sudden serotonin may show up. Tell me a little bit about how serotonin came into your work?

LS: Okay, again, I think, perhaps, we can flash back very briefly to that lit-
      tle diagram of Bernard Brodie and remember that the neuron that he
      drew (to represent the brain) had a serotonin input. I forget whether it
      was a plus sign or a minus sign, but I believe a minus sign, and it also
      had a norepinephrine input with the opposite sign. There was algebraic
      summation between these influences because these were antagonistic
      transmitters. And, the algebraic sum, or however the algebra went, deter-
      mined the neuron's behavior. So, this was the very simple theme when I
      started to consider my own theory of behavior. I needed to analyze the
      opposite paradigm to the reward paradigm, the so-called punishment
      paradigm, and the experimental work started with my collaborators at
      Wyeth Laboratories, Irving Geller and Joseph Seifter. These investiga-
      tors devised a "conflict" procedure to measure punishment effects and to
      explore the pharmacology of the punishment system. This research was
      of practical interest to Wyeth because the conflict test was an excellent
      psychopharmacology screening method for detecting the anti-anxiety
      actions of meprobamate and benzodiazepines. Indeed, it turned out to
      be a very powerful predictive tool. But there was not a lot of understand-
      ing yet of the underlying biochemistry of either meprobamate or benzo-
      diazepines. Then one day a paper appeared: Irv Kopin, I believe, was the
      senior author. My group, and other groups in Sweden, I think, then did
      related studies, all showing that the turnover of serotonin was markedly
      diminished by benzodiazepines. "Ah hah," I said, looking at the Kopin
      paper, "Isn't that interesting? If serotonin is the opposite number of cat-
      echolamines, which facilitate behavior through reward processes, then
      perhaps serotonin acts as the chemical brake which inhibits behavior
      through punishment processes. By reducing serotonin turnover, benzodi-
      azepines release the brake and disinhibit the conflict behavior."
          We evaluated this idea by testing a large number of different seroton-
      ergic agents in the conflict procedure. The results satisfied me that, in
      fact, an important component of this admittedly very complicated sero-
      tonin system is to mediate behaviorally-inhibitory effects through a pun-
      ishment mechanism. But with this background, it was quite surprising to
      me, Arvid, to see you pioneering the development of a novel antidepres-
      sant drug that increased serotonin activity by blockade of its reuptake. My
      simple little theory, based on the Brodie model, would have said, "Well,
      this drug of yours should rather have been a nice anxiety generating com-
      pound, hardly an antidepressant!" And so, it's a good lesson again to
      remember that the brain certainly possesses the necessary complexity to
      account for the complexity of behavior. We must, perhaps, analyze one
      factor at a time, and then try to study the interactions between different

factors, but we should always be prepared for surprises. And so, the question of serotonin's role in the action of antidepressants is, I think, a wonderful problem.

AC: But you were nearly right. I begin to sense that you found that serotonin and anxiety, the control of anxiety, are close to each other, somehow. Then you sort of turned it upside down, but still, you were pretty close, weren't you?

LS: Well, I think that there is a component of the serotonin system that is involved in punishment. Punishment, however, may be distinguished from anxiety, and so I am not sure if there aren't also some serotonin systems that might increase anxiety. Afterthought: interestingly the chief adverse effects of Prozac and other SSRIs include anxiety and nervousness. But I definitely think that serotonin acts generally as an inhibitor of behavior. There is serotonergic inhibition of sexual behavior and of aggression. There is serotonergic inhibition of feeding; thus, many good anorexics are serotonergic. So, there seems to be a theme that behavioral inhibition, not necessarily brain inhibition, but behavioral inhibition, may have a common serotonergic basis. And it would be a wonderful synthesis and resolution if there was some way to connect behavioral inhibition to antidepressant action.

AC: Yes. Larry, you have been in the area of mood control and you have been in the area of anxiety, so tell me a little bit about schizophrenia now.

LS: Oh yes, schizophrenia. Schizophrenia, of course, is the elephant that all the blind men put their hands on. To some, schizophrenia is like a snake when you grab the tail; to others, it's a wall when they press against the side. Schizophrenia is a fascinating problem and interesting experiment of nature in producing a distortion of some of the most important higher functions of the brain. Unfortunately, I don't think investigators have yet put their finger on, in a really precise way, what the fundamental deficit in schizophrenia is. I think we need a more insightful clinical and behavioral analysis of schizophrenia in order to move the pharmacological and biochemical analysis. Perhaps we should talk about some of the ideas we have already discussed in terms of potential fundamental deficits in schizophrenia.

The schizophrenic symptom that was particularly attractive to me, as one of the blind men with a career-long interest in reward, was anhedonia. This symptom, of course, is one of Bleuler's fundamental symptoms, and to me, the anhedonia immediately says impaired reward function. And so, shortly after the powerful catecholamine toxin, 6-hydroxydopamine was discovered, I got what I thought was a wonderful idea: Schizophrenia might be a neurodegenerative disease caused by an endogenous toxin, since it's a long-term disorder with a chronic downhill course in many cases. Again, the anhedonia was what I focused on as well as a lack of purposefulness in the behavior, in other words, I focused on that behavior and thinking as not goal-directed. All of this implied to me a degenerative disorder of the brain reinforcement system. Clinical observations of euphoria in early schizophrenia additionally suggested a paradoxical initial disease phase involving a toxic stimulation of catecholamine reward functions. Such catecholamine hyperactivity could explain the acute antipsychotic effects of phenothiazine drugs, which, of course, are dopamine blockers. Put another way, early psychosis may represent a reward system out of control. But I was mainly interested in the chronic, deteriorating, longer-term phase of schizophrenia and conceived the hypothesis that through some enzymatic error in the schizophrenic brain, certain dopamine and particularly norepinephrine neurons might secrete 6-hydroxydopamine rather than their natural transmitter.

6-hydroxydopamine is a very toxic material. Perhaps acting as a false transmitter or metabolic product, 6-hydroxydopamine would be taken back up into the catecholamine nerve ending and would destroy it. I had the audacity to write a little theoretical paper, which incidentally was considered only for two weeks in the editorial offices of *Science* before acceptance. The paper included some interesting experimental results: if we gave rats 6-hydroxydopamine intraventricularly, we produced a catatonia as well as big deficits in self-stimulation and other reward behaviors. And chlorpromazine, which was known to protect against the neuronal uptake of 6-hydroxydopamine, prevented these deficits. So there were several pieces of data here to propose a 6-hydroxydopamine theory of schizophrenia.

This publication gave me my fifteen minutes of fame. I was invited to speak everywhere, Arvid, but to my surprise, I quickly found out I was often invited to be criticized and to be shown wrong. I was still a relatively young man, and I believe what I didn't quite realize was that a lot of people looked at schizophrenia as a lifetime research occupation. They apparently were not ready for a solution at that time. In the early seventies, a solution to the schizophrenia problem might perhaps put an untimely end to many grants and research careers. And so, I traveled to many places and took heavy criticism for this audacious speculation. We also did some post-mortem work and discovered – consistent with the theory – some enzyme deficits in the brains of schizophrenics. These findings were not replicated, however, and I think there may be a lesson here for some of the work that we see in the meeting today. With the new brain imaging procedures, etc., whenever one has a new machine, a new tool, or a new method, inevitably one makes some comparative measurements on schizophrenics. Of course, by chance, some differences will appear, and these will get published. Then they have to be chased down later.

AC: Is there a possibility that through oxidation there could be formed some toxic metabolites of catecholamines? This is still an area, of course, that is quite active, even though, perhaps, the 6-hydroxydopamine pathway isn't so much looked upon now, but you have the oxidation pathway to form the very toxic quinones. And actually, we have in post-mortem brains of schizophrenics seen an elevation of these substances, so yes, you may have been right. Just like Brodie was right; although not exactly the way or not precisely in the sense that you formulate.

LS: Yes, and I think the other thing that is interesting along these lines is that the formation of neuromelanins may provide a protective pathway to dispose of these dangerous quinones. Incidentally, the names of the important catecholamine cell groups, the locus coeruleus (blue body) and the substantia nigra (black substance) are due to the neuromelanin content of these aggregates of dopamine and norepinephrine cell bodies.

AC: So, Larry, what do you think? Should we now move into what you are working on now, this fascinating work on what single cells can be doing in terms of reward and all that?

LS: Yes, that may be worth discussing, and this will take us into my current research. I begin by recognizing an important difference between voluntary and involuntary behavior. Only voluntary behavior can be controlled by rewards. This is because involuntary or reflex behavior is under the powerful and complete control of input stimulation; therefore, reflexes cannot be affected by rewarding outcomes or consequences. Reward processes permit successful behaviors to be built up and strengthened (reinforcement) and unsuccessful behaviors to be weakened or extinguished (non-reinforcement). Thus, these processes may have been decisive in the evolution of intelligent behavior.

Next, there is the very awkward question of the substrate of voluntary behavior. Most people think that complicated circuitries underlie all voluntary behavior; they assume, when the rat presses the lever that a lever-press circuit has fired off. But no one has yet found such a circuit, and I am not sure, if I were a young PhD student, that I would want to do a thesis where I had to identify such a circuit. In my opinion, current conceptions of how reward works are most unsatisfactory. These conceptions tend to emphasize the hedonic qualities of reward, and they assume, in effect, that the "good feelings" generated by rewards can somehow reorganize and strengthen response circuitries. So what we have here is a very casual, almost lay, type of notion.

And without tangible changes in behavioral circuitry to measure, how would one begin to assess the hedonic effects of reinforcement? After thinking about this difficult question for a long time, I found it useful to consider an alternative formulation. Incidentally, behavior is only arbitrarily broken into discrete responses; rather, like our stream of consciousness, behavior seems to flow continuously in constant interaction with the environment. If so, we may need a different conception of the behavioral substrate, perhaps some brain structure or more widespread collection of neurons that is spontaneously active. Such spontaneous neuronal activity could produce a continuous stream of behavior. If this idea were correct, then rewards might really act, not to rearrange brain circuitry, but instead to change the firing patterns of individual brain cells.

There is a way of testing such an idea. One could determine whether or not the activity of an individual neuron can be affected by reinforcement. Can one reward a neuron for, perhaps, firing off in a bursting pattern? The immediate difficulty is: how would one reward a brain cell? Our solution was based on the fact that cocaine is one of the most powerful pharmacological rewards known; the behavior of all animals tested, including humans, is reinforced by injections of this drug. Our cellular reinforcement experiments were performed in hippocampal slices to isolate the test neurons from the rest of the brain. We puffed minute injections of cocaine through the recording micropipette directly to the hippocampal cell whenever it performed the "correct" response, firing off in a bursting pattern. To our surprise, rates of bursting were progressively increased, not only by cocaine, but also by our good friend, the reinforcement transmitter dopamine. Dopamine was effective in a certain part of the hippocampus (CA_1), whereas opioids (such as dynorphin) seemed to be effective in a different part of the hippocampus (CA_3). Also, it was very significant that, just as in the case of whole-animal behavior, the burst-increasing effects of dopamine and dynorphin were observed to be "activity-dependent". Thus, the drugs increased rates of bursting only if given when the target cell had recently been actively bursting. If the cell had been firing in single spikes or was silent, then the microinjections were ineffective or even tended to suppress bursting rates.

AC: So, now you have some very intriguing evidence that a single cell can have a reinforcing mechanism. May I ask you a somewhat philosophical question? Do you think a single cell could have a mind?

LS: A mind? My own personal, perhaps unsophisticated, view on the mind-body question perhaps, being alluded to here is: how can objective things like the brain and its cellular activity be translated into subjective things, such as the mind. My own treatment of the brain-mind problem is to say that it's really a structure-function distinction. The mind should be thought of as a function of the brain, much as blood pressure is a function of the cardiovascular system. If this analogy is correct, then the fact that structure, brain, has functions, mind, is not a great puzzle and does not seem to constitute a philosophical dilemma. But I am not sure that everyone would be satisfied that subjective experience can be treated merely as a brain function, and thus solve the problem. However, if one accepts my definition, and if one also assumes that a neuron can exhibit a reinforcement function, then one might wish to assign a subjective correlate to that cellular function. If so – and I say this with some difficulty – then maybe a cell does have a mind! I see what you have tapped into here.

But all this makes me a little bit uncomfortable because I was brought up in a very behavioristic tradition; to me mind is almost a naughty word. Perhaps we should not be so rigid in our behaviorism and it may be time to consider seriously such concepts as mind and consciousness. Perhaps someday we can do the correct brain imaging and image the mind.

AC: That brings me to my last question. The area that you have pioneered has been considerably important for drug development, so from your perspective can you tell me a little bit about what do you think is going to happen, in terms of drug development, in the next, let's say, the next five years or so?

LS: Arvid, you do know how to ask difficult questions! I thought the question that was coming was: in this age of binding technology and molecular biology, what is the place of the older behavioral technologies which played such an important role in the development of many of our current drugs. Are we losing an important art with the somewhat diminishing interest in behavioral technologies? I do have a concern about that. Science follows fashions. Perhaps both of us can agree that the advances in molecular biology are wonderful and will help us to identify many of the receptors that we are interested in as academic pharmacologists. And in terms of practical drug development, molecular biology will produce some very interesting and wonderful natural protein hormones that might be advantageous. But molecular biology has to work with pharmacology to produce smaller molecules that might be useful as drugs which can be easily administered.

Maybe I shouldn't back off the question of new developments, but it's hard to confine oneself to a five-year time period because it takes so long to bring out a new drug. We still have a problem in the antidepressant field, where the drugs act too slowly, but fortunately, work such as yours with zimelidine has brought us a new class of antidepressant drugs that are largely free of many bothersome side effects. These side effects inhibited the use of antidepressants particularly in mild depressions because these patients are so fussy anyway, and if you poison them with anticholinergic and antihistamine effects and so forth, then they don't stay on their medications. And so, the selective serotonin reuptake inhibitors, I think, are producing a revolution in the treatment of mild depression.

After many years of looking for ever more specific dopamine blocking agents, the recent recognition that a relatively nonspecific agent, clozapine, may be more effective than other anti-schizophrenic drugs is interesting. The search for new clozapine-like agents should advance the treatment of schizophrenia. Also, there is a lot of interest now in the biology of memory. An increase in the elderly population makes the treatment of Alzheimer's disease, senility, and other important ailments of memory more pressing; indeed, in depression, memory deficits are a common and most troublesome symptom. Hopefully, we will soon see advances in memory enhancement by new drugs.

One of the most exciting new discoveries may move us a little bit out of psychopharmacology proper into a more generally metabolic area. I am very excited about the new protein, leptin, which controls feeding behavior and induces satiety. Leptin evidently is a protein signal from the fat deposits that tells you how much fat you have and how heavy you are. This signal is compared with the setting in the brain which tells you what your ideal weight is. If you have too much fat, you will release a lot of leptin; then, you will eat less. But if you are not quite fat enough and release too little leptin, then you will eat more. There also are effects of leptin on fat metabolism, temperature, blood sugar regulation, and so forth. So, in the area of feeding and weight control, a new hormone has been discovered with a target, very importantly, in the CNS. How it affects some of the other eating disorders, such as anorexia nervosa, may turn out to be very interesting.

AC: Well, thank you very much, Larry.

LS: Thank you so much, Professor Carlsson.

Clinical Scientists

ROBERT A. COHEN

Interviewed by Thomas A. Ban
Baltimore, Maryland, November.2, 2000

TB: It is November 2, 2000. I am Thomas Ban. We are in the house of Robert Cohen* in Baltimore to interview him for the archives of the American College of Neuropsychopharmacology. Could you tell us where and when were you born, something about your childhood, early interests and education?

RC: I was born in Chicago, and as I mentioned to you before we started this interview I was run over by a light truck at the age of ten and had a fracture of my femur very close to its head. The truck ran over my abdomen and I was in the hospital for ten weeks, something that would be impossible now. At first the doctors were quite concerned as to whether I would make it or not, but actually the only serious thing that happened was the fracture. After two weeks in the hospital it was clear that I was going to recover. But the recovery was rather slow and this hospital was the hospital in which I was born. The nurses and interns had spoiled me in the hospital. They spent a lot of time with me, joking with me, talking to me about various things. And by the time I left the hospital I decided that I wanted to be like them; so I began to think about how I could possibly become a doctor.

TB: How old were you when this happened, ten?

RC: Ten.

TB: So, it happened in 1919, right?

RC: My family was a typical family of that time. My grandparents had come to the United States from Prussia, around the 1880s. We were two boys and five girls, and like many other Jewish families the girls went to high school and the boys went to college. I knew that I was going to go to college from the time that I can remember. My mother had hoped that I would be a lawyer, but I rebelled and became a doctor. After graduating from high school I went for a year and a half to Crane Junior College, which was the Municipal College of Chicago. When I was admitted as a junior at the University of Chicago I registered for a new course in physiology, which was given by Ralph Gerard. Gerard had just come back from a National Research Council scholarship in Europe, where he had worked for six months with Dennis Hill measuring the speed of the nervous impulse.

---

* Robert A. Cohen was born in Chicago, Illinois in 1909, and received a PhD in physiology and a medical degree simultaneously in 1935 from the University of Chicago. He served at Chestnut Lodge Sanatorium in Rockville, Maryland, from 1947 to 1953, then until 1981 was a senior administrator at NIMH. Cohen died in 2009.

This was a fascinating course with no formal lectures. The first day, when Gerard had come into the laboratory to a relatively small group of about twenty students he was wearing a rather dilapidated lab coat with many acid holes in it, and smoking a big fat cigar, he asked us: "What is life?" And we began to try to give our answers to this unexpected question. And whatever we answered he asked: "how would you prove it?" Then he asked the students to criticize each other; that, to make a long story short, stirred up my interest. Looking back at it, he really opened a new world for me. In the laboratory we saw an assortment of animals. While he was moving around he got us talking and ultimately we had to choose our research project. There were two requirements. One, we had to get his permission to start it, and two we had to get his permission to stop it. My project was to measure the blood pressure of a frog. We made a little hemostat to register the blood pressure, then gave some adrenaline and found sometimes that the adrenaline made the blood pressure go down instead of up. We never found the answer why. We also found the paper by Roy Hoskins, which indicated that it could have something to do with the biochemical state of the nervous system at the time the adrenaline was given.

Gerard then became my counselor in my courses. In some way I feel grateful to him, because certainly what happened to me would not have happened with anyone else. But he also deprived me of an education because he advised me which courses to take. He decided that maybe one course of philosophy would be useful, so I had a course in philosophy. I had also a course in English history, because my father had been born in London, and I wanted to know something about English history. And I took one course in anthropology from Edwards Supeer, who was a distinguished anthropologist. All the rest were courses in science and languages, i.e., German and French, in order to get a PhD.

I finished the first year of medical school education before I graduated from college. During my first year of being in medical school, I had already taken many of the courses that my other colleagues were taking, so I began to do research then; Wade Marshall and I shared a laboratory. The people at Washington University had just demonstrated the shape of the nervous impulse and Wade was building a machine to reproduce that. And I was trying to see whether it was possible to restore conduction in nerves if one used a hydrogen acceptor rather than oxygen.

TB: Am I correct that we are in the early 1930s at the University of Chicago and that the findings of your research were to become your first paper?

RC: Yes. We demonstrated that it was possible to restore conduction with metadine (3-phenyl piperidine) and we published it in a paper.

TB: Do you remember the journal it was published in?

RC: Probably the *American Journal of Pharmacology*.

TB: And what did you do after that project?

RC: I became interested in studies of nerve metabolism and moved over from the laboratory that was on the east side of Gerard's office, to the metabolic laboratory on the west side of his office. There was a girl there that I was very attracted to, I must say, and she was also doing metabolic studies and between us we shared an apparatus. Mabel had it Monday, Wednesday and Friday and I had it Tuesday, Thursday and Saturday. And ultimately, in 1933, we got married. She was a year behind me in school, but we both finished at the same time in 1935. Let me go back for a moment. Before graduating I was seriously wondering whether I should get my medical degree. Nineteen-thirty-four was the depth of the Depression. But Dr. [Anton J.] Carlson, who was the Chairman of the Department of Physiology, strongly advised me to get my PhD in physiology and go on to complete my studies for an MD as well. Jobs were very hard to get in those years. Dr. Carlson was the President of the American Association of University Professors, and he thought that one would be better off having an MD and a PhD. One of the advantages of working for a PhD was that if you became an assistant that paid a thousand dollars a year, and the tuition in those days at a medical school was three hundred and seventy five dollars a year. So, when Mabel and I got married, we had an income of two thousand dollars a year and only seven hundred and fifty went to medical school. We could live very comfortably on twelve hundred and fifty dollars, which we did. We got through medical school owing the University only six hundred dollars at the end. Everything else was paid for.

One of the courses I assisted in was Dr. Nathaniel Kleitman's. About three years ago, Dr. Kleitman died; as you can imagine, he was one hundred and five years old. He was working on sleep. He and Aserinsky were the ones who described rapid eye movement (REM) sleep first. One day Dr. Kleitman told me to give the lecture on the physiology of behavior. I was able to read about everything that he recommended and in two hours I gave a digest of that. I thought at that time, well, wouldn't it be interesting if somehow or other we could do studies of brain metabolism in human beings, but I had no idea how this was going to come about. This caused me to look into psychiatry as a possible field where one might get involved in research. But the University of Chicago didn't have any psychiatry at that time. Roy Grinker was Assistant Professor of Neurology and the University had sent him to study psychiatry in Austria. He was analyzed in Vienna by Freud. He was to come back to the University and start the Department of Psychiatry. This is what he actually did, but he soon left the University and went to Michael Reese Hospital. He arrived at Michael Reese Hospital to take over the neurology service where I was an intern at the time. After his arrival all the members of the Neurology Department had resigned and Grinker took over the service and established his new Department of Psychiatry.

By the time I returned to Chicago from my internship, Margaret Wilson Gerard, the wife of Gerard, had been analyzed and became the first child analyst in Chicago. We had spoken to her and she recommended that I come East to get training in psychiatry. So I applied at Johns Hopkins where Adolf Meyer was the Professor and was accepted there. Mabel came as an intern at Baltimore City Hospital. We were thinking then of going back to Chicago after we finished our training. During that first year, we were going to the Medical Society meetings, and were fascinated by Dr Joseph Gesell's talk, and I thought that I ought to at least find out something about psychoanalysis. So, I decided that I'd leave Phipps Clinic and go to Sheppard Pratt Hospital where Dr. Gesell was a psychoanalyst. He was also a graduate of the Union Field Seminary and had a PhD in psychology. So I suggested to Mabel, who was thinking of internal medicine, that she ought to have at least a year also at Sheppard Pratt. We started out at Sheppard with some misgivings. Dr. Meyer was a little bit angry with me at first because I went to Sheppard Pratt. But then, when he would come as a consultant they always had me take him around. Later, he wrote me a letter saying that "we were sorry to lose you, but I see that you are not lost." We stayed at Sheppard Pratt a year and were planning to go to Chicago to continue analytic training. Back in Chicago I went to the Institute for Juvenile Research and Mabel went to Michael Reese Hospital. But we were troubled by the situation in Chicago, because there seemed to be a great deal of hostility between the two groups in psychiatry. The group in Washington seemed to be more congenial, so after a year, we came back to Sheppard Pratt Hospital.

I had joined the Naval Reserve. The recruiter from the Naval Reserve came around while I was at Hopkins and told us about the glories of serving in the Navy and said that if a war should start, they'll call the whole group so we would serve together and that seemed like the reasonable thing to do. But in July 1941, I got a letter from the Chief of Naval Operations asking me to report for duty at Norfolk Naval Hospital, in September of 1941. This was three months before the war started. It turned out that the Chief of the Psychiatric Service at Norfolk, Dr. Kennedy, became the Senior Psychiatrist in the Navy. So, this was in a sense a great opportunity for me. Lawrence [Coleman Kolb] whom I had known from Phipps Clinic, he was in neurology when I had been there, reported for duty a couple of months after I did. And Donald Dodge, who had been chief resident at New York Neurological reported for duty also. The three of us really had a marvelous year together. Our training was not very much, but each of us had had experiences that the others did not. And we got along extraordinarily well. We turned out a tremendous amount of work. It was on that basis that Dr. Kennedy, Chief of Psychiatry, assigned us to jobs that he thought we were particularly interested in and would make the most for ourselves, and the Navy.

And then, the last year and a half of the war I was assigned to the OSS, which was a special unit that was examining people who were going overseas. There I became acquainted with a very large group of psychologists, many of whom were very gifted academically, so I got acquainted with psychology at that time. Mabel didn't follow me around. She had gone to Chestnut Lodge to practice while I was gone and when I came out from the Navy I decided to go to Chestnut Lodge too. I was there for a year. Part of that time I did half time practice and then became interested in the treatment that they were attempting to do, with very sick schizophrenic patients. I met Dr. Felix at that time, because I was a member of Frank Braceland's examining team on the American Board. Felix was very interested in psychoanalysis. He thought that as Director of AMA he ought to know what psychoanalysis was about and so he went into psychoanalysis with Frieda Fromm-Reichmann. And since I had also been analyzed by Reichmann – I can't see any other reason why – he asked me in the summer of 1952, whether I would be interested in coming to the National Institute of Mental Health to set up the psychiatric research department.

TB: You were a psychiatrist with a background in physiology. By that time you had also published several papers.

RC: Yes. At the time I had some doubts whether psychoanalysis was something I wanted to spend the rest of my life doing. So I asked him what he had in mind, what sort of research. "Well we will have a building and there are going to be a hundred beds that you can have and you can do anything you want. The salary will be fifteen thousand dollars a year for you, and we might be able to get one or two other salaries and people" – but he wasn't sure about that. "You can go anywhere in the world that you'd be interested in going; the government will send you; you can invite anybody you want to have come as a consultant and the government will pay for it. The job is full time; no teaching, certainly no practice. The building should be ready by March of 1951. We promised that we would open."

And so, I agonized about it. It was not about the job itself, which seemed to be a fantastic opportunity, but I wondered about many things, including that I was making somewhere close to thirty thousand dollars. That didn't bother me because Mabel was in practice and we didn't need to have two incomes, and she said if you want to go, don't hesitate for that reason. But I wondered how we would get anybody else to come who wasn't in that position, where money was no object. So I talked and agonized. The Lodge was going very well then. We'd brought together quite a good staff of people. So, first, I thought "It won't work" and I said, no, I would not come. But Felix did something which I later learned was very clever as a way of recruiting; if somebody takes a long to time to make up his mind and says no, he'll have some doubt about it if you ask him again. So he asked me again. I felt a little bit as if Columbus had asked me to help him discover America. Would I have said, "Well, things are going so well here in Genoa that I can't come?'"

So I went and took the chance, and the one thing that I did learn is that nobody I ever hired came for less than he was already earning. I actually reported for duty on December 30, 1952. I talked to a number of senior people who were being called up at the time to serve in the Korean War, and to a lot of residents at very good places who were being called to active duty, because I thought, between the two, we'll get good people and if they stay for two years some of them will do good work and can stay and maybe some of the others will get so involved that they'll stay too. Then, Eisenhower ended the Korean War and all the senior people called up and asked, "Well, I don't really have to come, do I?" And I said, "of course not." So I started with great anxiety but determined to give it a try.

I remember the very first day, I reported as I said before, on December 30th, the very end of the year, Edward Everett and Josephine Sams, his wife, and I were sitting in an empty office; most of the people were away for the holidays and they came in and talked to me about what we were going to do and about what they would like to do. I always had a special relationship through the years with Ed Everett, who died tragically, and his wife. Ed was just a second year resident in psychiatry at that time. The first years were very very difficult, trying to bring together a more mature staff, and I had to wonder what are we going to try to do?

TB: I understood that you were invited by Robert Felix to set up the research department in psychiatry. Were you in charge of clinical investigations?

RC: Yes. Seymour Kety originally had the idea that he would bring together both the clinical and basic research staff, but he found that he was having difficulty in recruiting people. When I was introduced to Seymour, he was serving as the Scientific Director for Neurology and Psychiatry. Wade

Marshall, who I knew way back from Gerard's days, was there as the Lab Chief in Physiology; and John Clausen was there, whom I'd known at the Institute for Juvenile Research, as chief of Social and Environmental Studies. And then I became acquainted with David Shakow and told him that we needed to get some psychologists. He became very interested in helping me. I had known a whole group of psychologists from my OSS days and I would approach one after the other but they'd all say, no. And Shakow, who was trying to help, would be just as disappointed as I was after a little while; we had picked five people who we thought would do just wonderfully and would fit in, but they said no. So I got the idea that we should get Shakow himself and suggested Seymour offer him the position of joint Lab Chief in Clinical Investigations, to get him to come. And since Seymour had the same difficulty I had in getting experimental psychologists, he offered the job to Shakow. He accepted it and built up Psychology in the Institute. I gave extra money to John Clausen, who was already there in Seymour's division, to stay.

And then we tried and tried to find a Senior Clinical Psychiatrist. I'd had my eye on David Hamburg for a couple of years and finally he agreed to come. Then, in 1954, I had gone to visit hospitals in Europe through the World Health Organization (WHO). I was sent to different places, and among them was Joel Elkes in Birmingham. I was just fascinated that he had an idea about how one would bring together biology and psychology. He had a lot more background in chemistry than I did, and so I was hoping that he might come. Actually in 1956 when he was here in that famous meeting that Jonathan Cole and Ralph Gerard arranged, Joel agreed to come to become chief of the laboratory that, tentatively at that time, we called Laboratory of Psychosomatic Medicine; it included Ed Everett, Irv Kopin, Bob Butler, who later became the Director of the Aging Institute, and Phillip Cardin, who had worked with the Wolfes at Cornell. Then when Joel got back to England, where he was just setting up an experimental psychiatry unit, they said to him, "How can you do this? Here, we built a clinic for you and now you're leaving." So he wrote back to us and said that it just wouldn't be possible.

And then, one day Seymour came in and said "What would you think if I took that job?" I couldn't think of anything that would be better, and he brought Lou Sokoloff with him. Before that, on the same trip in which I'd met Joel Elkes, when I reached Paris, I found a letter from Ed Everett who was the acting Chief of that group. He and Charles Savage were trying to find out how and where LSD work was done. Most of the work was on animals, and Ed had gone to the laboratory of Bernard Brodie to get some help finding out how LSD produced its effect. He wrote to me that there was a pharmacologist named Axelrod in Brodie's laboratory, who would be just the right person for our laboratory. Enclosed was also a letter from David Shakow about a psychologist he met, so I wrote back from Paris to him: "go ahead offer them the jobs." This was my contribution to hiring Julie Axelrod.

TB: It seems that you brought together a remarkable team that set the foundation of the work at the Institute. It was also you who found Joel Elkes who was to come eventually on board. You were also behind the meeting that was organized by Jonathan Cole and Ralph Gerard in 1956 on issues related to clinical methodology in psychopharmacology.

RC: In 1957, I felt that we had reached the end of the beginning. David Hamburg was now the head of Adult Psychiatry and Fritz Redlich the head of Child Psychiatry. Seymour Kety was head of what we used to call the Laboratory of Psychosomatic Medicine, and was to become the Laboratory of Clinical Sciences. Joel Elkes came back for a visit in 1956–57 and said that now he could come. We had gone over to St. Elizabeths and I had talked to Jay Hoffman, who was the assistant director there, about getting a unit for him. Then Bob Felix and I went over to see [Winfred] Overholser and he said, "how about taking a building?" I didn't want a building, but Felix says, "Wonderful," and so we set it up.

TB: So that was the building where Joel Elkes' Clinical Neuropharmacology unit was set up?

RC: Yes. For the first two years we used to have a dinner meeting once a month to talk about the program. I thought that we worked very well together. Then my old friend, David Bodian, came and got Seymour to go to Johns Hopkins and take Adolf Meyer's old job. David Hamburg went out to Stanford University and John Clausen went to the University of California at Berkeley as Director of the Institute of Human Behavior. A year later, Seymour returned and said that he just couldn't see himself staying at Johns Hopkins, and asked me about coming back. I said "It would be wonderful if you did." So he came back. Then they got Joel Elkes a little bit later at Johns Hopkins, and Seymour went to McLean and Harvard in Boston.

TB: How did the departure of all those senior people affect your work?

RC: Actually what happened was that the younger people who stayed took things over. After Kety left, we thought that we should offer Julie Axelrod the job but after Julie said no, Irv Kopin took over. After Joel left, Floyd Bloom was there, and after Dave Hamburg left, Lyman [C. Wynne] was there and they took the jobs and did very well. I was sorry later to see Lyman go, but by that time, Bunney, Murphy and Goodwin had begun working. Bunney had done some of the first clinical studies after Julie

traced the effect of imipramine to the uptake of catecholamines in applying his findings in basic research to psychiatry. The Institute moved ahead
rapidly with biological research. And, then, I decided to leave. It was not
that I had lost interest, but I no longer felt confident about my knowledge
in making appointments. I'd been there for twenty-nine years at that time.

TB: You jumped way ahead to 1981. Could we get back to the late 1950s or
      early'60s?

RC: It was in 1957, as I said before, when we got that senior group together
      and I thought it was the end of the beginning. Everybody seemed to
      be deeply involved in the opportunity to do their research. We had an
      extraordinarily good relationship with Jim Shannon, who was the Director
      of NIH. And, of course by the end of the 1950s our horizon broadened.
      The year I joined Bob Felix in 1952, NIMH's budget was something like
      twelve million dollars. Seymour had a million dollars of that and I had a
      million. Seymour and I were members of the senior staff and we would
      go over to his office to talk about the Institute, as well as our program. I
      remember during those early years Dr. Felix went to Congress one year
      and Lister Hill said to him, "Dr. Felix, how much do you think you will
      come to ask us for in the years ahead?" And Dr. Felix said, "Senator Hill,
      I can foresee the day when I will ask you for twenty-five million dollars."
      He was just shaking inside. He hadn't cleared this with Shannon, and he
      didn't know what Shannon would say, but that was our horizon.
          And, gradually, our horizon spread. I thought we would have this small
      group of people and if they stayed together for five years or longer, we
      would make a very solid contribution as a group. Later on, it became
      clear that we were going to have vast amounts of money, and with the
      increase of money instead of having a relationship with each other we
      were having relations with people in Europe and on the West and East
      Coast. The idea of groups working together really went by the wayside.
      We gave up on that and tried to support the productive groups that we
      did have; we'd follow where the results would go in the direction that the
      research seemed to push us.

TB: I understand that with the money available in the late 1950s and early'60s
      activities grew rapidly in the laboratories and were extended to extramu-
      ral programs. Could you tell us about the different kind of activities the
      Institute became involved with and about some of the outstanding labo-
      ratories and programs?

RC: Actually, it would almost be a question of saying what we didn't do. After
      the Clinical Center had been open ten years there were seven clinical
      directors and at the anniversary each director gave an account on 10

projects. And we unanimously agreed that Julie Axelrod's was one of the most outstanding programs. This was before he got the Nobel Prize.

TB: So Julie Axelrod's was one of the most outstanding programs. Didn't you also have an important program on aging? Who was in charge of that?

RC: Jim Barron. And the psychopharmacology program also did very well.

TB: Were you involved in establishing the Psychopharmacology Service Center (PSC)?

RC: Not directly.

TB: But weren't all programs in some way under your direction?

RC: Yes. I supported the Psychopharmacology Service Center, but I can't say that I established it.

TB: But they had your support.

RC: Well, I supported it, and brought them together and did things to try to keep them contented.

TB: The group you brought together in the PSC was instrumental in developing the methodology in clinical investigations with psychotropic drugs. They also played an important role in establishing the American College of Neuropsychopharmacology. And the group you brought together at the Institute set the foundations of research at NIMH that was to lead psychiatric research during the second half of the 20th century. In the late 1960s you became director of Behavioral Research at the Institute. Could you tell us something about your activities in those years and especially in the 1970s?

RC: It would be difficult to put into words my activities in those years, but by the end of the 1970s, as I told you before, I reached a point where I felt that I could no longer contribute to the further development of the Institute.

TB: Is there anything you would like to say in general about your experiences in the Institute during 29 years?

RC: I never had a moment feeling that Shannon wasn't completely behind me.

TB: Didn't you serve on some of the committees of the Institute after you left?

RC: Fred Goodwin asked me to continue to serve on the promotion committee and I was very glad to do that until that committee was moved outside of the Institute.

TB: What did you do after you retired from the Institute?

RC: When I left the Institute I was asked to come back to Chestnut Lodge as the Director of Psychotherapy, which I was sort of interested in doing. They were running into problems, because the younger doctors who were engaged in psychoanalytic training didn't want to give medications to their patients at all, and they thought that since I was a very senior person I would be able to get them to use medication.

TB: Didn't you write a book in the 1980s on Frieda Fromm-Reichman?

RC: I wrote some papers, yes.

TB: You also wrote chapters in *Comprehensive Psychiatry* about manic depressive illness and schizophrenia. Are you still involved in writing papers?

RC: No. I felt that these last years have been difficult years for me. I can't hear well with my hearing aid, and I really can't go to meetings because I certainly can't follow. I can't hear well enough anymore.

TB: But during the 1980s you were still active?

RC: Actually for the ten years after NIMH I was quite active. But really for the last four years I'm not.

TB: Are you fully retired now?

RC: I really had to retire.

TB: You were born in 1909? So you are 91 years old. You've had a very distinguished career that started in physiology.

RC: Ralph Gerard had a very profound effect on both my wife and me. I think my wife's sister also got a PhD and MD in his lab. I have not told you yet that my first wife, Mabel died in 1972, after we'd been married thirty-nine years. But in 1974, two years after Mabel died, I married again, and I have been married twenty-six years now. Alice, my second wife, was in the Administrative staff at NIMH. My daughter from my first marriage is Professor of Pharmacology. She just presented a paper at a conference on cholecystokinin.

TB: So she is in the footsteps of her parents doing research. You did some early research in brain metabolism.

RC: One funny thing is that at the time when I was still directly involved in research and wrote my paper on hyperthyroidism and brain oxidation, they discovered that I had a carcinoma of the thyroid.

TB: When was that?

RC: It was in late 1956 or '57, something like that. I was fortunate that they were able to remove it. I really have had the experience of being a patient in the last years. After I retired from Chestnut Lodge when I was eighty-two, I had a good year and, then, I've had one thing after another.

TB: Could you tell us something more about your activities at Chestnut Lodge after you left NIMH?

RC: My work was quite interesting. Of course, by the time I returned to Chestnut Lodge the people I knew from before had left. David Rioch went to Walter Reed as Director of Neurological Research, and was quite productive. Bob Gibson went to Sheppard Pratt Hospital. He was also President of the American Psychiatric Association at a certain point in time. Otto Will went to the Riggs Foundation, as Medical Director and Alfred Stanton became Medical Director of McLean Hospital.

TB: What have you been doing since you retired from Chestnut Lodge?

RC: In the last years I've been reading, just reading.

TB: Is there anything else you would like to tell us? During the years you have been involved with many well know people. You also had some famous teachers. Would you like to mention some of them? You have already referred to Ralph Gerard.

RC: I had Frieda Fromm-Reichmann and Harry Stack Sullivan as my teachers, and what I remember is that when I finished discussing a patient with Frieda I had some idea of what I should do next, and when I finished discussing a patient with Sullivan I had some idea of what I had not been doing in working with the patient. While at the Phipps clinic I had Adolf Meyer as my teacher and I can remember whatever Meyer said made a very deep impression on me. During my year at Phipps, five mornings a week the whole staff attended a meeting that Dr. Meyer chaired, and each morning one of us would give a report on our work with a patient. He always made the closing remarks. And I also remember that he sometimes invited us to his home for tea on Sunday afternoon and even for dinner once or twice during the year.

TB: So he had a close relationship with the students and residents. Did you have any contact with the late Horsley Gantt while at Johns Hopkins?

RC: I had some contact with him.

TB: Did you ever take a course in administration?

RC: No, I worked my way up.

TB: In spite of that you have become a most distinguished research administrator in psychiatry, receiving numerous awards for your achievements. Now, if my recollection is correct, during the presidency of Jimmy Carter you became involved with the hostages in Iran.

RC: Oh yes, I went over to Iran and actually I still hear from one of the former hostages, every Christmas. Two of the hostages have died since.

TB: You were involved with them in the capacity of a psychiatrist?

RC: Well, yes. I guess I was the most experienced, well, certainly pretty close to being the most experienced psychiatrist to go over. It was a very moving experience. They were an impressive group of men and women.

TB: So, you were involved with the State Department in those years?

RC: The State Department organized that very impressively. Before we went over, I knew whom I would see and had talked to their wives or parents and seen the letters that they had written home. Each of us had been assigned a particular person we would see. And, then, after we got there, each evening the medical staff got together to report what had transpired. We also had group therapy sessions. I thought the State Department did an extraordinarily good job on that.

TB: During the many years you have been involved with psychiatry there were several paradigm changes in the field. You started in an era when psychiatry was dominated by Adolf Meyer's teachings. Then it was psychodynamics, and while you were at NIMH biological psychiatry became dominant. Would you like to comment on that?

RC: Well, I would like to see the two, the psychodynamic and biological, brought together. It seems to me very sad that we aren't paying the necessary attention to the psychodynamics of people now that we have so very much more knowledge of physiology. I'm sure there are people who are trying to bring psychodynamics and biological psychiatry together. Eric Kandel is one of them. It seems to me that the lessons Adolf Meyer taught are still, in a sense, a guiding principle.

TB: What about drugs in psychiatry? When the new drugs were introduced, did you feel that they had a major impact on treatment?

RC: Yes, and I tried to follow the literature. By the way my wife's nephew played an important role in the discovery of Effexor (venlafaxine), one of the newer antidepressants.

TB: Let me just ask one more question: What would you like to see to happen in the future in the field?

RC: I'd like to see psychodynamic therapy and pharmacotherapy brought together.

TB: On this note we should conclude this interview with Dr. Robert Cohen, one of the most distinguished research-administrators during the second half of the 20th century, who was instrumental in setting the foundation of research at NIMH. Thank you, Dr. Cohen for sharing this information with us. Thank you very much.

THOMAS DETRE

Interviewed by Benjamin S. Bunney
San Juan, Puerto Rico, December 9 13, 1996

SB: I'm Steve Bunney and I'm interviewing Dr. Thomas Detre*. Tom, how did you get started in medicine?

TD: My father and several members of my family were physicians. I was interested in medicine ever since I can remember. My interest in psychiatry was kindled by the remarks made by one of the priests in a Catholic high school I attended when he said that at the turn of the century a degenerate Jewish physician, Sigmund Freud, developed a pansexual theory of human behavior called psychoanalysis.

SB: Where was that?

TD: In Hungary. I went home, asked my father where I could read up on psychoanalysis and he gave me a few books by Freud and Ferenczi. I found the ideas fascinating but too speculative. I remained interested in psychiatry, however.

SB: And then you pursued medicine?

TD: I then pursued medicine, but only after the Second World War in 1945 because Jews were not admitted to medical schools when I got my BA. Two years later, in 1947, when the Communists were about to take over the government, I decided I did not want to live in another dictatorial regime. I left the country, emigrated to Italy, and graduated from the University of Rome in 1952.

SB: And then?

TD: And then, in 1953 I came to the United States on a lovely day in May and found out that the only internship I could get was at the Morrisania City Hospital in the Bronx, New York, but that was a very good experience. It toughened me up.

SB: How old were you at that time, Tom?

TD: Twenty-nine. I was accepted into Mount Sinai Hospital's psychiatric residency program a year later, but found it had too many pretensions of an academic institution without being one, and moved to Yale for the rest of my post-graduate education.

SB: What date did you arrive at Yale?

TD: July 1955.

---

* Thomas Detre was born in Budapset, Hungary in 1924, and received his MD from the University School of Medicine in Rome in 1952. He trained in psychiatry at Yale from 1955 to 1957, and stayed as a member of that department until 1973 when he became chairiman of the department of psychiatry and director of the Western Psychiatric Institute at the university of Pittsburgh.During his tenure at the University of Pittsburgh he rose to the position of Senior Vice Chancellor of Health Sciences as well as President of the University of Pittsburgh Medical Center. Detre died in 2010.

SB: And you were there for how long?

TD: I was there for 18½ years. When I left I was Professor of Psychiatry and Psychiatrist-in-Chief of Yale New Haven Hospital.

SB: When did you first become interested in neuropsychopharmacology?

TD: At Mount Sinai. I began to read about a very interesting psychotropic drug called reserpine, which for some reason now is out of fashion, though not necessarily for a good reason. Since it was unclear what reserpine was good for, I proposed to start an open trial in psychiatric patients. The chief resident joined me, to the consternation of the faculty, because Mount Sinai was then a very psychoanalytically oriented program. We presented our findings at a meeting of the New York Academy of Medicine and described an interesting observation, namely that when psychotic symptoms subsided following the administration of reserpine, another set of symptoms emerged which actually preceded the onset of the psychotic episode, a phenomenon called rollback. For example, when reserpine was given to severely depressed patients, after the symptoms of the psychotic depression subsided, they became extremely anxious, which made perfect sense since severe anxiety ushers in most depressive episodes. Although few believed this was possible, my observations have subsequently been confirmed.

SB: To go back to schizophrenic disorders, were you feeling that you were seeing the prodromata after the psychotic symptoms subsided?

TD: Exactly.

SB: This is interesting, because as you know right now, there's a big push to try to identify prodromal symptoms as soon as possible in order to see whether or not early treatment will prevent psychotic episodes. It would be interesting to go back to your observations to see if this would help us to determine the early warnings signs.

TD: I want to mention that the talk was given by the chief resident, not by me, but that was then the "convention."

SB: Yes, that's an old tradition actually.

TD: As I mentioned, Mount Sinai Hospital at the time was not particularly friendly to biological psychiatry and psychopharmacology, so with the help of a distinguished colleague, I got an interview with Dr. Fritz Redlich, who, as you recall, was once upon a time chairman of the Department of Psychiatry, and later Dean of the Yale Medical School. He was kind enough to accept me into the residency program. To my surprise, however, the situation at Yale was not very different from Mount Sinai. As I sat in the midst of my first teaching conference at Yale, presided over by the famous Jules Coleman, and the resident presented a schizophrenic patient, I proposed that instead of treating this young woman just with psychotherapy, we might want to give her some chlorpromazine. Jules Coleman just stared, but one of my fellow residents, who later became a good friend, turned to his neighbor and said, "This guy is for the birds." That was the attitude. Things got even worse when I became a resident, and later chief resident of the Yale Psychiatric Institute, where to the consternation of everyone, I suggested that the era of neuropsychopharmacology had arrived.

SB: Was Danny Freedman there at the time?

TD: You know, there was a peculiar dichotomy in many departments of psychiatry, not just Yale, but Stanford, Harvard, Columbia, and elsewhere. People interested in biological psychiatry could do anything they wanted to do in the lab but that was not necessarily acceptable in the clinical arena. Danny was very ambivalent about whether to start a career in clinical research or basic research. Eventually, he left Yale and spent about two years in the intramural program at NIMH. When he came back he stayed in the lab and I stayed in the clinic. Whenever a new drug came out he studied the mechanism of action and I started to do clinical trials. At some point we did an open trial on amitriptyline and after it appeared fairly effective, I suggested to my residents that we should do a controlled clinical trial. Even though they felt that they were being forced to use drugs, they declared that it was immoral to start a controlled clinical trial, because it would deprive patients of the benefits the drug might provide.

SB: I assume the reason Danny came back and you were able to run a service, with what appeared to some colleagues as a rather untraditional approach to the management of psychiatric patients, was that Dr. Redlich was able to embrace both sides?

TD: Redlich believed, quite correctly, that every language ought to be spoken and all flowers should bloom. He actually enjoyed the dialogues and the disputes among us, feeling that this provided an intellectually stimulating climate, and it did. This was indeed one of the hallmarks of his leadership style.

SB: Let's talk a little bit about the research that you have carried out over the years.

TD: Well, I started in New Haven looking at schizophrenic patients. I was particularly interested in the long-term effects of psychotropic drugs after the patient left the hospital and when adherence was no longer ensured by nurses and doctors. Of course, it turned out that the compliance was absolutely miserable. And there was little to be gained unless patients could be persuaded to adhere to a maintenance regime. As you are aware, the resistance to drug therapy at the time was not limited to patients, however. Many psychiatrists felt drugs were ineffective and deprived the patients of the "real" treatment, i.e. psychotherapy, as did the rest of society. So it was difficult to persuade patients to take medications until the public-at-large had a better understanding of the value of pharmacologic treatment, and it was also accepted by the medical profession. In an attempt to overcome this attitude, I started a joint patient/family psycho-educational program. In the course of studying a host of antidepressant drugs I discovered to my consternation what a bad idea it was to combine a monoamine oxidase inhibitor with certain other drugs, particularly amphetamine, as it produced a spectacular rise in systolic blood pressure. Although the inpatient service I directed at Yale New Haven Hospital had only 30 beds – it expanded several years later – we did a large number of clinical studies.

SB: Do you think the side effects of these drugs contributed to poor "adherence?"

TD: Absolutely. More patients were willing to take drugs and tolerate their side effects when they felt sick, but became less cooperative once they felt better. But then this change in attitude can be observed in other medical conditions as well. Having to take medication tends to be disturbing to one's self-image. It is a constant reminder that you are impaired or weak, as it were. Perhaps you remember the famous study of mothers who were told that their children could be protected from the cardiac damage caused by rheumatic fever by giving them flavored oral penicillin – which is obviously not a psychotropic drug – and six months later, over 40% of them were noncompliant. So we cannot even say that inadequate adherence is typical only of psychiatric patients.

SB: So you left Yale then, in?

TD: 1973.

SB: To become chairman of the Department of Psychiatry at the University of Pittsburgh.

TD: Yes, I left because I wanted to develop a department that would be dedicated to clinical research, not to the exclusion of basic research, but where clinical research would have the highest priority. I had a large number of my colleagues from Yale accompany me, which made my task easier. My former colleagues at Yale were also pleased, because some of the people who left with me were viewed as obnoxious. Together we established the department, which I had the pleasure of chairing for nine and a half years.

SB: People that are now in the ACNP whom you took with you include David Kupfer.

TD: Right.

SB: It must have really been a challenge, as chairman, to essentially build a department from scratch. So, how did that progress, in terms of doing what you had in mind?

TD: My view was that clinical research will never stay in the forefront unless it is backed up by a solid neuroscience program. That however could not be my agenda for the first five years, but it became my agenda in the second five years. Then I realized that unless the medical school improved further our own efforts would fail.

SB: So you took a different job?

TD: Yes, the Chancellor proposed that I head up the health sciences. I accepted his offer, but at his request I remained director of Western Psychiatric Institute and Clinic. My life had changed, but I continued to be very interested in psychiatry, managed to keep up to date with developments in the field, saw a few patients, and did a little teaching. I eventually had to stop because in addition to dedicating myself to improving the medical school and the other schools of the health sciences, I also became the President of the Medical Center.

SB: As Senior Vice Chancellor for Health Sciences at the University of Pittsburgh, you then had the opportunity to begin to build the basic science arm, as well as the clinical arm, and then to link the two of them.

TD: Yes. I think they are probably better linked here than at many other universities. In order to strengthen neuroscience in the Faculty of Arts and Sciences, I helped the university to establish a Department of Behavioral Neuroscience, and Ed Striker became the first chairman. You probably know him.

SB: Very well. And that comes under the medical school or the graduate school?

TD: The Faculty of Arts and Science. I felt strongly that all of the university should be involved in neuroscience, and the best way to accomplish this for the benefit of both the Medical School and the Faculty of Arts and Sciences would be for them to recruit jointly and offer joint appointments to encourage collaboration throughout the campus. Indeed, in a relatively short time, a strong interaction developed between the departments of Behavioral Neuroscience, and the School of Medicine's Departments of Neuroscience, Psychiatry, and Neurology. I assisted with the recruitments, hoping to select not just creative scientists, but ones who were not territorial and wanted to cooperate. Today about two-thirds of all recruits in the neurosciences have joint appointments in departments and schools of our university, which I believe is the future, since no department, or even school today, can be its own university.

SB: So, translational research was something that you had in mind all along when you began to set this up.

TD: I might add, of course, that a medical school is not a national science foundation. No matter how seductive we are, how well we teach, and what good role models we are, 80% of our graduates are going into private practice and it is important that we teach them how to remain up to date and to evaluate what they do.

SB: If I remember right, looking at the recent statistics of the University of Pittsburgh, the Department of Psychiatry now has more grant awards from the National Institutes of Health than any other department in the country.

TD: But that is strictly David Kupfer's fault.

SB: However, you brought David Kupfer when you came, so . . .

TD: Yes, but one cannot take credit for what others have accomplished.

SB: If you take responsibility for recruitment and have an eye to pick the right people, some credit is due.

TD: Perhaps what is most important is that the whole medical school has improved. You probably recall from one of your earlier visits that it was not very distinguished and ranked very low in federal funding, but now it is in 10th place. It is not as good as Yale, maybe never will be, but it's okay.

SB: Well, you keep us working hard. Tom, let's talk about the future for a moment. You've lived through some remarkable changes in the history of neuropsychopharmacology and the treatment of psychiatric patients. What do you see coming down the road?

TD: Well, I believe that rational drug design will eventually replace what has been a rather serendipitous way of finding new drugs, but I am not persuaded we are there yet. We will probably be able to design drugs that are cleaner in their mode of action.

SB: In terms of side effects?

TD: Not just in terms of side effects, but affecting the central nervous system a little more specifically than the so called dirty drugs we have today. Our hypotheses are often based on one receptor or one neurotransmitter and revised again as new receptors and neurotransmitters are identified. What concerns me, and we have talked about this in the past, is that just when a host of new biologic entities are ready to come down the pike the federal government, dedicated to a short term science policy, has stopped supporting training programs for clinical pharmacologists, who are also trained in molecular biology and genetics. I believe it should be one of the goals of the ACNP to campaign to ensure that we have an adequate number of clinical pharmacologists.

SB: So you're proposing that there be support for the training of these individuals, as well as research support to carry out the investigations?

TD: Correct, but I think the training of this new type of clinical pharmacologist is a very urgent national task.

SB: You get no argument from me on that.

JOEL ELKES

Interviewed by Fridolin Sulser
San Juan, Puerto Rico, December 12, 1995

FS: Joel,* welcome to ACNP History Task Force. It is quite a thrill for me to interview you as the first President of the ACNP. Now, the task force, the History Task Force, has imposed some rules, which we can follow, or if we like, we need not follow. So, one of the first questions they want me to ask you, is about your early educational experiences and the determining factors in your entering medical school.

JE: Well, as you probably know, I was raised in Lithuania and I went to secondary school in Lithuania; my father was a very prominent physician there. So I had the example of my father, who had himself been educated in Koenigsberg (now Kaliningrad, Russia), across the border in Germany, and had a really deep regard for both the practice of medicine, in which he was superb, and the science of medicine. I had always engaged, at least in my early days, towards the middle of my school years, in a dialogue between physics and medicine. I was deeply interested in physics. I spent my first prize monies on works describing the new physics and still remember the awe with which I'd viewed of collision paths of particles in a cloud chamber. I really wanted to go into physics, but I didn't have the mathematical equipment for that. I was kind of shy of mathematics. But then, at the same time, in discussing things with my father and friends, there was much talk about the sciences compounding medicine and physiology, of course. But the term biochemistry was still an unknown. The sheer concept of biochemistry – a chemistry of life no less – was still a strange concept. So, we talked about chemistry and life and life processes, and I remember discussing this and thinking to myself, well, maybe I can sort of ride into medicine by way of chemistry and physics, and get an idea of the sciences serving medicine and still keep my beloved physics with me. Then the main decision point came, and because I had such a superior example of physicianship in my father, I decided to go into medicine, by way of physical chemistry, organic chemistry, and surface and colloid chemistry. At all times I was pulled by physics, and this continued for quite some time, after I entered

---

* Born in Koenigsberg, Germany, in 1913, Joel Elkes graduated from the University of London with a medical degree in 1941. He joined Alastair Frazer in the department of pharmacology at the University of Birmingham, and in 1945 he was put in charge of the Mental Disease Research Unit in the Department. In 1951 Elkes became the founding director of the Department of Experimental Psychiatry at the University of Birmingham. In 1957 Elkes moved to the United States to become the chief of NIMH's neuropharmacology research center at St. Elizabeths Hospital in Washington. From 1963 to 1974 he was Psychiatrist in Chief at Johns Hopkins Hospital and head of the Department of Psychiatry and Behavioral Sciences at the university.

medical school. So, the answer is, I went to medicine because I had a secure example of good physicianship and a good person, in my father, and because I also hoped that medicine would lead me to a sort of relationship of science to life and nature. So I was becoming a physician, and also becoming a scientist serving medicine.

FS: What I was wondering about is how you then, after you finished medical school in London, chose psychopharmacology. This was in its infancy at that time. Maybe that was the reason for your choice?

JE: Well, that is a complicated question again, because very little was known about the effects of drugs on the mind at the time I was a student at St. Mary's Hospital, London. Quite honestly, I didn't see that as a tremendous interest, then. But while a student I became interested in immunology: There was a giant in the field at St. Mary's. He influenced me.

FS: Immunology?

JE: There was Sir Almroth Wright, the father of the typhus vaccine, who was a model for George Bernard Shaw in *The Doctor s Dilemma*. There was also my Dean, Sir Charles Wilson, who later became Churchill's physician. But "psychiatry" was a tiny, tiny fragment of the curriculum, taught in far too few lectures and demonstrations. This excited me tremendously. I went after psychiatry and read avidly, and began to try to connect, in my confused mind, physical chemistry, immunology, and mental function. How do chemistry of the body and brain relate to each other, how does it connect with mental function? The drugs which were then existent, were very, very ordinary drugs. But we did not precisely know how they worked.

FS: Joel, let me interrupt you. I always felt that your three heroes, whom you mentioned in your ACNP lecture, had something to do with this. You mentioned Einstein and physics; you mentioned Goethe; and, then, you mentioned Ehrlich and his receptors. Now, most people will understand why Einstein; they will understand why Ehrlich; but Americans do not know Goethe. Why Goethe? I know why, but I think Americans should also know why.

JE: Well, Goethe was to me an extraordinary example of what a human being, a person, can achieve on this planet. He was a poet, a master of both prose and poetry; he was Minister of State for the Duke whom he served; a theater director; and, as a hobby, almost, a scientist. Goethe studied the origin of plants; he studied light and the theory of colors. This rare combination of humanism, scientific creativity and the spirit filled me with immense admiration. It's just as simple as that. He was an example.

FS: So if my assumption is correct, that had something to do with you trying to get into pharmacology, combining chemistry, physics, and psychiatry at the same time?

JE: Oh, yes, whatever psychiatry was at the time. I read avidly. Freud, of course, his view that the future would produce physical markers for mental events, impressed me – something like that – I'm paraphrasing. But the drugs didn't really come into view until right after medical school, by which time in 1941, I went to Birmingham, England, to follow my friend, Alastair Frazer to the Department of Pharmacology. This Department was an extraordinary because from an early modest beginning, it grew to a large, significant, influential department, and had a very strong grounding throughout. Why? It happened because Frazer was a self-taught and self-sufficient physiologist. He was interested in fat absorption and the physics of the chylomicrons, tiny particles that flood the blood after a fatty meal. I became interested in the protein/lipoprotein covering of these particles, which stabilized this natural emulsion in the blood stream. When I started to work on lipoproteins, it was known that lipoproteins were built into the architecture of membranes and I started to think about the stability of the membrane surrounding the chylomicron and thus found myself back in physical chemistry. This work proceeded during the War. We learned of very specific molecules, the nerve gases, the anticholinesterases, which had a high affinity for the nervous system.

FS: That was your entry to the brain?

JE: That was one entry to the brain. On the other hand, I'd already worked in physical chemistry and the structure of biological membranes, lipoproteins. Suddenly I realized that the nervous system was full of lipoproteins. It was myelin, a beautiful paracrystalline structure ubiquitously distributed in the nervous system. I was fortunate, as my first PhD student, Bryan Finean, was a crystallographer who undertook the arduous task of studying the X-ray diffraction structure of living myelin. We decided to plunge into that field, the structure of a naturally occurring lipoprotein, which probably held special bioelectrical properties in the nervous system. Francis Schmitt had studied dried myelin; his classical work was a guide to studying living myelin and that became a challenge. Finean and I constructed a special chamber for irrigating a living sciatic nerve preparation which made it possible to shoot X-ray beams through a living structure while the environment of a segment of nerve was being changed systematically. We studied the effect of gradual drying, and irrigation with alcohol and ether of the crystal structure. The changes were orderly, repeatable, and to some extent reversible. The X-ray diffractive diagrams were clear and quite, quite beautiful. To this day, I cannot really tell you what possessed me to do this. I suppose it was the vain hope of seeing the penetration of molecules of an anesthetic into the molecular structure of myelin. However, suddenly I was in the nervous system! I hoped it could lead to visualizing the effects of drugs. At that time there was no real neurochemistry. There was Quastel's great work on the effect of barbiturates on glucose metabolism in brain homogenates. There was Richter working on cognate problems. My dream of specific attraction to certain receptors had to wait. We began to map the cholinesterases in certain parts of the brain. It was an indirect, confusing, and confounding journey. But I was into the brain. I was also an outsider, reading wildly, edging towards a neuropharmacology of behavior. There were very few people I could talk to at that time. I chose the anticholinesterases and the role of acetylcholine. I also read Sherrington.

Also, as it happened, I saw for the first time, sitting safely in the back of the auditorium, a demonstration at the Physiological Society in Cambridge by Lord Adrian, the great Adrian. He touched a vibrissa of a cat. There was a loud 'humph' on the loudspeaker. He touched another. There was silence and I sat there in the back, totally awed by the precision of the phenomenon, and I went up to Lord Adrian, at the time, and told him of my interest. He said, "Well, you're not really in physiology, you are in pharmacology." And I said that I really felt that pharmacology could lead us to physiology, understanding the way the brain does it naturally without the aid of chemical prostheses: This gradually became a main theme in my thinking: pharmacology as an approach to physiology. We started working on the cholinesterases and their regional distribution. At that time, acetylcholine was the main molecule in the central nervous system. This was due to Sir Henry Dale's influence.

FS: Joel, this is still a long way to psychiatry, but it didn't take you very long. It was in 1951, a milestone in your career, when you established the Department of Experimental Psychiatry in Birmingham, which is said to be the first of its kind in the world. Tell us a little bit about it.

JE: Well, before I do, I must refer you to several developments which took place before 1951. The first was that my late beloved wife Charmian and I started to work, for the first time in my career, in a mental hospital setting. I became very interested in the effect of drugs on the brain from my wide reading. About that time, we were in London, and heard of the effects of drugs on catatonic stupor from some French colleagues.

FS: Was this about 1948 or '49?

JE: About 1949. We started to look around for the syndrome in our own hospital and identified some 22 cases. We began to study the effects of Amytal (amobarbital), amphetamine, and mephenesin on the syndrome. We studied effects on mental function, on speech, and on other psychological responses, and also on blood pressure and foot temperature. These catatonics had a very striking syndrome. They were characterized by slate blue legs, arms, hands, and were non-verbal, not giving any indication of being present and aware. Given Amytal in doses that would put you or me to sleep, 350 or 400 milligrams, they came out of the stupor. This effect was very dramatic: they would talk; they would draw; they would write and they would communicate; and then, like in an Andersen fairy tale, they would relapse into a deep sleep. We'd measure foot temperature and would find that there was correlation between vasodilation, foot temperature, and psychomotor response. The process lasted for about three-fourths of an hour. Giving amphetamine in doses which would send you or me into wild excitement, these people deepened their stupor, and at the same time, there was sharp vasoconstriction and a sharp rise in blood pressure. We also had mephenesin, which had just been introduced as a muscle relaxant by Frank Berger; the catatonic rigidity was strikingly reduced but there was no psychomotor response. In other words, there was specificity in the drug response effects, and we wondered whether what we were dealing with was a state of hyperarousal. This was one piece of work which established us in the mental hospital culture; however, there was nothing between the patient and the laboratory, we needed another intermediate point.

The effect of drugs on the electric activity of the brain and the conscious animal suggested itself quite early; but no technique to do this was available. It is at this point that Philip Bradley entered my life as my second PhD student. Philip had had a background in zoology in the University of Bristol. He had worked on insects. We wondered whether a technique for implanting and recording in the unanesthatized animal was feasible. Philip said "yes," and for two years worked on developing techniques for recording electrical activity in the conscious and unrestrained animal. Bradley's cats became quite famous. They lived happily in the lab for up to nine months. No infection: I might say that the implantation occurred before the advent of penicillin. Prophylactic use of sulfonamides was the rule. The results were very striking. We began with the anticholinesterases, acetylcholine blockers and amphetamine. We studied cortical and sub-cortical activity and looked for correspondence between electrical activity and behavior. We found that with cholinergic and anticholinergic drugs there was no correspondence between electrical activity and behavior. With amphetamine there was correspondence, and the effects depended on intact connections to the mid-brain. This brought to mind Morruzzi and Magoun's work on the waking brain. At the same time, Marthe Vogt presented her findings on the presence of norepinephrine in the areas of the brain implicated by our experiments. Yet it was so tedious to do this work at the time. You dissect areas of the brain, you homogenize the various regions, you incubate the eluate in the Warburg Manometer, and then, you test the eluate against a guinea pig ileum for potency.

FS: This is interesting, Joel. It is somewhat parallel to the studies that my teacher, Walter Rudolph Hess, did in Zurich. You know, if I remember correctly, he worked on the conscious cat in 1950. So it is quite parallel.

JE: Yes. Geoffrey Harris, my colleague at St. Mary's Hospital and later a founding father of neuroendocrinology, visited Dr. Hess at the time although we ourselves had no contact with him. In any event, the results were very striking. We wondered what we should name our little unit. They wanted to call it Chemical Psychiatry, and I said, "No" and stuck with the term Experimental Psychiatry because I really believed that the experimental method is necessary to make psychiatry a science. In 1951, the University graciously named me head of a small department with that name. The department comprised: neurochemistry, represented by our work on the anticholinesterases; there was also electrophysiology, represented by Bradley's and my own work on conscious cats; there was animal behavior; and later ethology, represented by Dr. Michael Chance, a member of our department; and there were the clinical studies in catatonic stupor. We thought we had the footings of the field in place.

FS: Joel, another milestone that happened there was the first controlled trial with chlorpromazine. Could you elaborate on that?

JE: Again, I can only recall the occasion. We had just founded our Department of Experimental Psychiatry and we had a research facility at the Winton Green Mental Hospital. About this time there came to my office, Dr. W. R. Thrower, clinical director of Menley and James, a big pharmaceutical company. He said this was not a routine visit. He was very formal and unlocked his briefcase, and out of it came a paper in French, which was the account of the action of a hitherto unknown compound, an antihistamine, on the behavior of schizophrenic patients. I read it with slight disbelief, and said I would like to know more about it. Dr. Thrower said that's why he came; Menley and James had acquired the rights for the substance and had a supply of it in their safe. They could make up tablets and placebos for a trial. Would we carry out a controlled trial? I went to Charmian again, and said "here is something" – I did not know the magnitude of it – "should we do a trial?" In her characteristic way, she said, "yes," because by that time she had established a base in the mental hospital. She quickly accepted full responsibility for the trial. We had colleagues whom we could interest in the projects; but it was she who designed the trial, as a blind self-controlled design, and selected the patients. (Twenty-seven patients were involved, with about 13 schizophrenics and others with affective disorders or organic syndromes.) Overactive behavior was the main criterion for selection; the trial lasted about 22 weeks. And one day, one Saturday morning, we trooped down into the boardroom of the mental hospital, and spread the data on a big oak table. The code was broken and the record emerged. No statistics were necessary in seven patients. These patients had benefited strikingly and relapsed on placebo. The trial noted side effects and weight gain, effects that were at the same time described by others. However, most importantly, we learned much from the conduct of the trial itself. Allow me to read from the copy:

"Perhaps we may be allowed to draw attention to one last point, namely, the lessons we feel we have learnt from the trial itself. The research instrument in a trial of this sort being a group of people, and its conduct being inseparable from the individual use of words; we were impressed by the necessity for a 'blind' and self-controlled design, and independent multiple documentation. Furthermore, we were equally impressed by the false picture apt to be conveyed if undue reliance was placed on interview alone, as conducted in the clinic room. The patients' behavior in the ward was apt to be very different. For that reason the day and night nursing staff became indispensable and valued members of the observers' team. We were warmed and encouraged by the energy and care with which they did what was requested of them, provided this was clearly and simply set out at the beginning. A chronic 'back' ward thus became a rather interesting place to work in. There may well be a case for training senior nursing staff in elementary research method and in medical documentation. This would make for increased interest, increased attention to, and respect for detail, and the availability of a fund of information, all too often lost because it has not been asked for."

FS: You know, someone with your mind must have had some very profound thoughts about chlorpromazine. It was long before we knew about dopamine D_1, D_2, D_4 or what have you, how a drug could affect behavior. I find it incredible; this was one of the milestones in psychopharmacology. Tell us the impact it has had on the evolution of the entire field.

JE: Let me track back a little, because by that time I had slowly developed the view that we were dealing with indirect effects of the drugs on families of naturally occurring substances.

FS: Yes, this is interesting. Let me tell you something quickly that might interest you. When I came to the United States with a suitcase in October 1958 and walked into Brodie's laboratory, there was Arvid Carlssson showing the uneven distribution of dopamine in the brain, showing an enormous concentration of dopamine in the striatal areas. From the uneven distribution of dopamine he got to the conclusion that dopamine is more than a precursor to norepinephrine. I think this was in keeping with your thinking.

JE: Yes, yes, we began to talk about regional neurochemistry. Seymour Kety thought about regional differences in cerebral circulation and I thought about regional differences of neurotransmitters and families of naturally occurring compounds that had arisen in evolution to modulate and guide the interaction of neurons, and regulate excitation and inhibition in the nervous system. I thought of regional field effects in the nervous system.

FS: At a UCLA symposium....

JE: At UCLA, yes, the concept of regional chemistry was getting through. By that time we began to think of "how do we create a conversation on the subject?" This is how the idea of these symposia on regional neurochemistry arose. I believe it was, 1954 or '56; Seymour Kety, Heinrich Waelsch, Jordi Folch-Pi and Louis Flexner represented the United States; Geoffrey Harris and Richter, and myself, the United Kingdom.

FS: I was wondering if you could make a few comments on using the drug as a tool to unravel mechanisms. I mean, it's obviously something you were thinking about.

JE: Very much so. Cholinesterase and anticholinesterase has opened up the whole area of acetylcholine synthesis and its role in normal functions. So, to come back, to a general statement, I really feel that pharmacology, as we know it, will lead us to a deeper understanding of the body's natural inner pharmacy. It may give us a footing for a natural healing system.

FS: Joel, I couldn't agree more with you. I think that using these drugs wisely as tools has contributed more than anything else to the dissection of mechanisms. Listen, this is wonderful. Now, comes the big jump, and I don't quite understand why you made this big jump over the ocean to Washington, DC in 1957. You were in England and all of your friends were there. You had your former wife there and everything was working fine.

JE: Everything was working wonderfully.

FS: Why did you come to St. Elizabeths?

JE: First, it came from a deep personal relationship with Seymour Kety, Bob Cohen, and Bob Felix and their openness to ideas. I found it extremely hard to leave England. The University, the Medical Research Council, the Rockefeller Foundation could not have been more generous and rewarding; but the field was developing very fast in the United States, and I wanted to be part of it. When we started, our department started getting visitors every week. Wonderful conferences at which the idea of families of naturally occurring compounds was expressed. As far as I remember, I first expressed it in an invited paper to the newly founded Mental Health

Research Fund in 1952 and developed it further in our paper in 1957. Let me quote again:

"Perhaps rather than thinking in unitary terms, it may at this stage, be advisable to think in terms of the possible selection by chemical evolution of small families of closely related compounds, which by mutual interplay would govern the phenomena of excitation and inhibition in the central nervous system. Acetylcholine, noradrenaline and 5-hydroxytryptamine may be parent molecules of this kind; but one has only to compare the effects of acetylcholine and succinylcholine, or noradrenaline with its methylated congener to realize how profound the effects of even slight changes of molecular configuration can be. The astonishing use which chemical evolution has made of the steroids is but another example of the same economy. It is likely that neurons possessing slight but definite differences in enzyme constitution may be differentially susceptible to neurohumoral agents. Such neurons may be unevenly distributed in topography close, or widely separated areas in the central nervous system, these differences probably extending to the finest level of histological organization. Phylogenetically older parts, and perhaps, more particularly, the mid-line regions and the periventricular nuclei may, in terms of cell population and chemical constitution be significantly different from parts characteristic of late development."

I cannot describe to you the intensity with which I saw, in my mind's eye, these naturally occurring molecules distributed regionally in the brain. When, much later, I saw the Swedish fluorescent photographic evidence, confirming their uneven distribution, I experienced a shocked feeling of awe. The idea of a regional neurochemistry took root. In those years I had, peripherally, become active in neurochemistry. I was organizing secretary of the first international neurochemical symposium, which took place at Magdalen College, Oxford in 1954. Other symposia followed, the third being held in Ravenna, Italy, convened by Seymour Kety and myself on the theme of 'Regional Neurochemistry.'

FS: Now I come to your center at St. Elizabeths. It was you who catalyzed the development of that center, the organization.

JE: Well, there was nothing there.

FS: There was nothing there?

JE: Nothing, nothing there at all.

FS: It was just walls?

JE: It was just the William A. White building, a 300 bed chronic hospital.

FS: It was like an old chronic hospital!

JE: Yes, we came in with a budget to Dr. Shannon with Bob Felix, Bob Cohen, and Seymour Kety, and we put our labs in the basement, and the administration at the top between patients, who were all around us. That was the beginning of what became the Clinical Neuropharmacology Research Center. I was the first director of that center. In fact I remember there was helluva timetable getting it done. As a matter of fact, Seymour sent me the floor plan of the basement at St. Elizabeths to England, the catalogues, and said "please design labs, because we need it now." I designed the labs in England. And then, we came to present it to the director of NIH, Dr. Shannon, one Sunday morning and he approved it readily, actually increased our budget. I could tell you a good story about that one.

FS: So, this is how it started.

JE: And then we recruited the various people. One of my first recruits was Hans Weil-Malherbe.

FS: This is another thing that I think is very, very significant. You have always been able to recruit superb people.

JE: Well, I brought Weil-Malherbe from England. He started his own lab. He was very early in the amine story and he started to collaborate with Julie Axelrod.

FS: It was about the time when I came to Brodie's lab.

JE: And then we had Fellows, many, many, too numerous to name.

FS: And Max Hamilton.

JE: And Max Hamilton spent time with us and wrote his famous Lectures on Methodology while he was a Fellow at St. Elizabeths.

FS: And, Paul Bender was there.

JE: Oh, yes. I can't remember all the names.

FS: Joel, what do you consider as the major accomplishment in your unit? You were there from 1957 till '63.

JE: Till 1963.

FS: This is a tough question to ask.

JE: At the fundamental level there were really three accomplishments. There was Floyd Bloom's work with Nino Salmoiraghi on the electrophysiological response of individual neurons to different transmitters, providing chemical evidence of homogeneity at the unit level. And then, there was Weil-Malherbe's work on the amines, which then linked up with Julie's work.

FS: You're right, yes.

JE: Then there was work on the effect of metabolites on animal behavior, which Steve Szára did. He showed that tryptamine derivatives had a differential effect on conditioned behavior. There was Fritz Freyhan's fine work on the whole concept of what he referred to as Comprehensive Psychiatry, which included drug effects, but also emphasized the active social support system and the analysis of the factors which played a part in the recovery of the individual patient. Mainly, a culture was created and conversation proceeded. It was a wonderful, heady, exciting time in the middle of a very chronic mental hospital. There were people coming virtually from all over the world and there were talks and discussions and excitement. At the same time, there was also always and always, which is what we had hoped, the presence of the patient. For example, you go to the canteen for lunch and there's a schizophrenic hallucinating under a tree. You're never very far away from the problem that brought you here. And, gradually there developed a sense of place, a sense of belonging. Gradually, I realized that, my God, together we created something pretty wonderful.

FS: You know, Joel, what impresses me about this whole thing is that you never imposed yourself on these people and you've never put your name on the papers. You supported them. You discussed the importance of their work, but you did not impose your name on papers like Floyd Bloom's. It's amazing, you know. You were a gentleman.

JE: One is a chief. One is a good gardener. The institute is a sort of green-house, one which identifies plants, grows them, and one makes sure that people have everything that they need. I'll give you an example that comes to mind. There was Richard Michael. Richard Michael, a very good neuroendocrinologist, is now in Atlanta, Georgia, but at that time he was a pupil of Geoffrey Harris. He needed radioactive estradiol to implant into the hypothalamus to show the effect of hormones on sexual behavior, which was very specific in terms of both the hormone, the location of the hormone and its uptake in certain cells of the hypothalamus. He gave me a hard time trying to find this damn radioactive estradiol, but we did. We got the stuff. When he published his paper, it was really quite a remark-able paper; he showed the distinct contribution of certain cells of the hypothalamus to sexual behavior. My job was to cultivate talent. I did it in Birmingham. I did it at St. Elizabeths and the Research Center, and then I hope I did it again at Hopkins.

FS: Joel, I think this is a matter of style, and this was the Joel Elkes' style. That leads me to the next step in your career. In 1963, you went to Hopkins and it was there where you got a stellar group of pre-clinical and clinical neuroscientists put together. This was quite unique, you know.

JE: Well, again, I was just fortunate. For one thing, I was awed to step into the shoes of the ones who preceded me, Adolf Meyer, Whitehorn, and Seymour Kety. When I started, my office was next to Adolf Meyer's library, and I started reading his convoluted English and his more con-voluted German, but, my God, what clear concepts the man had. He struggled with the term psychobiology for years. His Salmon lectures were significantly published after his death. I felt that sounded right to me: Psychobiology – biology of mental life – was a good fit between me and the job. There was also a fit between my temperament and the total climate. This was not a shiny new institute. It was an old, old brick building, with old smells, and had animal laboratories in the building. On the third floor, there was Curt Richter who did all his magnificent work on chronobiology in rats. So there was a wonderful tradition. There were also some great people around already, Horsley Gantt, the only surviving pupil of Pavlov; Jerry Frank, the author of *Persuasion and Healing*; John Money, one of the best authorities on sexual behavior in man, and more and more junior colleagues.

These substantial figures were ranging from biology to psychoanalysis. The comprehensiveness was congenial to my view of psychiatry, and I wanted to convey the comprehensiveness to medical students to give them templates on which they could build. I named the department, Department of Psychiatry and the Behavioral Sciences; I intended to start students off with a course in Basic Behavioral Sciences. However, there was no time in the curriculum for behavioral science. So we organized a course on Saturdays. Four strands formed the core; Human Development, Human Learning, Human Communication and the Social Field. The course was shot through with biology at every stage.

The other thing which we did, was to recruit the Chairmen of the other departments, to teach in our introductory course: Alan Barnes, Chief of Gynecology and Obstetrics, Robert Cooke, who was Chief of Pediatrics, colleagues from Harvey's Department of Medicine, and Blalock's Department of Surgery gave introductory lectures in our course which was really an introduction to medicine as a whole. Suddenly, psychiatry became alive and connected to other departments. I gave the introductory lectures myself; the response was encouraging. The students noted the change and responded magnificently. Residents suddenly shot up. There was a tremendous competition for the few residents' posts that we had. Wonderful people appeared. Sol Snyder, Joe Coyle, and Ross Baldessarini were residents at Hopkins.

FS: You obviously transferred your enthusiasm and your views to these people. I think this is one of your major contributions: nurture of people, your support of people.

JE: Yes, but, you know, that brings me back to my youth again, and my parents. They were extraordinary, nurturing people. They made me feel wanted and secure, and at the same time, there was always, always, the questioning spirit, the wish, to understand, the 'why'? That's what really ensued; somehow, invariably everywhere, in Birmingham, at St. Elizabeths and Hopkins. There were some fine, fine conversations in my youth.

FS: Joel, I am rushing a little bit, but I have to come to questions that the ACNP wants me to ask you. If you look back on fifty years in psychopharmacology, who were the scientists who had the most impact on your work, who would you single out?

JE: This is a hard question. Sherrington, one of the giants in early neuroscience, is one; Lord Adrian, who had tremendous depth, and inordinate experimental skills, is another.

FS: Was there anybody in the clinical area?

JE: In the clinical area, Adolf Meyer, because of the comprehensiveness of his approach. I'm hard pressed to answer this question, because there were so many, but among my contemporaries.....

FS: Seymour Kety, obviously?

JE: Seymour represented again, a wonderful blend of comprehensiveness, precision, and humanity. You know, I've known scientists, great scientists. They impressed me by their ideas, but when I'd got to know them often they were a little disappointing. Seymour had a tremendous influence on me as a person. He was gentle, he was human, he thought clearly, and had a contagious Woody Allen sense of humor. Then there was Heinrich Waelsch, the Dean of neurochemistry at that time; he had a continental acerbic sense of humor, a delight. He had a tremendous style....

FS: He was at Columbia.

JE: He was at Columbia. He did all of the work on ammonia and the brain. Heinrich Waelsch, Seymour Kety, Jordi Folch, and myself with Geoffrey Harris and Derek Richter convened the first Neurochemical Symposium at Oxford in 1954. We gathered together the leaders of neurochemistry when it was first beginning. Nino Salmoiraghi and Floyd Bloom came into my life late, absolutely wonderful workers. Floyd was always seeing the big picture. His brilliance and his imagination were always showing. Ross Baldessarini, as resident, was showing a balance between being a gifted psychotherapist when he was a resident, and a damn good biochemist in the lab. And I could go on and on, but to answer your question, the giants in my life mentioned above influenced me by the way they thought, more than anything else.

FS: Now, you have to put your modesty aside for the next question. The ACNP asked me to ask what you think, Joel, were your greatest contributions to the field?

JE: At the conceptual level, very early, the concept of families of neuroregulatory compounds, their uneven distribution in the central nervous system and the key role this concept of regional neurochemistry played in understanding the mode of action of psychoactive drugs, and how the brain does it without drugs. Secondly, the role of pharmacology as a gateway to physiology, to understanding how the brain works naturally, without the chemical prostheses of drugs; pharmacology as a way of exploring the phenomena, the layering, the organization of mental life, and giving us an insight into schizophrenia as a disorder of information processing in the brain.

FS: We, today, start talking again about the cross-talk in the brain, you know.

JE: Yes, it's in that paper that Bradley and I wrote that we talk about it. And, in the CIBA symposium paper, I'm quite specific about the interaction between drugs and families of naturally occurring compounds. Another contribution was the importance of understanding the interaction between environment, the social setting, the action and even the dose of a drug; the same drug in the same person in the same dose can produce different effects according to changes in the environment which precede, accompany or follow the administration of the medication. Thirdly, providing a setting where intelligent conversation between neurochemistry, electrophysiology, behavior and subjective experience could take place, and where experiment interacts with clinical experience. This was the Department of Experimental Psychiatry. I tried to be a good gardener and cultivate transdisciplinarians.

ALFRED M. FREEDMAN

Interviewed by Thomas A. Ban
New York, New York, November 3, 2000

TB: This is an interview with Dr. Alfred Freedman* for the Archives of the American College of Neuropsychopharmacology. We are in the apartment of Dr. Freedman in New York. It is November 3, 2000. I am Thomas Ban. Let us start from the very beginning. If you could tell us when and where were you born, say something about your education and early interests?

AF: I was born in Albany, New York, a small town at that time, although it was the capital of New York State. I was born on January 7, 1917. That appalls me when I realize soon I will have my 84th birthday. My parents were immigrants from Eastern Europe. My mother was born in a small town near Vilnius, that we always called Vilna. The small town she was born in, which we called Smargon (although the name on the current maps is Smargoni) is actually in Belarus at the present time. Anyway, she came here when she was about eighteen or nineteen years old in the early twentieth century. My father was born in Poland in a small town, Wisocki Modiuvetz. He studied to be a Rabbi in a city, Lomza. My Polish colleagues would tell me it's pronounced "Womza." He came here around the same time as my mother, and they met and got married. They lived and had small businesses in Massachusetts, which did not succeed. So finally they ended up in Albany, running a small grocery store. I was the third child. I had two older sisters and we lived above the grocery store.

We lived in an, I would say, rather poor mostly Irish and Polish immigrant neighborhood where I picked up a few words of Polish that I still remember. Anyway, I attended public school in Albany. Right next door to the school was the public library and that was heaven for me. Every Friday they used to have a storytelling hour, which I attended. After that hour I would get a lot of books to read for the next week, and that was a very happy occasion. That was my life until I was ten years old. I did very well in school. As a matter of fact, I entered a citywide achievement test when I was in the 5th grade and received the highest grade in the city! By that time my father had been doing very well in real estate investments, and so we moved from the south end of Albany, which was really the poorest part of the city, up to Pine Hills, which was one of the posh

* Alfred M. Freedman was born in Albany, New York, in 1917; he earned an undergraduate degree at Cornell University in 1937, and then studied medicine at the University of Minnesota, graduating in 1941. Freedman trained on the children's service of Bellevue Hospital in New York City, staying on as a staff psychiatrist, from 1948 to 1955. After working in several different pediatric posts, he became chairman of psychiatry at New York Medical College in 1960, from which post he retired in 1989. Freedman died in 2011.

neighborhoods. And there I finished the 7th grade. After that I went to the junior high school, which was some distance away.

Unfortunately, when I went to junior high school in the fall of 1929, my father's investments all went bad and he lost quite heavily. So actually he again opened up a grocery store not far from our home on Pine Avenue. These were very hard times. He had to work very hard. My mother also worked in the store and it was very difficult. I was in high school but I spent all my available time helping out in the grocery store. My greatest interest was in mathematics and science. When I graduated I got a medal for my achievements in mathematics and science. I particularly liked chemistry. I remember it as my very favorite subject. The mathematics I had at high school was limited. We did have advanced algebra, but I remember very well our poor teacher. It was really a bit beyond her, what she had to teach, but we used to help her out by making suggestions. She was very grateful for that. I was amazed when I got to college and found all those bright kids from New York City, who had studied calculus in high school.

It was the Great Depression when I went to high school and we had a very marginal sort of life in those years. I remember that I started driving the truck for the store when I was fourteen years old and was picked up once by the police. Fortunately, in my father's good times, he became very friendly with a superintendent in one of his buildings, who became a policeman; so he, fortunately, got me off. I remember in those years driving hurriedly to the bank to make a deposit before the bank closed at 2:00 o'clock, in order to meet the deadline of the checks my father had written to pay the bills that he couldn't delay anymore. So it was a difficult time. I used to work in the store after school, as well as on Saturdays. On Sunday, we kept the store open for half a day and I would run that myself to give my father and mother a little time off. In addition to the grocery and meat market, we got the idea of having newspapers and magazines in the store, which my parents allotted to me to handle. All the money that came in from the papers and magazines was put aside for me to go to college. In the meantime one of my sisters had started college at Cornell. My parents worked very hard to make sure that there was enough money for her to finish.

TB: The re were three of you, right?

AF: There were four of us. I also had a brother, five years younger than me. There was actually another boy in between the two of us, who died when he was six months old.

TB: Both of your older sisters went to college?

AF: All four of us. My mother was unceasing in her efforts. She wanted us not only to go to college, but become doctors or lawyers. For the girls graduate school would have been fine for her. Anyway, I realized very soon that as far as college was concerned, in Albany there was a Normal School for teachers that later became a college, and is now the basis of the State University of New York in Albany. It used to be right next door to the high school but later on it moved away from there. So that was always a possibility for me if I didn't win a scholarship to Cornell. They had statewide scholarships in those years that were distributed by county. Albany County had three and I won one of those three. Then I won an additional state tuition scholarship that with the other scholarship was the basis of my going to an Ivy League College.

There were several things, I might say, that shaped my development in high school. One was my devotion to chemistry and physics. Also, there were two books that were very important to me. One was *Arrowsmith* by Sinclair Lewis, which introduced me to the whole idea of devoting one's life to research. I remember the experiments he was doing on bacteria and his research in the Caribbean. That book had a great impact on me. The other one was Paul De Kruif's *Microbe Hunters*, which described the lives of those who made important contributions to the progress of bacteriology and the elucidation of the cause and cure of disease. They were Koch, Pasteur, Walter Reed and many others. After reading that book I wanted to become a researcher.

TB: Did any of your teachers have a major impact on deciding your career choice?

AF: I think the teacher who seemed most interested and encouraging, was my history teacher. Her name was Ms. Bradt. They were all friendly, I got top grades, but I never got any particular encouragement. And I remember that we had a man who taught us chemistry. His name was Job, Mr. Job. He was a rather aloof man but a good teacher. As long as you did your work that was okay. But he wasn't a person to say, "Oh, that's very good, what are your plans, you might think of studying biochemistry." No, there was nothing like that. I didn't have any of my teachers give me encouragement. It all came from myself.

TB: So it was your decision entirely without any encouragement?

AF: Well, as I said, my mother was very enthusiastic to have me and my brother become doctors and my father joined her in that. He was busy in the store all day and when he came home he had a bite to eat and would fall asleep at the table. So he didn't say very much in that regard until I had become successful, and then he wrote to me, "You did it all on your own." Anyway, my sister graduated from Cornell in 1933, and I graduated from high school in the same year. And, of course, that was a very important year, not only because of my graduation, but also because of my perturbation in regard to going to college and about my future life. And, as you know, that was also the year Hitler came to power.

TB: Yes, in the spring of 1933

AF: To go back a little in time, we were all very impressed in 1928, when Franklin Delano Roosevelt became Governor of New York. He was very popular and impressive, though my father said they elected a cripple as a governor and had to install elevators in the executive mansion to accommodate him. But Roosevelt was truly a charismatic figure. He always drove around in an open car in Albany; he'd sit in the back with a chauffeur in the front. And I remember standing on the main street one day when they were driving along. People started clapping, and saying hurrah. Men took off their hats and waved them. He had a cigarette in a cigarette holder, and tipped his hat. I had followed the election in 1928, when Al Smith ran against Herbert Hoover. We had listened on the radio to the Democratic Convention in 1932. It was quite a battle between Roosevelt and Al Smith who was bitter because he looked upon Roosevelt as his protégé. It was Smith who persuaded Roosevelt to become Governor.

Anyway, eventually Roosevelt became President and that was important for me because of the various programs he introduced to do something about the Depression. And then Hitler came into power. It was very troublesome. He was a threat to the world, but particularly to us Jews. I was studying at Cornell but my funds were very inadequate. My parents had some money that they gave me, but I depended mostly on my two scholarships. As a result of Roosevelt's efforts, they formed what was called the National Youth Administration (NYA) that gave money for young people to get jobs. So I got a job cleaning the aquarium in a research laboratory under a man named Myron Gordon. I was 16 years old when I went to college, and being from a small town and a family that was, in many ways, out of the mainstream, I was very poorly prepared for college. I really felt very lost. At times, during my first year, I felt like giving it up and going home. It was a feeling of being a burden on my family; they had difficulty making out anyway. But, in any event, I persevered.

TB: So you worked in an aquarium while in college?

AF: Yes. But some time during the first year my job in the aquarium was changed from cleaner to becoming a translator. What actually happened was that one day Myron was sort of groaning over some stuff, and he asked me whether I knew German. When I told him that I did, since I had German in high school, he opened a scientific journal, pointed to a word and asked, "Do you know what this is?" I did. Soon after that incident he said, "Forget about cleaning the aquarium; you can translate German for me. Here, take this home. I want you to translate this article and this will be your job here." This was very nice, because I was able to work at home instead of going at night to the aquarium. He gave me a dictionary and I would translate the articles he had.

Myron Gordon's research was essentially on the genetics of melanoma. He found that by crossing two breeds of fish, *Xiphophorus Helleri*, a sword-tailed fish, and *Platypoecilus Maculatus*, a tropical fish, one of the hybrids got black spots that would develop into melanomas. I found all this fascinating. I became taken up with this, because the articles were about melanomas, crossbreeding fish, and genetics; the material was scientifically stimulating. I was avidly reading the books Myron Gordon had in his library. One of the classics of the time on the topic was Ewing's *Neoplastic Disease* and I used to read on melanoma and other stuff in it. I was really taken by the topic, and more or less decided that if I go to medical school I'm going to work on cancer and I'm going to find a cure for it. Then, one day, I remember him talking to me about his correspondence with a man who had been doing similar work in Germany, and saying, "Imagine in a letter I got in 1934 or '36 from this man in Germany; he closed his letter instead of 'best regards,' by writing 'Heil Hitler.'"

TB: What did you major in?

AF: It was a pre-med major. But I was determined that I was going to complete a major in mathematics, physics and chemistry. I took calculus in my first year and I did very well in it as I recall, and became very interested. During my first year I didn't get involved in any extracurricular activities; I was busy translating and with my studies. But they had a series of lectures every year by some distinguished person and I attended those. There was a lecture I particularly remember, given by Eddington, a very famous astronomer, cosmologist and scientific philosopher. He talked about atoms, and atomic energy and that opened a new world to me. I ended up getting a flat 100 in my freshman chemistry, that was quite spectacular, and I got very high grades throughout that year in all the different subjects. But I decided that medicine was not for me; I wanted to study physics and become what we called in those days an atomic scientist. So when I went home and told my parents that I was going to give up medicine and was going to become an atomic physicist, they were dismayed. And I remember my father telling me that for thousands of years the men in our family had been Rabbis or teachers, and he was the first one who did not finish his rabbinical studies and became a businessman because his father, my grandfather, a Hebrew teacher, moved to the United States. He didn't have much appreciation for me becoming a professor of physics, and my mother felt kind of bad about it also. Anyway, by the end of the summer I decided to go back to my original plan and study medicine.

TB: So you went back and continued with your pre-med courses.

AF: One always wonders what would have happened if one had done it in the other way, if I would have become an atomic physicist. It was 1934, just the early days that new field was opening up. It would probably have been very interesting too, because the following year Hans Bethe, a famous physicist, came to Cornell after leaving Germany, and organized a whole unit of Nuclear Physics. Later on he moved to Los Alamos and was involved in making the atomic bomb. So I might have been involved in making the atomic bomb.

TB: But you decided to prepare for medical school.

AF: Yes, and it was tough going. But I succeeded and had even some fun. I can't look back and say, "oh, those wonderful college days." It was stressful with a lot of tension. I was also concerned about how my parents were making out. They had many crises in their business, and when I got those checks for my scholarship, I foolishly endorsed them and sent them home. My father was furious and sent them back. But what I did indicated my own anxieties in regard to the home situation.

TB: Did you continue doing well at school?

AF: I did well in school, as you might expect. I had problems with some courses, like comparative anatomy. I think I only got a B in it, but I had As in chemistry, physics, and all the other subjects. I had to take Freshman English and it turned out, Professor French, the man who was teaching it, and who was my advisor, had been somebody my sister knew. He was a very nice person. I enjoyed his course and did very well. Actually, I also took second year English which was not required. He was very encouraging and invited me once to his home for dinner. He liked the essays I wrote, particularly when I just wrote of my own experiences or life, rather than trying to be another Shakespeare or Hemingway. So he was a very important person in my life. He encouraged me to do things I could do. I actually did complete a major in chemistry and in physics. I had to take sort of a short course in biochemistry, but I took the regular course and also took physical chemistry that was not required, and instead of taking the short course in physics, I took two years of physics. The physics teacher was very impressed; he was very good to me and encouraged me in my activities.

I must say, in retrospect, I had social phobia. I was very timid and very shy. I found it very difficult and it would not occur to me to ask anybody to do something for me. A third person who became very important for me, was a doctor that I met. Actually, this was the period of time when the civil war broke out in Spain. I was very taken up with the Spanish Civil War, and was desperately eager for the Loyalists to hold out against

Franco. And there were on the campus various things going on, which I entered, supporting the Loyalists. And through this connection, I met a couple. One was a doctor. He was the head of pathology at a center for tubercular patients. He was born in Germany and had been in the army as a doctor in World War I. Then, by 1922 or so, he decided to come to the United States. His name was Max Pinner. So when I was introduced to Max and he said that he was a pathologist, I replied, "Oh, that's interesting. I've been doing reading on cancer". He said, "Oh, really. What have you been reading?" I replied, "I've been reading Ewing's textbook on cancer." So he asked, "Oh, what are you interested in?" Then I started telling him about melanoma and he became very interested and friendly. Actually, they had me to their house and I saw a lot of them.

Then, in the fourth year, it was time to apply to medical school. And, as I said before, I had a bit of social phobia. Anyway, I was very timid. It didn't occur to me to go to Professor French, or to the professor of physics, or to Max Pinner and say, "I'm worried about getting into medical school." I just could not go and tell them, "You know I'm Jewish; I have no big connections; my father and my uncle are not doctors; can you advise me?" Instead of asking for their help I just went and handed in my application. But in spite of my high marks, Cornell turned me down, and so did all the other medical schools I applied to.

TB: Did all the schools turn you down?

AF: I only applied to schools in the East and I remember being interviewed at the New York Medical College and they looked at me and said "boy, look at these grades. Did you ever see anything like that?" They turned me down, though, because I was Jewish. One of my Jewish classmates whose uncle was a doctor on the staff there was accepted. You had to have connections in those years. I had none. And I had hoped to get into Albany Medical School, but there again, I had no connections and they gave me a hard time. My father and my mother were immigrants, so they were not impressed. I recall going to the University of Rochester and being interviewed by Dean Whipple, who was a very famous surgeon. He was very nasty and asked, "Why do all you people want to become doctors? Why don't you just work in the grocery store like your father does?" Anyway, that was a terrible blow. I didn't have money to travel back and forth, so I hitchhiked to Rochester. I remember, while standing at a crossroad hitchhiking back to Ithaca, of thinking the hell with all this, I should just leave and go Southwest and see what will happen.

TB: What did you do?

AF: In January 1937 I enrolled in the graduate school in Zoology, in the department that Myron Gordon was in, and I began my first research project there. In my readings on cancer, I had been really impressed that there were certain substances that caused cancer, so I thought I should try to see what would happen with the development of cells if I raised them in a solution of carcinogenic substances. I had taken a course in Experimental Embryology and learned about various embryology organizers. I was also familiar with the writing of a German named Holtfreter on this subject. So, with the help of a colleague in the Department of Zoology, we collected the eggs of early spring frogs. And then I got some cancer producing substances and raised the eggs in a solution of them. Meanwhile, someone told me about the possibility of getting admitted to medical school at the University of Minnesota. So, I applied and to my surprise I was accepted. All I had to do was take a pre-med examination. One of the women instructors in the laboratory carried on my work and when the eggs were hatched into tadpoles, she actually made sections of them and sent them to me in Minnesota.

Before I left I went to say goodbye to French, and when I told him the problems I had he was furious with me and said, "Why didn't you tell me your problems? Why didn't you ask me for advice? I'd have written a letter for you." If I had told him he would have gone over to see the Dean of the Medical School of Cornell in Ithaca, one of the two schools they had at that time, and could have solved the problem. Apparently, he was an advisor there with a lot of influence. The same thing happened when I went to see Max Pinner. He also said that he could have helped me to get accepted at New York University. It was the first time in my life in which I found myself unable to advance myself by asking for things. It happened again many times later in life. So many of the things in my life I achieved passively. Anyway, that was the end of my Cornell experience.

TB: And you left for Minnesota.

AF: Well, it was a long, long trip. I remember going out there by train. I had never been west of Rochester before. So that was a whole new world and I did not know what to expect. I arrived there in the evening and I spent the night in a hotel close by the railroad station. And then I went up to the campus the next day and looked for a place to stay. At Cornell, the dormitories were too expensive for my very limited budget. But by the time I went to Minnesota, the situation, thanks to Roosevelt, was somewhat better. Of course, medical school in Minnesota was a big bargain compared to New York. It was free for residents of Minnesota, and also those from North and South Dakota and Montana because they had no medical school. And it was about $300.00 for others. I also found a cheap place to live, right around the campus. It wasn't too bad. Compared to Ithaca, prices were very reasonable at that time in Minnesota. We were still in the years when there was a so-called numerus clausus for Jewish students. They would decide in advance how many they would take every year. As I discovered later there were three out of state Jewish students in my class. The other two were from New York City. One had gone to Brooklyn College and the other, I think to City College. It turned out that the Dean of the medical school was a very liberal man, who was troubled by the quota for Jewish students.

Contrary to my years in college where I excelled in school, in Minnesota I didn't devote myself to my studies in the first two years. I think in some way it was a sort of reaction to not getting into Cornell, or Yale or Harvard. I wasn't industrious in doing my work and neglected my studies, so I got Bs. It went on to the extent that instead of taking Part I of the National Board Examinations at the end of the second year, I did it sometime in the third year. To my surprise, it turned out that I got the highest grade in biochemistry for the country. I can't explain how it happened but it turned out that way. I did various things during those two years, as if I was trying to make up for all that I missed as an undergraduate. So even if I had to miss a class I went to the weekly concerts held for the students by the Minneapolis Symphony Orchestra and became a devoted follower of Dimitri Metropolis, its conductor. It was the time when the Spanish Civil War was winding up. It was also the time of the Munich Agreement and the onslaught on Czechoslovakia. I remember being very involved in those issues and going around the city in a car with a loudspeaker shouting, "Protect Czechoslovakia against the Nazis." And the group that I was involved in organized a big rally on the steps of the University auditorium. Unfortunately, it was the day after Chamberlain went to Munich and announced that there's going to be peace; that Hitler would have Czechoslovakia, or the Sudetenland. And I remember the professor of history got up and said, "Well, Ancient Bohemia will not die." It was very sad.

TB: So you got involved more in politics than in your studies.

AF: I liked histology in the 1st year, and in 2nd year pathology really turned me on. And I did very well in it. It was very funny. The other students thought I was sort of unusual, but on the other hand, I was a recognized expert on politics and international events. When sitting around at lunch, one or another would ask, "What do you think is going to happen with Hitler?" or "Is he going to take the rest of Czechoslovakia?" or things like that they had heard, but had not read very much about. So anyway, that was sort of interesting.

TB: What about in the 3rd year and later on?

AF: In the third year I was really taken with clinical work and became enthusiastic about my studies. So, in the last two years I did well, but I never made up for what I missed in the first two years. I also met an associate professor of physiology, in charge of neurophysiology, through some mutual friends, and told him that I wanted to devote my life to research. So he said, "Well, why don't you come up and maybe we can work out a project." He was doing research in traumatic or neurogenic shock, and being a neurophysiologist, he was interested in what role the nerves played in it.

At that time, the prevailing authority in traumatic shock was Professor Blalock at Johns Hopkins. He thought that the big danger was the pooling away of blood from the various parts of the body, that blood pressure goes down and not even blood transfusion could help in preventing death. And this associate professor I worked with had an idea to do a project on that. We bound one leg of a cat tightly so there could be no accumulation of blood in that leg, and then I was hitting the leg of the cat with an iron pipe, so that the cat would go into shock, its blood pressure dropped, and eventually it would die. And then by doing an autopsy we established that the accumulation of blood in the traumatic area was not different in one leg from the other, and concluded that in the pathological mechanism of traumatic shock pooling of blood never plays an important role. I actually had my first paper on our findings in this research. I think it was published in the *Journal of Physiology*. Then we did another paper together that was published in the *Proceedings* of the Society of Experimental Biology. And on the basis of these two papers, I was elected as an undergraduate to the research society Sigma Xi, which was a big honor. Very few students got elected to that prestigious national organization. I remember that at the dinner in honor of the new members, Bell, the Professor of Pathology, was the principal speaker. The main point of his speech was, "Well, what you have to do as a researcher is define your area very early and just stick to that for life. For example, I became interested in the pathology of the kidney, so I devoted my life to glomerular nephritis, nephrosis, and all kinds of things with the kidney." I thought to myself that's not for me. I'm going to be another Leonardo da Vinci.

TB: So you worked in neurophysiology while in medical school?

AF: That's right. And, the guy I was working with was Herman Kabat, who had his PhD in Neuroanatomy and Neurophysiology from Northwestern. I used to work with him on his experiments. He was interested in anoxia of the brain and the experiment of closing off the carotids for a short time, to see which cells were more sensitive to the lack of oxygen. He had a collaborator, a professor of neuropathology, whose name was Baker. At the time, Psychiatry was a subdivision of the department of medicine, and Baker was assigned the task of teaching psychiatry. He was a very uninspiring teacher of the topic. He handed out notes to read, it was a kind of one, two, three. If you had asked me the subject I would least likely want to pursue as a career at that time, I would have said Psychiatry.

TB: Could you tell us something about those notes?

AF: We got a list of symptoms for diagnosing schizophrenia and manic-depressive psychosis. He was sort of more interested in showing us possible pathology than talking about clinical symptoms. The one thing I remember in psychiatry was a psychiatrist in town who was in private practice. He was one of the originators of ECT, and was experimenting with it. We went to his office for a demonstration. I remember, he had all kinds of equipment and batteries. I think that was the most interesting lesson we had in our course in psychiatry.

TB: What about your clerkship?

AF: We had rather staggered clerkships. We were divided in four groups and I was in one where we worked all summer, and then I had the fall off, and I went home. Before leaving, Kabat, the guy I was working with in neurophysiology, told me that while I was in Albany I should visit Harold Himwich, the Professor of Physiology at the Albany Medical College who was working on the same sort of things in the brain.

TB: Could you just remind us what you were working on with him?

AF: I was working on anoxia of the brain, and its consequences on brain function. So when I was in Albany, I went down to the Albany Medical School and met Harold Himwich. Do you know him?

TB: Yes. I did know him.

AF: Well, Himwich was a bossy but friendly guy and when we met he said, "Yeah, I read your rotten paper." And then he invited me to spend some time in his lab before returning to Minnesota. He had an assistant at that time whose name was Fazekas, also a medical student, who later became Chief of Medicine at the City Hospital in Washington. I spent some time working with Harold on his projects. In those days, the belief and the conviction was that all metabolism in the brain was due to glucose. And he was working on that, not only in adult but also in fetal brains. Since the metabolism of the brain was at a lower level in the brains of the fetus and the newborn, in case of anoxia a fetus, or a newborn cat, could survive longer than an older one and would have less damage to its brain. Anyway, I worked on those experiments with him and Fazekas.

TB: For how long did you work with him?

AF: Just during my vacation in 1940. I had to go back to school and finish my studies. I enjoyed working with Harold Himwich, and the time I spent with Fazekas and a couple of the other people in the laboratory. Albany had a large Little Italy, and we used to drive there to some typical Italian restaurants with checkered tablecloths to have spaghetti and meatballs. It was a very pleasant time for me, I learned a lot from Harold Himwich, and the work he did was useful to the research I did with Kabat on traumatic shock and its possible prevention. Then, just before my return to Minnesota, I got a telegram from Kabat that took me a little while to comprehend. It said: "Adrian in oil, please come right away." And then I realized that he was talking about adrenaline in oil that he wanted me to work on. It was in the late 1940s when everything was tuning up for war. Research in traumatic shock and especially in its possible prevention became of special importance and Kabat thought that if we could show that brain anoxia, traumatic shock, could be prevented by the administration of adrenaline in oil the army would love it.

TB: So you went back to Minnesota after your vacation and continued your research with him?

AF: Yes, I did. We published a paper on our findings. Adrenaline in oil really did not work very well. In the meanwhile, I was finishing up my clerkship and headed for graduation. Minnesota was a very friendly place. I made a lot of friends and many times I've regretted not staying there, because I made good contacts with the clinical people. But, I think, with the war impending, I wanted to go back East and be with my parents.

TB: Where did you do your internship?

AF: I thought I'd like to go to New York to do my internship, and Max Pinner, who by then was Chief of the tuberculosis service at Montefiore Hospital, was ready to arrange an internship in his hospital. But I decided that I wanted to get a big city experience. So I became an intern at Harlem Hospital.

TB: Is here anything else you would like to tell us about your experiences in Minnesota?

AF: Yes. Prior to starting with my internship I had to complete my clerkship in obstetrics at the City Hospital in Minneapolis. I had never delivered a baby before, but on the day soon after my arrival to work, the resident I was assigned to, left me to have his supper. As soon as he went down on one elevator, another elevator came up with a woman yelling and screaming, she was about to deliver a baby. Fortunately I had a very good nurse there with me but by the time she got me into my gown and gloves the baby's head was already beginning to appear. She stood over my shoulder and kept on telling me what to do and how to take hold of the baby. Then I brought the baby out, tied the cord and under her supervision cleaned the baby's throat. That was a big moment. It was the first baby I ever delivered. I delivered a lot more after that. Anyway, it all went well. Then, when the resident returned from lunch he told me the big news that Germany had invaded Russia.

TB: What year did you graduate?

AF: In June 1941, and I started my internship on the 1st of July.

TB: So you moved in June 1941 from Minneapolis to New York?

AF: Yes, but I went to Albany to spend a few days with my family before starting my internship in New York.

TB: Could you say something about your internship?

AF: It was a very busy internship. We got very little teaching. I think it was a poor choice on my part, but in any event, I spent the year with a very friendly bunch of people. My zeal for research did not leave me and Harold Himwich told me that a friend of his, with the name of Bulova, was doing research at Harlem Hospital. Those were the days when all through the country, they had stations with various types of antisera for pneumonia and if someone had pneumonia they typed it to provide the most appropriate treatment. And Bulova dedicated his life to develop antisera for pneumonia. His ward was completely oxygenated with signs around, don't smoke and don't light a match, because the place could blow up. He had an associate who was a refugee from Europe who was doing some research that dealt with nucleoproteins. I told them about my interest in research shortly after I started to work with them.

As you know by that time Hitler had already taken over Czechoslovakia, and invaded Poland. So for a few months I attended to my duties at the hospital and was doing my research with Bulova. Our hospital used to send an ambulance to the Polo Grounds where the Giants football team played and all of us interns, who were interested in football, went with the ambulance to watch the games. And then, I vividly remember that on December 7, 1941 while sitting and watching the games, I suddenly realized that something extraordinary was going on. It started with an announcement, as I recall, asking Col. Donovan to call the operator. Then about 15 minutes later there was another announcement asking Col. Donovan's chauffeur to go to gate 21. While the game continued some people were paged, but I only found out, overhearing the radios on the street while returning to the hospital, that the Japanese had bombed Pearl Harbor. Although I signed up for a two-year internship I told the hospital that I was leaving after my first year. It was okay because I needed only a one-year internship to get my license. In the meantime I talked to Harold Himwich who had some contacts with the air surgeons.

TB: So, you left to become an air surgeon?

AF: Foolishly I didn't look into what it would require to become an air surgeon. Apparently I didn't qualify because my eyesight was poor. So I ended up in the Army Air Force, as it was called then. But I was just assigned as a regular doctor, and I would have done better if I had continued with my training and had some special skills. I worked in a dispensary and escorted troop trains as a medical officer. And on one of those trains, coming back from Colorado Springs to Illinois, I met Marcia. We became attracted to each other and six months later we got married. Before we got married I was sent to get further training in the army at Carlisle Barracks in Pennsylvania. Most of the medical officers in Miami were middle aged, and they picked me immediately as the youngest one, who was single and had no children, to go to Carlisle. So, I spent 12 weeks marching around in the snow and studying military tactics. When I got back to Miami Beach where I was stationed we got married. Shortly before my wedding I was asked by our commanding officer if I'd be interested in going to a laboratory school at Johns Hopkins. I grabbed the opportunity, because I realized that I would be stuck by remaining an ordinary doctor. So we went to Baltimore and after ninety days I returned from Baltimore to Miami as a laboratory officer. In the meantime Arthur Mirsky was made the Chief of the laboratory. So when I came back I got a job in the laboratory in one of the hospitals I was running the hematology service.

As soon as I began with my new activities, I started to look for a research project. I recall, that I read a paper in *JAMA* on heterophile antibody in viral pneumonia that was quite prevalent then, particularly in the army. So I decided, I'd study heterophile antibodies on random soldiers in the hospital, and discovered that it was the antibody of infectious mononucleosis. I wrote this up with Mirsky, and was going to send it to *JAMA* where I got the idea from. But Mirsky felt that we should send it to a military magazine because it would be better for my career. It was bad advice; the paper got buried and lost. By the time it appeared other people got all the credit for the discovery of heterophile antibody in infectious mononucleosis. Anyway, it was my research. I was in the laboratory for about a year before I was transferred to be in charge of a laboratory in Gulfport, Mississippi in the station hospital, which, at the time, had 1,000 beds. It was quite a big enterprise.

TB: So you moved from Miami to Gulfport.

AF: I had a fairly good size staff in Gulfport and while I was doing my job one of our soldiers, who just returned from the Pacific,. committed suicide by taking Seconal (secobarbital). So, I collected the gastric contents as well as some blood and sent it to the regional laboratory for analysis because we did not have the necessary facilities for that. I found out from the Surgeon General's library that there had been no reported cases of successful suicide so far with Seconal. I don't remember any longer whose drug Seconal was, but I remember that its advertisement said that was a safe drug insofar as suicide is concerned. And when I got my figures of the blood levels of Seconal in the soldier, I called the professor of Pharmacology at the Tulane University who confirmed for me that the level in the blood was high enough to cause a fatal outcome. So I wrote this up in a paper, and this time I didn't make a mistake but sent it to *JAMA*. In my paper I wrote that I was reporting a case of Seconal overdose with a fatal outcome. I also said that there had been no reported cases of successful suicide with Seconal in the literature. Then, in the next issue of *JAMA* a letter appeared saying that Captain Freedman's survey of the medical literature was inadequate. If he had looked at the coroner's reports in Los Angeles County, he would have seen that Aimee McPherson, a famous evangelist, had committed suicide by taking Seconal a year or two before my report.

TB: So during the time you were in Gulfport you reported on a case of fatal overdose with Seconal.

AF: Actually, in Gulfport, I became very friendly with the psychiatrist, who was from St. Louis. So, I used to spend time with him and he would show some of his cases to me. I was spending a lot of time on the psychiatry ward there and found it quite interesting. I also remember telling him that I might go into psychiatry eventually to study the biochemistry of mental illness.

TB: So is this how you got into psychiatry?

AF: I might have gone directly into psychiatry, but I thought I would get two years' credit for my pathology boards, for the work I did in the army.

TB: When were you discharged from the army?

AF: I was discharged in January 1946. I was officially on leave with pay from January and actually discharged in March.

TB: What did you do after your discharge?

AF: My intention was to go into pathology, and Dr. Pinner told me that I should contact his friend, Dr. Klemperer at Mount Sinai Hospital, who was the head of pathology there. When I met Dr. Klemperer he said, "Anybody that my friend, Max Pinner sends has a place in my laboratory." So after a brief vacation in Florida with Marsha's parents, I reported for work at Mount Sinai in New York. As it turned out, the place was flooded with veterans like me, and we were given work on a voluntary basis.

TB: So did you or didn't you have a job there?

AF: I didn't have a regular appointment; I couldn't even go and eat at the staff dining room. After going to the dining room a couple of times they told me, and also the others, that we should not come back. So I decided at that point that I was not going to spend my life in a mortuary doing post mortems, and started to look around for a job.

Harold Himwich by that time had left his job as professor of physiology in Albany and became director of research at Edgewood Arsenal in

Maryland. And when I called him, he invited me to come down to work with him. So we moved from New York and I did research with Harold on anticholinesterases, the German nerve gases. By blocking cholinesterase, the enzyme responsible for breaking down acetylcholine, these gases left the acetylcholine unchecked in the brain that led to death within seconds. Somewhere, along in there, I got the idea of trying to inject the DFP (di-isopropyl phosphorofluoridate) into an animal to see what effect it would have. And, lo and behold, when we injected it, the cat got grand mal seizures with a spectacular EEG. Harold became very excited about that and thought that it might be that the cause of epilepsy is a deficiency of cholinesterase or an excess of acetylcholine. So anyway, we did a whole series of experiments in this area of research. In the meantime I read a paper from which I learned that there is more cholinesterase in the brain after birth and was thinking that the acquisition of intelligence in some way might be related to changes in the level of acetylcholine. While working with Himwich I realized that I'd really prefer to work on humans rather than the cats and rabbits we were working on. It might also be a factor that several of my friends were going into psychiatry. So I thought, well, I should also train to become a psychiatrist. I actually wanted to become a child psychiatrist, and work on the biochemistry of the development of intelligence.

TB: So this was the time you decided to leave pathology for psychiatry?

AF: When I told Harold that I would like to get into psychiatry, he introduced me to Karl Bowman, who was professor of psychiatry at the University of California in San Francisco, and I was accepted to start my residency there. But in the meantime Harold told me, "Oh, I wouldn't go to California. The best place for psychiatry in the country is Bellevue. You ought to go to Bellevue." So I went up to New York, saw Sam Wortis and he accepted me on Himwich's recommendation. Instead of going to California we went to New York.

TB: When did you actually leave Himwich to start with your residency in psychiatry?

AF: In June 1948. Although I did not go to San Francisco we drove out to California in 1956 and '57; Marcia's brother was living out there. And when I looked at the city I said to Marcia, "Oh, God, what a mistake I made." I must say that San Francisco is a beautiful city, but so is New York. Anyway, I went to get training at Bellevue.

TB: So, you started your psychiatric residency at Bellevue in July 1948.

AF: I started as a first year resident at $18.00 a month. But fortunately that was the time of the GI Bill and I got enough to live on with some help from Marcia's parents. And Marcia was doing some work, too. It was okay. After

I started at Bellevue in psychiatry I looked around for some research to be done, but I must say there wasn't very much going on and the residency occupied a good deal of time. While a resident I spent some time in the EEG laboratory. I was given credit for my time in the army, so I only needed two years to complete my training. During my training I made contact with Lauretta Bender, who was in charge of the child psychiatry service.

TB: She was one of the pioneers of child psychiatry.

AF: Lauretta Bender was one of the outstanding child psychiatrists in the country, I would say. She, Leo Kanner, and maybe a couple of other people were well known even outside of the United States. She had invented the Bender-Gestalt test that is still widely used in the country. She and Paul Schilder had worked with psychotic children, which they diagnosed as childhood schizophrenia. I became interested in childhood schizophrenia and hypothesized childhood schizophrenia and adult schizophrenia were related. Later on I followed up the children they had diagnosed as childhood schizophrenia; I found that most of them were adult schizophrenics in hospitals or living in the community.

TB: So you worked with Lauretta Bender.

AF: She was very interested in neurological soft signs in schizophrenic children, and perceived childhood schizophrenia as a neuro-developmental disease, a "lag in development." I wrote a couple of papers with her on this topic. She also had written papers with her husband.

TB: Wasn't her husband Paul Schilder, the famous neurologist and psychoanalyst?

AF: Yes. I also became very interested in psychotic children who were damaging themselves. We had several head bangers. One of the kids kept on banging his head so hard that we put a football helmet on him, so that he wouldn't injure himself. I remember reading about Paul Ehrlich in high school and was fascinated by his idea of finding magic bullets for diseases. So I started looking around to find a magic bullet to treat these children. All we used in these children in those days were paraldehyde and sodium amobarbital that would knock them out. And that didn't seem to be very satisfactory to me. So, I started experimenting with various drugs and that's where my psychopharmacology really began.

TB: So, we are now in the mid 1950s?

AF: No. Actually 1951, before chlorpromazine appeared in the USA.

TB: And you were in those years in child psychiatry?

AF: I took my board examination in 1952 and became first, the junior, and then the senior psychiatrist on the children's ward.

TB: So, after taking the board examination in psychiatry you stayed in child psychiatry?

AF: Yes.

TB: You were in child psychiatry in the years when chlorpromazine and reserpine were introduced?

AF: Yes, but not exclusively. I started private practice and saw adult patients as well.

TB: And you were looking for magic bullets?

AF: Well, I did and when I attended neurology grand rounds I learned about a new antihistaminic drug that was found useful in patients with Parkinson's disease and other neurological disorders. The drug produced somnolence and had a pacifying effect. So I thought I should try it because it might be effective in some of the children I was treating.

TB: What was the drug you are talking about?

AF: It was Benadryl (diphenhydramine). I used it in a few children and it seemed to have beneficial effects. Besides Benadryl, I also used Phenergan (promethazine) and Miltown (meprobamate), soon after they were introduced.

TB: So you used Benadryl in a few children before you used chlorpromazine?

AF: Oh, yes, before we even knew about chlorpromazine.

TB: What about Phenergan?

AF: I used Phenergan after I heard about chlorpromazine. I think it was Squibb or American Home Products that had Phenergan, and I suggested to them that we should try Phenergan in children because it resembles chlorpromazine.

TB: It differs by one methyl group on the side chain.

AF: Antihistamines worked in psychotic children. I remember telling that to Himwich, who by that time was in Galesburg, Illinois. After I told him about our findings with Benadryl in children he tried it in psychotic adults and it did not work.

TB: So, you were one of the first trying some of the new drugs in children; you were pioneering pharmacotherapy in children.

AF: I was trying to develop it and I wrote a couple of papers on my findings with several drugs, as for example with Benadryl.

TB: Did Lauretta Bender show any interest in your findings with Benadryl?

AF: Oh, yes, she was very much interested in it. As a matter of fact, I was very amused to learn that even after I left the children's service, she continued to use it. The other day I was talking to a psychiatrist who worked with Lauretta Bender after I left and he told me that she continued using Benadryl, and not just her but also Barbara Fish and others.

TB: So it was you who established the place of Benadryl in child psychiatry.

AF: Yes. My original findings remained the basis for the use of Benadryl in child psychiatry. However, I must emphasize, I continued my work testing various drugs on psychotic children. In those early days I conducted controlled studies in collaboration with two colleagues. I checked the records and randomly assigned various drugs and placebo to the children. They were examined by my two colleagues who reported the findings to me and I collated the results. One of our studies showed clearly that chlorpromazine was superior to Benadryl, although I must say that Lauretta Bender was unimpressed with my findings and insisted that in her experience Benadryl was superior and never changed her mind. The Professor of Pediatrics at New York University (NYU) was very interested in the study and pressured me to have it published in the *Journal of Pediatrics*. That probably was a mistake. It should have been published in the *American Journal of Psychiatry*. However I continued my studies with various psychopharmacologic agents in children particularly as new drugs appeared on the market. This continued later at Downstate. I think I made a very important contribution to psychopharmacology in children.

TB: When did you leave Bellevue?

AF: I guess I left in 1954.

TB: Why did you leave?

AF: I thought that I had had enough of full time hospital work. So for a short time I was in private practice while working as an instructor in child psychiatry and doing research at the Columbia Presbyterian Hospital. I was the psychiatrist on the team that was studying the Riley-Day Syndrome that was to become known as familial dysautonomia.

TB: Could you tell us something about familial dysautonomia?

AF: This is an inherited disorder present almost exclusively in Jewish children. One of its most distressing aspects is severe vomiting that could lead to dehydration, changes in electrolyte balance and death. We used to meet once a month with the parents of these children. And one of the parents was a pharmacist, who came to me after one of those sessions and told me about the announcement of a French drug that was supposed to be very good for nausea and vomiting. He was wondering whether it could control the vomiting of these children. We were in need of a drug that could control vomiting in the children, so I asked him to bring me some written material on the substance. So he did, and he showed me a brochure on chlorpromazine. At that time chlorpromazine was already being evaluated in the United States by Smith, Kline & French (SK&F), and I decided to try it in children with familial dysautonomia as well as my Bellevue population of psychotic children.

TB: You tried it to control vomiting in familial dysautonomia with chlorpromazine?

AF: Yes, but before doing that I tried to find out what was known about the drug. So I learned that they used it first in general anesthesia. I also learned that there were clinical trials going on in several places with the drug, including on the adult psychiatric wards at Bellevue Hospital. After that I got hold of chlorpromazine, and in a comparative study I found it better than Benadryl or Phenergan in the control of vomiting. I thought that chlorpromazine might also be good for psychotic children as well as other disturbed kids, so as I said before, I did clinical research on our Bellevue population with chlorpromazine as well as other drugs.

TB: So you were also among the first or might even be the first using chlorpromazine in children. You did this work at the Columbia Presbyterian Hospital in New York.

AF: But also at Bellevue with disturbed children. It was about that time that Richard Day accepted the position of Professor of Pediatrics at Downstate Medical Center of the State University in Brooklyn and was looking for a psychiatrist to work on the ward. I was ready to take a full time job again, so I decided to apply for the job and I was accepted. I was working in his department from 1955 to the end of the 1950s.

TB: As a child psychiatrist.

AF: Yes, I was the child psychiatrist in the Department of Pediatrics and continued my research in psychopharmacology in children. Then, Dick got me interested in erythroblastosis fetalis in premature babies. I succeeded in getting a large grant from NIH to study brain damage in prematures. In our study we matched a large cohort of premature infants with full term controls in Bedford Stuyvesant, a very impoverished black neighborhood in Brooklyn, and found brain damage in a larger proportion of premature infants than in their full term matched controls. We continued this study for six or seven years and published several papers on our findings. One of the important findings was, as I already mentioned, that prematures had more brain damage than the others. Another important finding was in the follow-up of these kids. Bedford Stuyvesant was a very impoverished neighborhood where the children were growing up in an environment deprived of any intellectual stimulation. The only newspapers these children saw were the newspapers they slept on. And what we found was three years after they were born it became evident that the difference in cognitive development between the brain damaged and matched non-brain damaged prematures growing up in this intellectually deprived environment disappeared.

These findings led us to look into how we could enrich the development of these kids; how could we do something for them? Actually the work we did became noted, more than I had realized. And even about three or four years ago when I saw Julius Richmond, past Surgeon General, who is a Harvard Professor Emeritus, he said, "Oh that paper you wrote with

Helen Wortis, that showed the terrible effects of impoverishment, of poverty on the growth and development of children, I always use it and quote it." When I expressed surprise he sent me a recent paper of his quoting our paper. We developed a program on how to enrich the development of impoverished children that we started in Brooklyn, and that continued in New York after my departure from Downstate to join New York Medical College. To extend our program we collaborated with people who eventually set up a whole consortium dedicated to this issue of preventing the effects of impoverishment and deprivation on the development of children. Our findings stimulated interest in developing programs even outside of the United States. Some colleagues gave us credit as a precursor of Head Start. We had a colleague, Reuven Feuerstein in Jerusalem, who developed a whole enrichment program, with whom we were in contact. So that was one of my major efforts in the five years I spent at Downstate.

I was also involved in other activities at Downstate. I recall that I was running an annual symposium on childhood schizophrenia. It was originally organized by Carl Hirschberg but I took it over when he got sick, and I ran it for about three or four years. I actually just started to put the material of the program together in a book when I was approached by New York Medical College to become Chairman of the Department of Psychiatry there.

TB: What year was that?

AF: Well, it was the end of 1959. I think it was in the winter. Some of my friends encouraged me whereas some others discouraged me from taking the job. I was told that it's not the best Medical School in New York, that I would not be able to get support and that there was no real budget for the Department. And some of the things I was told were true. There had never been a full time Chairman of the Department of Psychiatry at New York Medical College. The previous one was a part time chairman who had a huge private practice. But I thought of the possibilities of building a Department there and decided to take the job. And so I begin there in September 1960. I brought over the research projects we had been doing on child development at Downstate and addressed myself to the task of building a Department. The New York Medical College was then in the Flower Hospital at the corner of 106th street and 5th Avenue. Our primary teaching hospital was the Metropolitan Hospital. Both the Medical School and Metropolitan Hospital were in East Harlem, which was, and still is, probably the most impoverished area of New York with the highest incidence of drug abuse, particularly heroin addiction and severe alcoholism. So I decided that we should focus on drug abuse. And it just happened that at the time the city had approached a number of the teaching hospitals and medical schools about doing work on drug abuse, and they all turned it down. It was considered sort of dirty work. But we accepted the challenge and set up a detoxification unit at Metropolitan Hospital for adults and adolescents. There was great publicity at the time about drug abuse in adolescents. And so we set up a ward for adolescents. When I started, neither Metropolitan Hospital nor Flower Hospital had an in-patient psychiatric service. So the addiction services in those hospitals gave me a base to operate from.

I also inherited a very small outpatient clinic that had very few patients because, as it turned out, the nurse who received the new patients felt that anybody who didn't speak good English could not profit from psychiatric care. Since most of the population in the area were Puerto Ricans who had little English, she turned them all away. Anyway, we changed that and in about a year our Outpatient Clinic visits went from about five thousand up to about seventy thousand. That was a very active service. And we developed several programs, over the years, for drug abuse. First, as I said before, we set up a detoxification unit, then we realized that a detoxification unit alone does nothing but get the patients out to get them back again; it was a revolving door.

So we became very much interested in community mental health. We felt that the community approach was very important, not only for drug abuse, but for all psychiatric disorders. So, even before President Kennedy made his address in 1963 about the importance of community mental health we already started a community mental health program. I had a team working in East Harlem. Then we started to develop educational programs for neighborhood groups, particularly for schools, in regard to drug abuse. We were very active. I participated in a White House Conference on drug abuse that was run by Robert Kennedy. It was a very rewarding period, particularly in the Kennedy era. Marcia, my wife, who is an economist, a labor economist, worked in those years on the transition from school to work, in juvenile delinquency and other similar areas. She was a consultant to Robert Kennedy and I will always remember that in the middle of the night, suddenly the phone would ring and they'd say "This is Attorney General Kennedy's office, is Marcia there?" Usually, instead of going and looking up records, they'd call Marcia as the expert, and she would tell them. Then we'd go back to bed. So anyway, it was a very exciting period of time for all of us.

There were those two programs in drug abuse, but at the same time, we had an interest in community mental health that was reinforced by Kennedy's address. And we applied for a grant to build a new Mental Health Center. We already had two wards in the hospital for drug abuse and we now managed to get, with some maneuvering, two more wards for adult psychiatry. The Dean was helpful in spite of the fact that he had to take some beds away from other services. I remember the Professor of Obstetrics and Gynecology telling him, "You'll turn over any wards over my dead body." Then, a reporter from one of the newspapers went to Kings County Hospital and wrote a huge expose about how miserable the treatment was there. Mental hospitals were overcrowded and the city had to respond. This gave me an opportunity to put in my two cents and they told me that they were going to build a Psychiatric Hospital at Metropolitan Hospital, but then there was no money for it. This was in the Kennedy era after passage of the Comprehensive Community Mental Health Centers Act. We applied for a construction grant and got it. So we built a Psychiatric Institute with a Community Mental Health Center. And then we put in for a staffing grant, which we were awarded. Now we were in business.

Since we were involved in drug abuse and interested in finding some treatment for opiate addicts, Ab Wikler invited me to Lexington for a discussion. He thought that the opiate antagonists were the answer. He had the theory that drug abuse is a conditioned response. He thought that the initial effect of a drug, like heroin, was reinforced by subsequent use, and especially when in the withdrawal period the discomfort disappears by taking another dose. He was providing some evidence for his theory in animal experiments. The conditioned aspects of addiction to heroin and other drugs in Wikler's theory were lasting effects if left untreated. For example, let's say someone from East Harlem was arrested for a crime and up in Sing Sing would be withdrawn from all drugs he was using. But then, two or three years later he is discharged, and when passing by Harlem, his old neighborhood, on the train he would suddenly develop withdrawal symptoms so severe that he rushes off the train to look for some heroin. So anyway, I thought Wikler's theory made a lot of sense, and he was working at that time on cyclazocine, an opiate antagonist. I became interested in this opiate antagonist and we agreed that I would try it out.

It just happened that Max Fink, who had been in St. Louis and was very unhappy there, came to me and asked if I had a job for him. So he joined me, and although his life-long interest was ECT, he agreed to work on drug abuse, while of course, he continued his research with ECT. We started a program on cyclazocine and the substance proved to be an effective opiate antagonist. The theory for cyclazocine treatment was that if you could prevent any response to heroin over time, the conditioned response would become extinguished. Cyclazocine worked all right as an opiate antagonist but it had side effects, like vivid hallucinations in some subjects, that prohibited its continued use. We also noticed that some individuals had high spirits and euphoria while on the drug. We thought cyclazocine might be an antidepressant and decided to try it in adults and also in children. I used antidepressants in children and especially Tofranil (imipramine), in spite of the commonly held belief at that time that children had no depression. But the idea of using cyclazocine in depression was abandoned because of the hallucinations produced by the drug which could not be overcome.

TB: Did you study Tofranil in children?

AF: I did.

TB: It was probably the first study on children.

AF: Probably.

TB: And you also did some early clinical studies with opiate antagonists.

AF: Yes. And the men taking cyclazocine told us that it acted as an aphrodisiac. They said, "I'm getting up in the morning with an erection like I haven't had since I was fifteen years old." But we figured that heroin inhibits sex, and by using an antagonist the effects of heroin were wearing off and that was what they experienced. So, anyway, we weren't getting any further with cyclazocine, although we felt that it was working. Then we discovered naloxone, and Max Fink and I did a series of experiments with naloxone. In some of these experiments we injected heroin first and saw no response. Then we did the opposite, injecting heroin followed by naloxone. The heroin rush disappeared after the injection of naloxone. So we felt that it should be an effective drug and started to use it in drug addicts.

TB: What period of time did you do the work with opiate antagonists?

AF: We're getting into the late 1960s. In those years I felt that drug abuse has a biological basis. It seemed that from all practical purposes every young boy in East Harlem was trying heroin, but only a small percentage of them took it again and became addicts. It was suggested that there might be social pressure on the particular child that becomes addicted. Another hypothesis was that a child who has a stable family relationship or a close relationship with a teacher or a priest would be able to resist further use. But I felt that there must be a biological aspect to drug addiction, a vulnerability or susceptibility to drug abuse, so I was looking around for various sorts of biological approaches to treatment at the time. When I saw Wikler and when Max joined me, I think it had to be in 1965 or '66, we started an active program in the pharmacological treatment of drug addiction.

TB: So you found that naloxone was an effective agent.

AF: It seemed that naloxone would be an effective agent, but its effect only lasted three to four hours. So we started looking for ways of prolonging the effect of naloxone, by mixing it with other substances. I remember that the ALZA Corporation on the West Coast, specialized in modifying drugs so that they would have longer periods of action, but they had nothing to offer that would prolong the effect of naloxone. In spite of the problem of its short duration of action, we continued using naloxone. But then Endo Pharmaceuticals that made naloxone was sold to DuPont, and DuPont decided that there was no money in naloxone, and to our consternation, stopped manufacturing it. So we contacted one of the science writers at the *New York Times*, and he wrote a column on "The great possibility of a drug for drug abuse, that's being eliminated by DuPont." The next morning after the column appeared I got a call from DuPont that they could give me another drug that we could use instead of naloxone. So then naltrexone came along, that was longer acting than naloxone. We were among the first to use it, and this takes us well into the 1970s. And, during the 1970s we also found ß-blockers useful in the treatment of addiction.

TB: So you had Max Fink working in your department.

AF: Yes, and I should have mentioned that when I became Chairman, I made two important recruits. One was Lothar Kalinowsky, who was instrumental in introducing ECT and other physical therapies in the USA, and the other was Silvano Arieti, a distinguished psychoanalyst. Lothar turned out to be a wonderful friend. I have enormous regard for him and his wife. Soon after Kalinowsky joined the department there was a meeting in New York organized about Sakel's insulin coma therapy with invited participants from all around the world. And during the meeting Lothar told me that there were two people among the guests who wanted to travel around the United States. Then he said, "You know they need about five hundred dollars each, and I have a man who will donate it but he wants to give it in a way that he can take a tax deduction, so can you handle that for him?" I said, "Sure, no problem, have him make the check out to the Department of Psychiatry." And then I said, "Why don't you ask him for money so we can have distinguished psychiatrists from abroad give lectures here?" So Lothar said, "Don't be ridiculous, he'll never do that." The man's name was Goldman, a former patient of Kalinowsky who was grateful to him, so I said, "You tell him we'll name the lectures 'The Goldman Lectures.'" So Kalinowsky went to Goldman immediately and called me at midnight all excited, and said, "You were right, when I told him that this Dr. Freedman has this crazy idea of having lectures from distinguished psychiatrists from abroad and thought maybe you'd support it, he responded, 'well, that's a good idea. If you like, I'll give you five thousand dollars to start with,' and when I told him, I'm sure you wouldn't be interested, but he wanted to name the lectures The Goldman Lectures, he responded, 'Oh! I'll give you ten thousand dollars every year.'" So every year, we got the money as long as Goldman lived.

TB: When did this happen?

AF: Mid 1960s. It happened soon after Lothar Kalinowsky joined me and became a professor in the Department. The Gracie Square Hospital where he was doing most of his work was having troubles and they were talking about selling it, and the New York Psychiatric Institute he was affiliated with never really did very much for him. We became very dear friends and the Goldman Lectures were wonderful. We invited famous psychiatrists from Europe and Asia to lecture and we not only paid them for their trip, but we gave them extra money to travel around the United States. We had prominent psychiatrists like Pierre Pichot from France, Hanns Hippius from Germany, and Paul Kielholz from Switzerland here. We also had Manfred Bleuler from Burghölzli and Martin Roth from the UK.

TB: At the time you became chairman we were still in the psychodynamic era of psychiatry in the United States.

AF: I had psychoanalytic training and got a certificate in 1955 from the William Alanson White Institute. And I was a member of the American Academy of Psychoanalysis. But I always adhered to an integrative approach, that behavior is based on the dynamic interplay between environment, experience, and biology. I'm very committed to that approach.

TB: Dd you promote integration in your residency program?

AF: Yes, of course. We had no residency training program when I arrived but within a year I got one started, and it proved to be very successful. We put great emphasis on our undergraduate program, and for several years our students ranked number one in the National Board Examination in the country. So we had a very good teaching program. Before I moved to New York Medical College I was thinking about editing a multi-authored book on child psychiatry. But then, I started to think of developing a comprehensive textbook of psychiatry that would be multi-authored. I invited Harold Kaplan to join me in doing it. So we started to look for a possible publisher. It was hard to find one because they didn't think a multi-authored text in psychiatry would work. After several publishers rejected it, Williams and Wilkins agreed that they would take it up. We understood that at first their committee had turned it down, but then they decided maybe it was worth a try. So they were only going to publish five thousand copies, but then, before it was published they decided to increase it to ten thousand. Eventually they sold somewhere around fifty-five thousand. The book was a smashing success.

TB: What year was the first edition published?

AF: 1967.

TB: 1967. If I remember well that year every psychiatric resident received a copy of it from Hoffmann LaRoche.

AF: That was particularly gratifying to me was that it became the textbook for the country. I remember Fritz Redlich telling me, "Your book is going to kill my book with Danny Freedman and also Larry Kolb's book." Both books remained in circulation of course, but we dominated the market. But in addition to the United States and Canada, the book was used all around the world by people for years to come. And in 1988, to leap ahead a little, when I was in Melbourne giving a talk, Professor Sing, who's now the Chairman of the department there, got up and he said, "I want to personally thank Professor Freedman for being an enormous help to me, when I was studying to take the Royal College Examination; his book came out at the time and I just studied it backward and forward several times, and, I passed without any trouble. I want to thank you for it". So, my identity for a long time rested on the book; it still does in many ways, particularly abroad as well as in this country. When I meet people they frequently say, "Oh, you're the Freedman of the *Comprehensive Textbook*.

TB: The *Comprehensive Textbook* has been very extensively used.

AF: I was especially pleased when I learned that it was well received abroad. Apparently many of the European psychiatrists thought a textbook by an American would be purely psychoanalytical and were surprised to see a textbook with chapters on biological aspects of psychiatry by Seymour Kety, on psychopharmacology by Jonathan Cole, on ECT by Max Fink, and other topics, edited by an American. It was a book that reflected my philosophy; it was eclectic with sections ranging from various psychoanalytic theories and community psychiatry to drug abuse. So the Europeans were impressed.

TB: It had an impact on teaching psychiatry, at least in North America.

AF: Another thing that happened during my first decade at the New York Medical College was that my very good friend Leon Eisenberg became Chairman at Massachusetts General Hospital and asked me to go to Harvard as professor. Well, I evaded the issue and foolishly decided not to take the job. So, anyway, that's another one of those things. But I was involved in so many new things at the time; we were building a new building, I had many programs, I had just recruited Roy John from Rochester.

TB: What years are we talking about?

AF: 1967–78

TB: So you also had Roy John?

AF: We had him for about, probably ten years or so.

TB: So you had a program in neurophysiology?

AF: Yes. We had many programs including a program in psychology.

TB: Then in the early 1970s you became a national figure.

AF: In 1970, I became President of the American Psychopathological Association, after serving for years on many of their committees, and just as my term was ending in 1971 I was elected President of the ACNP. During my Presidency. I was trying to make substance abuse a legitimate subject of psychopharmacology and I don't think I succeeded very well, even though I spoke about it in my Presidential address and I turned out a volume with Seymour Fisher on drug abuse. I was also trying to democratize the ACNP, get more people involved and maybe to have regional meetings organized several times a year. I guess some of that has occurred over the years. And then, in the fall of 1971, I was approached to run on petition for President of the APA. Previously, the APA had been a closed corporation; and the hierarchy would select the person, usually someone who had been Secretary or Vice President, to become the President.

He, always a man in those years, was proposed on a single slate and elected without any opposition. At that time there were lots of things going on about the Vietnam War, and also the gays were beginning to assert themselves and were looking for recognition in the APA. So the Committee of Concerned Psychiatrists was formed. It was actually that Committee which approached me about running for President. And, my immediate response was, "Don't be ridiculous!" First of all, I didn't want a job that would take me away from work that I thought was more important. Secondly, the medical school had just set up a sabbatical program and I was the first to be granted one. Third, I had plans to do a study on alcoholism and drug abuse that year with WHO in Europe and I was looking to travel around Europe from Paris. Thus, the school had approved a sabbatical program and I would have a year abroad. So I said repeatedly, "No, I can't do it, I'm just not known enough around the country." But every time I turned it down somebody else would call asking me again and again to accept it.

Then I got a call from Lester Grinspoon, and he said, "Look you don't have to worry about your sabbatical, because you'll never win, but it's very important for the movement, for the cause, for you to run. You'll get forty five percent of the votes, and then you'll be able to do what you were planning to do, and you'll have also done a great service." So I said, with my luck, I'll probably win and I won't be able to go on sabbatical.

Anyway, that's the way it turned out. And on the first ballot I won by two votes. I was running against your fellow Hungarian, whatever his name was,[George Tarjan], at UCLA in California with Jolly West. Anyway, Jolly West and the others demanded a recount, and I won by three votes. I increased my margin by fifty percent. So, anyway, I became President in May 1972 and that was in Dallas.

The APA has been an important part of my life. I had been active for a long time in the local APA before I became President of the District Branch of New York that was probably the largest in the country. And then I became a delegate to the Assembly for the area of New York State before I was elected President. So I had been active in the APA, but then as President Elect, I became even more active.

TB: Did you take your sabbatical while President or after your presidency?

AF: No, I never got a sabbatical. I had to give it up and then the school cancelled it. It turned out that a lot of the people on the faculty were supported by city money, at the city hospital, and the city said, "if you don't work you don't get paid." So that meant that the school would have to pay for sabbaticals for all these people who were paid from Metropolitan Hospital money. They decided they couldn't afford it.

TB: So now we're in the early 1970s when you became President Elect of the APA.

AF: It was a little rough at the beginning, because I was an interloper in the old boys' club. But everybody was quite helpful, especially Walter Barton, the Executive Director at the time. During the year I was President Elect I went around the country lecturing to district branches and meanwhile I kept the ball rolling in the department. In May 1973, in Hawaii, I became President and my presidency ended in 1974 in Detroit. We achieved during my presidency a number of things that I think are noteworthy. First of all we started with a reorganization of APA because I felt there was unrest in the Assembly, a feeling that they were being denigrated. We had our first conference about the reorganization in the Keys, in Florida, the "Key Conference" It took several years' negotiations, so before the reorganization was completed and the Assembly received more powers we decided to have multiple slates and not just one slate for election. The APA has since had another major reorganization, but that was necessitated about two-years ago by the tax laws.

TB: Having a multiple slate for electing officers was in important step in the democratization of the APA.

AF: Another major achievement during my presidency was on the status of homosexuality. In December 1973 the Board of Trustees, passed a resolution to delete homosexuality from the *Diagnostic and Statistical Manual* of the Association (*DSM II*) and declare that homosexuality was not a disease. We had very strong opposition from the psychoanalysts to pass this resolution. One of the leading psychoanalysts, Irving Bieber, who spoke up, was a member of my department. They were quite aroused because they had published papers and books about homosexuality being based on having an aggressive mother and a passive father. There was also another psychoanalyst who spoke up, and I found that quite surprising because it was well known that his son was homosexual. I guess nobody asked him whether he considered himself a passive father. But to make a long story short, the psychoanalysts were so upset that they organized a referendum that was defeated by a majority vote of sixty against forty; that was a major victory.

It might be of interest that one of my sons, who lives in Washington and is the Washington correspondent for the Hearst Newspapers, informed me that in 1999 the *Washington Post*, when identifying the most worthy story for each day during the 20th century, selected as the most worthy story for December 13, 1973 the APA's declaration that homosexuality is not a disease. That was the most important story for that day for a hundred years! I brought this to the attention of the Board at the Board of Trustees meeting and spoke also about it to Jim Krajeski, who's the Editor of *Psychiatric News*. And the next thing that happened was that his Associate Editor called and asked me to write it up for them. So in September, there was a historical note written on it by me, I don't know if you saw it. That was another important achievement during that year. There are also several other things that happened during my presidency.

TB: Tell us about them.

AF: In my presidential address I dedicated a large section to the integration of the different approaches in psychiatry, and I made a point about ethical issues and the abuse of psychiatry.

TB: Weren't you in the Soviet Union on a mission to try to find out what was going on?

AF: Oh yes, I went to the Soviet Union in October or November 1973 and we visited the Serbski Institute that was thought to be the place where most of the abuse went on. We were fighting all through our visit with the Russian psychiatrists but with some of them I became good friends. One of those psychiatrists whom you probably know was Marat Vartanian.

TB: Yes, I worked with his brother Felix when I was consultant at WHO.

AF: After my Presidency I was elected to the Board of Psychiatry and Neurology and served there for eight years. I was working closely with Marc Hollender on the Board and we were involved in a lot of educational programs. It was called to our attention that there were very few women in psychiatry and that it was difficult for women to get residency training because many of them were married and had young children. So we developed a program, a mother's residency program; instead of three it was four years, they could take the summer off and could stay home when their child was sick and so on. And the people covering for them were not resentful. Actually the program worked out very well; we got a lot of very, very fine women. A couple of them were trained in Pediatrics but had to stop practicing because they had two or three children. And then when they heard of this program they decided to get trained in psychiatry and eventually became child psychiatrists.

TB: Didn't you get also involved in the APA with international affairs?

AF: Yes, and after my Presidency I became chairman of the Committee on International Affairs. We organized joint meetings after our annual meetings with sister organizations. We had a meeting in the 1960s and 1970s with the Australians after the annual meeting in San Francisco, and with the Irish after the annual a meeting in New York. I also remember organizing with Pichot a joint meeting of the American and French societies. I was the Chair of the Committee on International Affairs when in 1977 Sadat made his trip to Jerusalem and made a speech in the Knesset, saying, "We should make peace, we are after all, all brothers." I was fascinated by his speech and we decided that we would go to Egypt and to Israel, survey the situation and see whether we could help in making advances. So, we went to Egypt with great enthusiasm and we were warmly welcomed. We attended Sabbath services at the Great Temple and Synagogue in Cairo. And then, we went to Israel, came back to Egypt, went again to Israel and everything looked wonderful, but ultimately it didn't quite work out. The project continued until interest in our activities was lost and we couldn't raise any more money.

TB: Was this about the same time you became involved with the American Committee on the Prevention and Treatment of Depression?

AF: That started much before. In 1972, I attended the CINP Meeting in Copenhagen and went out to dinner with Pierre Pichot to the Tivoli Gardens and while we were walking to find a restaurant we ran into Paul Kielholz and Hanns Hippius. So we decided to have dinner together, the four of us. It was at that dinner that Kielholz invited me to attend, in January 1973, the meeting of the International Committee for Prevention and Treatment of Depression (PTD) in St. Moritz. Fritz Freyhan was the chairman of the American PTD Committee for many years and after his death I succeeded him.

TB: I remember that very well because I was a member of that Committee.

AF: I was also on the executive committee of PTD as well as on the jury of the Anna-Monika Foundation Award selecting the most important contribution of the year in the understanding or treatment of affective disorders. All those were very rewarding experiences that slowly came to an end after Paul Kielholz died in the mid-1980s. I did a lot of traveling and lecturing around the world. I was elected a visiting professor to Australia and New Zealand and that was a great experience.

TB: Where did your support for the visiting professorship came from? I'm asking this because I had a visiting professorship in 1975 to New Zealand that was supported by Pfizer.

AF: It was awarded by the Royal College of Australia and New Zealand and supported by Roche. I traveled with my wife and we stopped off in Jakarta. I lectured there and we were entertained. From Jakarta we went to Bali and then all around Australia starting in Perth. I also had the opportunity to run a big workshop for WHO in Changsha, China, on psychiatric education that gave us an opportunity to travel around China.

TB: When was that?

AF: In 1982. We also made other visits to China. And we went to Japan, where I became good friends with Professor Nishizono. Then, in 1993, I went to Japan and China, as a consultant for WHO. In the early 1990s I was appointed Honorary Professor of Psychiatry at the Hunan Medical School in Hunan, China.

TB: Weren't you interested also in psychiatric diagnoses in the early 1980s?

AF: Yes, in the 1980s we published a small volume that was rather critical about many of the *DSM-III* diagnoses. I felt *DSM-III* was proliferating too many diagnoses, and that rather than splitting disorders further and further it would be important to integrate diagnoses, bringing them together. I was also involved, at Pierre Pichot's invitation, in a conference in Paris that dealt with the French translation of *DSM-IV*.

TB: If I remember well you were very much involved in editing journals in the 1980s.

AF: I had been on the editorial board of several journals. One of them was *International Journal of Pharmacopsychiatry*.

TB: That was to become *Neuropsychobiology*.

AF: And I was also on the editorial board of the series *Modern Problems of Pharmacopsychiatry*. Then I was approached by Elsevier about whether I would like to edit a new journal that they would support, and so I started *Integrative Psychiatry*.

TB: What year was that?

AF: In 1982.

TB: It was an excellent journal.

AF: I tried to promote the biopsychosocial model, the integration of experience and structure into one whole. I continued with *Integrative Psychiatry* until I retired in 1989 or 1990. But then, I became interested in continuing it, and so we started again around 1992 but unfortunately I had to stop because of health problems.

TB: Weren't you also involved with the International Society of Political Psychology (ISPP) and the journal of that Society?

AF: I was not a member of the ISPP but I had several friends there, particularly one man who had been in the State Department, who approached me to become editor of the journal of the Society. It was not really a journal, but I was interested and turned what they had into a real journal. I must have been editor-in-chief of that journal for several years until 1989 when I retired. In appreciation of my services to the journal ISPP established an Alfred M. Freedman Award annually, for the best paper that was presented at the annual meeting of the Society.

TB: What about your research in the 1980s?

AF: One area of particular interest of mine during that period of time was combined treatment with psychotherapy and drugs. I delivered a paper on that at one of the St. Moritz meetings, in which I pointed out that combined treatment of depression with psychotherapy and antidepressants is superior to either of these treatment modalities alone. Later on Gerry Klerman and Myrna Weisman wrote several papers on the superiority of combined treatment with psychotherapy and drugs in depression. And I was doing research with Turan Itil, who also joined me shortly after Max Fink left, in several programs. He set up a computerized EEG laboratory in Valhalla.

TB: In Valhalla?

AF: I have not mentioned that the medical school, in the early 1980s, decided to move the school to Westchester, Valhalla. This was the time that Roy John left. We lost our old facilities and it took a long time to develop new ones in Westchester. But we still continued with several research programs and I even extended our activities to studying psychotropic drugs in medically ill patients. I received a grant for that, and it was Mike Bloomenfield who carried out the research in the program. We also did a study with ß-blockers and found them of some use in narcotic addiction.

TB: What did you work on with Turan Itil?

AF: I had several projects with Turan Itil. One of them was related to the AIDS outbreak in those years. We became interested whether one could detect by EEG, early changes in the brain that would indicate whether dementia or other mental changes were going to develop. And we found that one might be able to detect by EEG early changes that predict the development of mental changes in patients with AIDS. At the same time other people in the Department were using psychological tests that would predict the development of mental changes in the same patients, and the findings from these tests corresponded with the EEG findings.

TB: Did you have any other projects with Turan?

AF: I was also working with him on natural substances, using his expertise in quantitative EEG and my connections in China. It was in the course of this research that we identified Gingko Biloba as a possible remedy for the treatment of Alzheimer's disease. We tried to get a grant for testing it but did not succeed. Finally, Turan found that Schering, a German corporation, was interested in it.

TB: How did you proceed with Gingko?

AF: We conducted a multi-centered study with Gingko in Alzheimer's disease. It was a very carefully designed study, and Le Bras, who at the time was still Turan's son-in- law, wrote up the findings.

TB: When was that?

AF: We published the paper in 1997. To my knowledge it was the only double-blind carefully done and properly analyzed study on Gingko. And our findings indicated that Gingko would probably delay development of Alzheimer's by six months. It's not enormous, but still significant. And further work is going on to try to isolate the various constituents of Gingko. I'm no longer involved in that.

TB: Yes, but you were instrumental in getting the substance from China and opening up that research.

AF As a matter of fact, originally I was the principal investigator.

TB: Were you involved in any other research in psychopharmacology after Gingko?

AF: I would have done more, but in late 1989 I diagnosed myself with cancer of the breast and was operated on. Then, by the time I recovered from that I was diagnosed with cancer of the prostate. That inhibited my activity a great deal for a couple of years and when I thought I was improving and getting better, in 1994 I had a reoccurrence of my cancer of the prostate. So all these interfered a lot with my activity, but we still, in between my breast cancer and my prostate cancer, went to Casablanca and made a trip to Morocco. We were invited by a good friend of mine, Driss Moussaoui.

TB: Isn't he the chairman of the Department of Psychiatry in Casablanca?

AF: Yes. I first met Moussaoui when he was still a very young man working with Pichot. He came to New York and Pichot told him to drop in to see me. It was in the middle of winter, he had no coat and he had very light shoes on. I tried unsuccessfully to persuade him to borrow one of my coats. Then, when we got to Paris some months later, Pichot sent Moussaoui to meet us at the airport at five o'clock in the morning. He has remained a very good friend. We exchange e-mail regularly. He is a very, very nice guy. Then when we came back I was tentatively diagnosed with cancer of the prostate, but the first biopsy was negative. But then, my PSA was increasing and when they did a more extensive biopsy they found cancer in both lobes. I elected to have X-ray treatment, because at that time I was already seventy-three. The surgeon said he had operated on older people but I was of the opinion that if you're over seventy you should not have surgery. I don't know whether that was a mistake or not. Then in 1993 we traveled around the world. We started at a meeting in Dublin on psychosocial rehabilitation. Then we attended a meeting of the PTD in Prien, near Munich. From Germany we went to attend WHO meetings in Fukuoka, Beijing and Changsha; and then we went to other places in China. In the next year, in 1994, I was invited to a meeting outside of Thessalonica in Greece. From there we made a tour of Anatolia, sponsored by the American Museum of Natural History. It was on that train tour that it became obvious that my wife, Marcia, had some heart troubles; she couldn't climb the hills. After we returned home, her heart condition was diagnosed, but still she remained active. So we went to Santa Fe to the Opera and then visited friends in the mountains of Colorado. That all went okay, except Marsha had some trouble at the higher altitudes. She welcomed the experience, but realized that probably she would never make a trip like that again. Then after we came back, in December 1994, I was diagnosed with a recurrence of my prostate cancer. Still, in 1995 we went abroad again, and that was the last trip we made, because in 1997 I was diagnosed with lymphosarcoma of my thigh, and Marcia with Parkinson's disease. So, we've been quite inhibited in our activities. This is why I have not continued the work with Gingko and done no other research in psychopharmacology. I told Turan that I would like to see *Integrative Psychiatry* continued but I told him also that he would have to do all the work. But he got too busy doing other projects, so we closed the journal.

TB: You also founded, with Turan, the Academy.

AF: The Academy of Psychiatry - Academia Psychiatrica.

TB: Yes.

AF: That was flourishing, but again I was confined by my illness, and Turan had a lot of other things to do, so gradually, after great promise, the Academy sort of subsided. I am also Vice President of the American Division of an International Foundation for Mental Health and Neurosciences that was founded by Jean-Paul Macher in Rouffach. Do you know who he is?

TB: Yes. Are you still actively involved with Macher's Foundation?

AF: We just had a meeting in October.

TB: In Rouffach?

AF: No, here in New York. You see, we must have meetings of the American Corporation. I was president of the meeting in Rouffach a few years before and Macher already asked me to come back there next September.

TB: So they still have a meeting annually?

AF: They have an annual meeting, usually in September. Have you ever attended?

TB: Yes, I have attended several times.

AF: Wonderful food.

TB: Yes.

AF: And a good meeting.

TB: So what are your current activities?

AF: Well, I have maintained my interest in various basic science and clinical endeavors, but I don't have the hands-on relationship at present with any of the projects as I had with Gingko. So my interest has turned to areas of concern. One is the whole issue of capital punishment. I've been working on that with Abraham Halpern who's a forensic psychiatrist, and was a member of my faculty. We first started out when the American Medical Association (AMA) was changing its regulation for psychiatry that would open up many avenues for psychiatrists to participate in executions. We fought against that, and I was able to persuade the Board of Trustees of the APA that they should not approve the AMA resolution. I participated in the debates of the APA resolution at the annual meeting and we wrote several articles on our position. We were concerned about the resolution because we are opposed to capital punishment. I think it's primitive and barbarous to put anyone through that. But the possibility of abolition of the death penalty in the United States is very remote. There's too much support for it. Anybody like Mario Cuomo, the former governor of New York, who ran for reelection and stated "I'm opposed to capital punishment," was defeated. The American Bar Association in 1997 passed a resolution calling for a moratorium on the death penalty, which we thought was a great idea. They pointed out all the inequities, like discrimination; essentially poor people are sent to death without adequate legal representation. They also pointed out the big variations between the different states. Texas executes a lot of people. So does Florida; whereas other states have very few executions or none. So we thought that was very good issue, and we've been working on getting a moratorium resolution through the APA first. We started at the District Branch at Westchester and then the New York State and finally we got it approved by the Assembly last June. Then it went through the Council on Law and Psychiatry and just last week, at the Board of Trustees meeting, they approved it. But by the time it was approved, it had been rewritten to the extent that it will have to go back to the Assembly for final approval. This will be next week. So I hope it will all go through, and then we'll get started on the AMA and other societies to get them to approve of the moratorium idea. This is one area I've been involved in this last year.

     And I've been on the Ethics Committee of the APA, the Ethics Appeals Board, a sort of Supreme Court of the Ethics of APA, for many years. So I keep busy.

TB: So, it seems you are busy and are doing things you are interested in. It is remarkable that in addition to your varied activities you had time for publishing the most comprehensive textbook of psychiatry ever written. Is there any other book you have written or edited that you would like to comment on?

AF: Well, there's a volume I did with Seymour Fisher that I referred to earlier, on drug abuse, which was an attempt to get the ACNP more interested in drug abuse. I wrote a paper in it about the numbers game that Presidents like Nixon were playing. When politically correct they declare a war on drugs, and after spending a billion dollars on it, the numbers of those using drugs like heroin are slightly decreasing, say, two to three percent. Then, when everything quiets down they come back up again. There is an actual fluctuation in the use of drugs like heroin, and now we recognize that the billions of dollars that have been spent on drug programs have been a waste.

TB: During the many years of your activities you were the recipient of many distinctions.

AF: I got an award from the APA and from the University of Helsinki. Then I got a medal for my activities in political psychology. I also got the Wyeth Award from the World Psychiatric Association (WPA) for my contributions to international psychiatry. It was a nice award, because it had ten thousand dollars attached to it. The Mental Hygiene Association gave me an award, and the county executive of Westchester County declared a day in my honor. The New York tabloid the *Daily News* did a study of psychiatrists in New York City and they decided I was the outstanding psychiatrist in New York. Of course, in their usual tabloid fashion, they labeled me the "Super Shrink," the most distinguished "Shrink" in New York. So that was fun. After I received that award in the mid-seventies, my two secretaries bought t-shirts that said "Super Shrink" on it. I received many other awards that are listed in my CV.

TB: As one of the pioneers of psychopharmacology in child psychiatry, how do you feel about psychopharmacology today and about the future of it?

AF: Well, I think psychopharmacology has a promising future. I have appeared at various times, before groups that, even if not hostile, were not in favor of drugs. I usually tell them if they had seen Bellevue Hospital in New York in 1948, when I started my residency in psychiatry, they would have an appreciation of what the new drugs did. There was a pervasive smell of formaldehyde mixed with urine and feces that hit you when you entered the disturbed wards, with patients in camisoles wandering up and down babbling. It was really bedlam.

   We cannot emphasize sufficiently the enormous contribution psychopharmacology has made to the care of the seriously mentally ill. In my presidential address to the APA I emphasized that we have to pay attention to the hospitalized and seriously mentally ill patients. The new drugs made it possible to provide care in the community, but to do it properly we need to have support for it. So, there have been enormous changes already in this country and also in other countries in the treatment and care of psychiatric patients as a result of the introduction of the new drugs. There has also been steady progress in the development of new drugs. And we are now entering a new era! I'm just very sorry that I'm too old and too ignorant to participate in all the molecular and genomic developments that are taking place which are leading to a new era in which drugs may be designed to cure selectively specific syndromes or defects, either genetic or biological. Currently we see the same problem with psychotropic drugs as we see in cancer treatment, which I have become too familiar with; chemotherapy that doesn't act selectively on a particular cell may also kill the heart muscle as well as the cancer cells. So, to have psychotropic drugs that would act selectively would be a great achievement.

TB: So you foresee that we will have drugs that will act selectively on distinct mental pathologies?

AF: Another area that I have been concerned with and peripherally involved with is bringing the new treatments for the mentally ill to developing countries. I have been interested in training people in developing countries to recognize, diagnose and treat psychiatric syndromes properly with the use of new treatments and especially with the new drugs. This represents a difficult problem in terms of whom to train because in countries like Botswana and some other Third World nations there might be one trained psychiatrist for the whole country. The economic aspects of treatments would also need to be addressed. Many of those countries can't afford expensive drugs such as, for example, the new atypical antipsychotics; the teaching must get through that without some of these new remedies they can treat their patients properly. Haldol is still just as good of a drug as any of the new atypicals. It really works. I feel strongly that everyone should have access to treatment, and that optimal treatment could be provided with affordable drugs.

TB: So you feel that it would be important to teach people in developing countries about the proper use of psychotropic drugs without raising unwarranted expectations about unaffordable new drugs. I understand that you feel strongly that everyone should have access to optimal treatment.

AF: Oh, yes.

TB: Is there anything else you'd like to see happen in psychopharmacology or psychiatry?

AF: Well, I'd like to see the treatment of the mentally and physically ill based on the same principles. I would like to see that there is no discrimination, financially or otherwise in the treatment of the mentally ill. After all, WHO studies have shown repeatedly that depression and mental illness in general are becoming the leading cause of incapacity in work. So, I would like to see greater attention and greater respect, in regard for the mentally ill in general.

I am particularly concerned, as I always have been, with the issues of development in the child and the mental health of children. I'm aware that our knowledge of child development and the neuronal changes that take place in the brain during childhood and adolescence are still insufficient to identify factors that are significant in function and maturation. In the recent issue of *Science* I was very intrigued by an article which pointed out that it is now recognized that neurons can regenerate and proliferate, and that the failure of cells to proliferate in the hippocampus may be involved in the pathogenesis of depression. I found especially interesting the findings reported in this article that the antidepressant drugs as well as ECT stimulate the proliferation of cells in the hippocampus. If this is the case, then you have something to hang on to in depression research. The usual way of testing an antidepressant drug is really pretty far-fetched, but if you have something specific, like cells in the hippocampus, you really have something to go on. So that's the sort of thing that interests me a great deal. What can be done with genomes, that's also very fascinating. Genetics and psychiatry I think are going to be very important areas of research.

TB: So, on this note I think we should conclude my interview with Dr. Alfred Freedman, one of the pioneers of psychopharmacology in children. Thank you very much Al for your contributions to psychopharmacology and dedication to the treatment of the mentally ill and for sharing with us this information.

AF: Well, thank you very much. And particular thanks for your skillful interviewing technique. I am impressed with the breadth of the material you
were able to elicit while keeping me very comfortable. I give you full marks
as an interviewer. I am really very grateful to you.

LOUIS A. GOTTSCHALK

Interviewed by William E. Bunney, Jr.
San Juan, Puerto Rico, December 10, 1996

WB: I am Dr. William Bunney, Professor of Psychiatry and Human Behavior, University of California at Irvine. I am interviewing   Dr. Louis A. Gottschalk,* who is Professor Emeritus of Psychiatry & Human Behavior at the University of California, Irvine School of Medicine and the Founding Chairman of the Department. He is one of the premier neuro-psychopharmacologists in our field. Louis, I would like to ask you, could you tell us a little bit about your training?

LG: Yes. I was born in St. Louis, Missouri, and I went to university at Washington University in St. Louis. I attended undergraduate school there. As I reflect on it now, I had the good fortune of having some very inspiring scientific educators as an undergraduate. Then I went to the Washington University Medical School where I didn't realize it at the time I was being programmed by a number of Nobel Prize laureates. At Washington University undergraduate school, there was Arthur Holly Compton, a Nobel Prize winning physicist. At the Medical School, I was a student under Carl and Gerty Cori, Nobel Prize winning biochemists, and Joseph Erlanger, a Nobel Prize winning physiologist. I didn't know it, but I just seemed naturally to be molded and shaped into doing a lot of research.

Beginning as a medical student I had a position working as a research assistant, funded by the Josiah Macy Foundation, under some famous professors in the Department of Neuropsychiatry. There was David Rioch, whom I believe you know. The neuropsychiatry department was headed by John C. Whitehorn, who already back in those times had a neuro-biochemical view of the etiology and pathogenesis of neuropsychiatric illnesses. And another interesting person in that department was a man that did the first frontal ablation experiments in animals; his name was Carlyle Jacobsen, PhD; and he did these studies while he was still at Yale University. In any case, that's where I got my medical school training. I did internship in straight medicine at Washington University, Barnes Hospital. In those days – it may happen again – the departments of psychiatry and neurology were together in one department. So my residency was in

---

* Louis A. Gottschalk was born in St. Louis, Missouri in 1916 and earned his medical degree in 1943 at Washington University School of Medicine in St. Louis. He received a PhD in 1977 from the Southern California Psychoanalytic Institute. After postgraduate training in EEG and service at the child psychiatric clinic of Michael Reese Hospital in Chicago from 1949 to 1951 he spent two years (1951–1953) with the intramural psychiatric research branch of NIH. He moved in 1953 to the Department of Psychiatry, University of Cincinnati College of Medicine. There he remained until 1967, when he became founding chairman (1967–1978) and director of the Department of Psychiatry and Human Behavior at the University of California at Irvine. Gottschalk stayed at Irvine for the rest of his career. Gottschalk died in 2008.

neurology and psychiatry at Barnes and McMillan Hospitals at Washington University, St. Louis. Then, I think in 1947, I had to go into military service; and I was invited to transfer from the US Army, in which I was in the reserve corps during my internship and residency, to the United States Public Health Service, USPHS. As a matter of fact, I had a couple more years of accredited neuropsychiatric training while I was stationed at the United States Public Health Hospital in Fort Worth, Texas. This hospital, which was a so-called "narcotic" hospital, a 2,000 bed hospital on 10,000 acres, had been transformed into a neuropsychiatric hospital to diagnose and care for neuropsychiatric casualties resulting from military service during World War II. I was one of many psychiatrists from the USPHS and the Navy looking after these neuropsychiatrically disabled Navy and Marine Corps service people there. I had some more training in Chicago, Illinois in child psychiatry at the Michael Reese Neuropsychiatric and Psychosomatic Center. There I also ran the EEG, electroencephalography laboratory. In those days, in the late 1940s, it was still in style to get psychoanalytic training. I got that kind of training at the Chicago Institute for Psychoanalysis in child and adult psychoanalysis.

WB: You had some impressive mentors along the way, people who were really giants in the field.

LG: I was lucky; I really was. In Chicago, I worked under Roy R. Grinker at Michael Reese, and at the Institute for Psychoanalysis, I trained under Franz Alexander and Thomas French. I was lucky, and didn't realize it.

WB: What got you interested in psychopharmacology?

LG: I was programmed very young, I think, to do research, and when psychoactive drugs came along, I was right into neuropsychopharmacology, very interested to learn more about them. That was about the time chlorpromazine came along in, probably 1957 or something like that. And it was also the advent of the benzodiazepines. What happened was that after my training in Chicago, I went to the National Institutes of Health. I was, in fact, the first research psychiatrist at NIH. It was in 1951, and again I encountered David Rioch who was Chief of Neuropsychiatry at Walter Reed Army Hospital. In Chicago, I got interested in epilepsy and the trigger mechanisms of epilepsy in children. I took a group of epileptic kids who were on anticonvulsant drugs, in whom the anticonvulsant drugs were not being effective with regards to their epilepsy. I tried psychotherapy, play therapy or other types of therapy, and lo and behold, for many of them their seizures disappeared. And I wrote and published those findings. So when I went to the National Institutes of Health, while I wondered what kind of research I was going to do, I went to Walter Reed Hospital and found some more patients that had epileptiform paroxysms in their EEGs. I thought well, maybe I can find out what happens if you just have these patients free-associate while you are getting their EEGs. This idea came to me because I had had psychoanalytic training. I selected patients who had paroxysms of abnormal EEGs and I found out that some of those people, when they spoke about emotional things, showed more paroxysms.

At that point, it came to me that one of the most inexact areas in the field of psychiatry was dealing with interviews and the things that people said and the ways in which they said them. I decided it would not be a bad idea to try to develop more objective ways of arriving at accurate measures of anxiety or hostility as well as how schizophrenic somebody was. That diagnostic achievement is generally accomplished through the neuropsychiatric interview and the content and form of language. So it was there that I started to get into the measurement of neuropsychiatric states and traits from the content analysis of speech and verbal texts. And when I left NIH to become Research Professor of Psychiatry at the University of Cincinnati, some of the new drugs were being developed by the pharmaceutical industry and coming on the market. I got into try-ing to decide how to measure the effects of psychoactive drugs. I actu-ally did some early clinical trials to determine whether or not drugs like diazepam (Valium), or chlordiazepoxide (Librium), might indeed be anti-anxiety agents. We did placebo-drug studies, and we got five minute speech samples which would measure objectively, with a method I had developed, whether or not subjects were less anxious when they were on the benzodiazepines. And these were the early psychopharmacological studies.

WB: How did you come up with the idea of the five-minute speech sam-ple? I know this was something you developed and expanded on very successfully.

LG: It was. I can remember very clearly, at the time I was working at Walter Reed, interviewing epileptic patients and non-epileptic patients who had abnormal paroxysms on EEGs. And then I reflected that there are very sensitive technologies for measuring accurately many neurobiological phenomena, using biochemical measures and physiological approaches, such as recording brain waves, but we have no very accurate means of measuring the magnitude of various psychobiological states. There is, of course, the diagnostic interview, and the neuropsychiatrically focused diagnostic interview, which require a verbal dialogue. And at that point, I decided, hey, this is it! This could be a tough research field, but why not get into this area? I had also been an English major, as well as a biol-ogy and chemistry major at undergraduate school. And that background facilitated my getting into the measurement of neuropsychobiologi-cal dimensions. I thought it would certainly have some use if a reliable and valid testing procedure could be developed. The challenge was that the development of such a measurement procedure would have to go through many stages.

I should, here, give some acknowledgment to a person I met at the University of Cincinnati, Goldine C. Gleser who had specialized in meas-urement psychology. She had a doctorate degree, a PhD. She had also been a math major. She helped me on the statistical side of some of the problems to be solved in developing a measurement tool for detect-ing and assessing the magnitude of various psychobiological states. I do not think that I should get into more detail about statistical problems, but these will come up again, for I can see that the research areas I have gotten into, especially with drugs and other biochemical factors in neu-ropsychiatric illness, have followed me. In any case, I have continued to persist in working on the content analysis of language and have devel-oped a computerized method of doing this, because I sincerely believe that in time, instead of psychiatric interviews or the use of various adjec-tive check lists or other methods of measuring the magnitude of various psychological and psychiatric states, we will be using the computer, and we will actually use voice recognition. I am working on that now, but I've digressed a bit.

WB: No, I think that is one of the central issues, and you've made a major con-tribution with this. And, if I understand, this has to do with the diagnosis of emotions and has been used to follow behavioral change after medica-tions. Is this correct?

LG: Absolutely right. I have kept following those ideas. As I think about it now, I do recall some of the people at Washington University Medical School, James Bishop, a neurophysiologist, David Rioch, who inspired me. Those fine neuroscientists, the way they thought, and the way they pursued things, I think got transferred and internalized by me. But, any case, with regards to psychiatric drugs, I did get involved after a while in looking at the blood levels and the pharmacokinetics of psychoactive drugs, such as the benzodiazepines.

WB: This was in Cincinnati?

LG: This was in Cincinnati. And, I found that if you had too low a blood level, you did not get any definite antianxiety effect, but over a certain blood level there was this significant correlation between the anxiety scores, that is, a reduction in anxiety scores derived from my Content Analysis Scales, and the blood level of the benzodiazepine, as well as the half-life of the benzodiazepine. I also found that the some of the benzodiazepines produce cognitive impairment, or at least impairment of recent memory, and that's related to blood levels. And from that, I got into looking at the effects of some of the major tranquilizers on schizophrenia, like thioridazine and mesoridazine. I found that the blood levels of those drugs, up to a certain extent in some schizophrenic patients, did correlate positively with an improvement. About a third of those schizophrenic patients did not have a very favorable response to those major tranquilizers, but two-thirds did.

WB: Now, your Content Analysis Scales have had international acceptance, as I understand it.

LG: Yes, one might expect they would. The German neuroscientists got interested in that sort of methodological approach and they have borrowed and used my ideas. They published a number of books using my content analysis methodology. The Chairman of the Department of Psychiatry in Hamburg, Germany told me that he and his colleagues got a million dollar research grant from the German government to test and apply our content analysis methodology to their neuropsychiatric research. And, since then, their studies have been published. The procedure has been published in Spanish in Chile, and in many other languages, in Norway, Poland, Australia, Italy, the Netherlands, and Germany. And lately, people from other countries have also asked us whether we have a computer program in their language to do this. It is rather awesome that they would ask such a question, because computer programs are not readily transformed and adaptable to other languages.

We are currently working on a computer program that will handle the Spanish language because such a large percentage of the world's population speaks Spanish. But, yes, it has been shown that the norms that we have in normal individuals, free of mental or physical disorders, for anxiety and hostility, are not any different from the norms in Norway, Australia or Germany. I suspect and think there's a difference in a country like Poland. I have had a visiting professor that lived there who is coming to visit us again, and she found, and I am not surprised, that having suffered the ravages of war the norms there for anxiety run a little bit higher than the American norms. But, yes, there's been a great deal of international interest in our methodology.

WB: Is that translatable? Is that the issue?

LG: Yes, it is, but not the computer program.

WB: It's a major effort in itself to translate that. Are there specific hypotheses that you've tested in some of this work?

LG: Yes. Well, some hypotheses. I think an obvious one was that blood levels of a drug should relate to the clinical effect. That is, within certain parameters, true. But if the blood level is too low, we have found out the drug is not going to have an effect. Also, you can give too large a drug dose, and we did find that above a certain blood level a drug produces no more favorable clinical effect. That's for immediate effects of the drug.

And there was another hypothesis that I noticed at these meetings that has not had much effect yet in neuropsychopharmacology. That is, we got interested in the finding that thioridazine or mesoridazine in some people, produce adverse cardiovascular effects, cardiac irregularities. And at the time we were studying those phenomena and getting electro-cardiographic measurements and drug blood levels on patients, we got the idea to find out whether there are any differences in the psychoactive drug metabolites in people that get these cardiac irregularities. And lo and behold, we did discover that a metabolite that is not active psychoactively, sulfaridazine, does have an adverse cardiovascular effect. Those individuals that had the cardiac irregularities had elevated sulfaridizine at that time. We were excited about that, published the finding, and tried to get the drug companies to provide further financial support so we could study the biochemical basis for the adverse cardiovascular effect of sulfaridazine. But, they were doing so well marketing their drugs, that they would not fund it. But, I mention it now because the whole area of abnormal effects, side effects, I think, will be studied, perhaps, more and more. I think we are caught so much in the excitement about the favorable effects of drugs that the possibility that a drug's metabolites in everybody may be slightly different, except perhaps for identical twins, has not been focused on. We do metabolize these drugs slightly differently and subtle drug-metabolite effects are sometimes cardinal and important so they can influence or obscure findings. That might become more and more important but has not been followed up very much. So that was one of the hypotheses we had; namely that some of a pharmacological agent's metabolites which are not psychoactive, might have other somatic and biological adverse effects.

WB: Do you remember when you published your first paper, or presented it?

LG: Oh yes, I think that was probably out of medical school. It was in psycho-somatic medicine and not on psychoactive drugs. It was on vasomotor conditioning in human subjects. I did some of the research while I was a medical student. We found out by using classical conditioning that some people are very easily conditioned to have vasal constriction, and if you measure blood flow in the fingers with one or two faradic shock treatments to one hand some are and some are not conditioned. That got published, I think, around 1946 or something of that sort. We're pretty proud of it and it probably does have some importance, indicating that we are quite different in our capacity to be conditioned; that was a conditioned response to turning on a light. And some people who were conditioned just to a couple of reinforcements, continued to have vasal constriction if a light was turned on. No wonder some people get bad hypertension and some don't. There are probably genetic and other differences.

WB: Now, I know you're still active in doing some research. Can you tell us a little bit about what you're doing now?

LG: Yes, I'm still involved and I'm delighted that our own department has a brain-imaging center, and I know you are too, because we did do a fair number of studies on brain imaging and PET scans. We did look at the relationship of anxiety, hostility and dreams recently, with Ernest Noble, who was formerly at the University of California Irvine (UCI). We've done a study with PET scan, showing that people with the A_1 allele, who are normal and who have no psychiatric history of drug abuse, alcoholism or obesity themselves or in their family, have significantly different PET scans from people who don't have that allele. We would have never been able to do that if we hadn't had a PET scan in our own backyard.

Another study that I think is related to neuropsychopharmacology, which was published in 1991, showed that, of all things, manganese was elevated in the hair of violent criminals, compared to controls. I didn't think much of that paper, but we published it because there was no question about the finding. I didn't believe it the first time. I thought it was chance so we got another sample of criminals and controls and it showed up in the second sample. I was still pretty skeptical, being a Missouri boy from the Show Me State. So we got a third sample and it showed up again. The puzzling thing about the paper and the finding was that we had empirical findings without any hypotheses. Since then the Japanese and others have shown that manganese does lower the serotonin level in the brains of rats, and there have been a number of other studies replicating our finding. We are applying for a grant. It's going to the neurochemistry and biochemistry program of NIMH. I can't believe that one little element would be a big factor in the problems we're plagued with in our society, namely violence, but it may make some contribution. So we're into that. The research is going to have to be in an animal model, and I'm not unhappy about it, because we can control everything. That's one area.

Another area does relate to content analysis. There was an advertisement by the National Institute on Drug Abuse, soliciting grant applications on computerized neuropsychiatric testing software. Well, I thought, that was just built for us. What they want is software that will pick up cognitive impairment in people who have been involved in drug abuse. So we've gone far. Whether we'll get it or not is something else. One way or the other we're going to do that. We're into that area and I think we have a pretty good chance to get the grant. Who knows?

WB: Well, I often think, once a researcher, always a researcher. How many papers have you published?

LG: Well, I've got over two hundred papers and two hundred journal articles and about twenty-six books.

WB: Well, it's impressive in a fifty-year span and you're still going strong.

LG: I have a problem and I bet the Bunneys are going to have it too, namely, I wouldn't know how to retire. I think it's a problem.

WB: Now, who were some of the important people, not just in the beginning of your work, but along the way, that you interacted with working in the same area, where colleagues were important for you to communicate with?

LG: Well, over the years, I'm still going to flash back to some of those mentors, back at Washington U and in Chicago, who certainly were internalized by me. I was probably more carried away by them that they are with me.

WB: You still see the influence of psychoanalysis though. You have that concept internalized, which I also happen to believe in.

LG: Well, by internalized I mean that they're in the protein substance of my brain.

WB: I know what you mean.

LG: And the psychoanalysis thing, although I'm still a training analyst, I must say that I figure it's pretty much an art form, and I'm disappointed that it hasn't lent itself to an empirical approach. But it probably has influenced my willingness to listen to people for a long time, as it probably has influenced you. By internalize, I mean in a biochemical way. Oh, I think of various people in Cincinnati, Arthur Mirsky, a biochemically oriented researcher, and Maurice Levine for that matter, who made it possible for me to do research, and was encouraging. But at the University of California at Irvine, there were many people in the medical school who made it possible to do research and also try to run a department. As a matter of fact, if I hadn't been able to do research, I don't think I would have been able to tolerate the administrative problems. There have been a lot of people involved in looking at the relationship of pharmacokinetics and chemical response and I edited two books on the topic and these were both under the imprimatur of the American College of Neuropsychopharmacology. It isn't a big or very important area these days. Everybody can get blood levels now. I'm impressed with this particular ACNP meeting. But what carries me away here, is the genetics and its role in psychoactive drugs and so on.

WB: If you had to list one thing, what would you consider your biggest contribution to the field of science?

LG: It's hard to pick one thing, but if I had to, it's a preoccupation with the accuracy and the precision of measurement, whether it's a measurement of psychological states and traits from speech, or the accuracy of measurement from blood levels of psychoactive drugs, you know, ranging from radioimmune assay to gas chromatographics. I think I've been occupied with developing or asking for the best or most precise and ingenious methods of measurement. It seems to me a lot of big discoveries have been made from the microscope or the telescope. You were instrumental in bringing a brain-imaging center to UCI and I'm fascinated by that too. I can't say that the brain imaging center is my contribution, but I certainly go that way. And, I do question the accuracy of the measurements. So I think a tremendous curiosity and insistence on objective and accurate measurements is one of my contributions.

WB: Okay. Were there any times that you were tempted to leave science, to leave research, job offers that would have taken you, either, out of the field or into too much administration?

LG: No, just like today, I can't imagine life with retirement and not doing science. And, administration, I had a taste of it. It was fun to have the opportunity to develop a department and get it started, but I've avoided accepting positions of too much administration, because I thought it would take me away from science.

WB: Well, you were the founding Chair?

LG: Right.

WB: At the University of California, Irvine Department of Psychiatry.

LG: And, I notice that you, too, are able to keep your activities in the science area and avoid too much administration. It takes one to know one.

WB: Are you pleased the way things have turned out or unhappy?

LG: Oh, you mean in my career?

WB: Your career.

LG: I'm pleased the way it's worked and I would like to continue the present and the way it's working. I have a phobia of retirement and I think I'll keep going as long as I can, because it's such a fascinating field. I can't think of anything more fascinating.

WB: Okay, now where do you see the field in neuropsychopharmacology going in the future. What's in the realistic future? What's in the blue-sky future? What's your vision?

LG: Well, I think, in one area that I've made a very original contribution is the diagnosis of mental disorders and nervous problems from language. I think, eventually, that's going to be possible from just voice recognition.

WB: What do you mean by voice recognition?

LG: The way that my content analysis measure works is, the material is tape recorded and then the typescript is put on a diskette and into a computer program known as LISP, which comes up with content scores on twelve different scales.

WB: You mean, like anxiety and depression, that kind?

LG: Anxiety, how schizophrenic someone is, how much cognitive impairment and how psychotic. The trouble is that takes time. Somebody has to type what is said. I think it's going to be possible, in time, to take speech, even with hesitations because they get scored too, to directly program speech or verbal texts for the computer.

WB: Without the intermediate typing?

LG: Without the typing. Yes. And, that's being done now. The problem is that the computer has to learn somebody's language. We're getting new software. I got software a couple of years ago from IBM but it was very picky, finicky and imprecise. The new software is going to be broader and more accurate. The advances in computer technology are so fast I think that's going to be relevant. You may think what's that got to do with neuropsychopharmacology? Well, it's going to shorten some aspects of the diagnostic process. It's going to make it more precise. And combining that with the very amazing and encouraging advances in translating genetic differences to understanding differences between various organisms – subhuman and human – it's going to help us predict which people are especially vulnerable. And I do think there's going to be a more successful application of drugs and treatment for individuals, and it's going to be a combination of these things. Our technology is really going places. The biggest problem is going to be, can it be funded adequately. But that's another question. I'm a strong believer that we're on the right track. We're making tremendous advances, not just in psychiatric illnesses, but in software programs like this. Some of the illnesses are neurological, say, multiple sclerosis and so on, and the interaction of genetic and environmental factors is well attended to. So, I'm very optimistic that we're going to continue to see tremendous advances in our field here.

WB: You see more accurate diagnosis, a more accurate tailoring to active treatment modalities in the future, and, then, eventually, an impact of genetics.

LG: Right.

WB: Now, what have I left out?

LG: I think you've covered everything.

WB: Anything else you want to put on the record?

LG: No, I think you've covered things very well. I really don't have much more to say, except I'm riding high on the continuing opportunity to do research and very happy that, at least in my genes the Alzheimer's gene is absent or not playing a big part. I think it's very fortunate and I thank whoever is responsible for this.

WB: Okay. So, I've been interviewing, today, Dr. Louis Gottschalk, professor at UCI. He has had a distinguished career, spanning over fifty years from the introduction of neuroleptic drugs through to the present time. He continues, actively, in research. He's known many of the great people in the field of neuropsychopharmacology and it's been an honor to interview him.

LG: Thank you very much, Biff.

GERALD J. SARWER-FONER

Interviewed by A. George Awad
San Juan, Puerto Rico, December 12, 1994

GA: Professor Sarwer-Foner* is in a very special position for me in terms of my research interest over the last fifteen years. Apart from being chairman of the Department of Psychiatry at the University of Ottawa for many years before he retired, one of his major contributions was his early work on psychodynamic issues related to drug response. All of us owe him a great deal for recognizing what has now become an important issue, the role of extra-pharmacological factors in drug response. He has been a pioneer in that area. He combined psychoanalytic and psychodynamic views with psychopharmacology while participating in the early development of psychopharmacology on this continent. With this brief introduction, it is my pleasure to welcome Professor Sarwer-Foner, and to ask him to tell us what sort of training he had and what provoked his interest in the new psychotherapeutic drugs.

GS: Thank you George, it is my pleasure! Well, like many Canadians at the time, I had a choice, and that choice was that I could train in Canada, or train in the United States, or in both. I decided to train in both! I went down to Butler Hospital to work with David Graham Wright, who is now dead, and later with Douglas Bond at Case Western Reserve, as well as with Gregory Zilboorg and other well-known psychoanalytically trained therapists of neurotic patients, and characterological patients who would now be called personality disorder patients. I also worked with all the leaders in the use of psychodynamic principles in the treatment of psychosis. I think that I was probably one of the first, if not the first, Canadian trained in these principles when I came back to Canada in 1953 to join Dr. Travis Dancey at the Queen Mary Veterans' Hospital, that was part of Professor Ewen Cameron's very large and rapidly growing department of psychiatry. So I knew a lot about schizophrenia and about the dynamic factors of schizophrenia, and a fair amount about insulin coma, which was one of the main treatments at the time. Indeed, one of my first theories, that appeared later on in Rinkel's book about insulin coma therapy, was that the intense nursing care given to schizophrenic patients – absolutely dependent upon the love, so to speak, and devotion of the doctors

---

* Gerald J. Sarwer-Foner was born in Vilkovsk, Poland in 1924 and imigrated to Canada at age seven. He graduated in medicine from the University of Montreal in 1951. In 1953, after training at several American centers, he joined the Department of Psychiatry at Queen Mary Veterans Hospital in Montreal, one of the teaching hospitals of McGill's Department of Psychiatry. In 1971 he became professor of psychiatry at the University of Ottawa, and in 1974 head of the department. Currently he is professor of Psychiatry at Wayne State Univesity in Detroit, Michigan.

and the nursing staff in the insulin-induced coma – played a very large role in replacing some of the not altogether good mothering and fathering that some of these people had in their earlier lives. For me, this was one of the major factors in the effectiveness of insulin coma.

Now by the time I returned from the States the neuroleptic era had started, and my early involvement in it is related to a serendipitous accident. When I was a medical student at the University of Montreal I founded the undergraduate medical journal, and one of the things we did was ask some of the professors and some of the students to divide up the medical literature, the journals of the time, and summarize interesting articles for publication. I took the journals that the others didn't want to do, and in one of these journals was a weekly summary of scientific papers out of the University of Paris teaching hospitals. Among those papers was Henri Laborit's who was working with a phenothiazine compound. The Rhône-Poulenc company had thousands of these products, many phenothiazine drugs, and nobody bothered with them at the time. But Laborit was interested in neurosurgery and developed what was called the "lytic cocktail" in anesthesiology, in which he used antihistaminic phenothiazines to decrease brain metabolism so he could operate on highly vascular gliomas. Many years later he was amazed that I had read his articles; that became a bond of friendship between us.

Now, Laborit told Pierre Deniker, who was working with Professor Jean Delay in the department of psychiatry at Ste. Anne's hospital in Paris, that these compounds calmed people; they did not put them to sleep, but made them drowsy. He also told him that it might be worthwhile to test these drugs on inpatients. The result was the 1952 study by Delay and Deniker of 36 manic-depressive patients in the classic French medical style: looking at the signs and symptoms of what happened after they gave them the drug that was to become known as chlorpromazine. By then I was back in Montreal at Queen Mary Veterans' Hospital.

McGill University, at the time, was a very large training center. It was to become one of the three largest training centers in the world in the years that followed. The other two were the Menninger Clinic in Topeka, Kansas, and the Maudsley Hospital at the University of London, in England. They were all about the same size. Each had between 153 and 156 residents in psychiatry from all over the world. Heinz Lehmann was in charge of research at the Verdun Protestant Hospital, one of the teaching hospitals affiliated with McGill, and he was given chlorpromazine to try. He wasn't the first in North America who was given chlorpromazine. Bill Winkelman, Jr. of Philadelphia had been given chlorpromazine earlier and started to work with it sooner, but he published later. Heinz was working at the time with a young resident called Hanrahan; he gave these drugs to Hanrahan and went on holiday. Hanrahan used them and reported to Heinz that there was something special about them. The rest is history; Heinz published the first North American paper on chlorpromazine.

Now, everybody knows that. But what most people don't know – and that is pertinent to my career – is that if Heinz hadn't published, the first paper on chlorpromazine would have been published by Hasan Azima and Bill Ogle, who were working at the Allan Memorial Institute. Their paper was published three months later. Azima was from the old Persian royal family. His mother was a Persian princess before the Shah took over, and he was a most cultivated gentleman. His wife, Fern, is a very well-known psychologist now, but I am speaking about the time when they were at the beginning of their careers. Bill Ogle was a Canadian Army Corps officer in World War II who was hit in the mastoid by a German bullet that pierced his tank's armor. Fortunately they had a neurosurgical unit that saved his life. He became my research assistant when I set up my research department at Queen Mary Veterans' Hospital. Reserpine had just appeared on the psychiatric scene at the time. Nate Kline in New York had worked with Rauwolfia serpentina, and then with reserpine. I had done some work with Rauwolfia serpentina and chlorpromazine, and was just starting to study reserpine.

Because of the setup at Queen Mary's Hospital, we could study drugs with a high ratio of nurses and doctors to patients. Dr. Dancey, the head of the service, had a humane approach to research. He believed that we must study what each patient was suffering from, and look at not only the diagnosis but also their behavior. So it was easy to set up a very careful study of the dynamic factors and to follow every single patient in psychotherapy with three or four independent observers of the drug effect. The patients were selected not because of the disease they had but because they had a measurable disorder of affect. They had to have a disordered expression of emotion that was measurable. It could be the negative symptoms of schizophrenia, agitation, anxiety, depressive affect, manic affect, inappropriate affect, or no affect, but it had to be something that we could describe clearly and then follow meticulously. When we began to do this of course Ogle and I found how the drugs influenced people.

My approach to psychopharmacological research was based on ego defenses. I did not think that the drugs were going to create basic biological changes although in some very aggressive patients, they might tone down the aggression by modifying energy levels. I felt that the drug would change the ego defenses of the patient. Many years later Mortimer Ostow was the first formal analyst who tried to deal with impasses in analysis by adding drugs. He published on this, but my papers with Ogle and my other collaborators were the first publications on how drugs affected ego defenses and how this translated into changes in symptoms and signs. To give an example: one of the first patients we had was a very vigorous, strong and handsome man. He was a well-known parachutist, who used his extroverted masculine energy to prove that he was a man, but underneath this he wasn't so secure. When he was given reserpine, it knocked down his energy, and the minute he didn't have much energy his blood pressure dropped and he developed the most amazing left-right hallucinations and delusions. He felt that the left side of his arm was getting big and turning blue and he would say, "Look, don't you see my blue hand; don't you see it?" The left side was his sister's side, the feminine side, and he saw it as getting bigger and out of proportion because he felt that we had removed his energy and his manhood. Passivity equaled femininity and activity equaled masculinity, and we had inadvertently taken away his defense against these underlying doubts by giving him this drug. We stopped the drug and continued psychotherapy; he very rapidly remitted. When Roy Grinker heard me present these data he rushed over and grabbed me and said, "This should be published in the *Archives*." And it was. So, as a result, at a very young age of 29 or 30, I had the beginnings of an international reputation.

We also started to work on what was later called the "target symptom" approach to psychopharmacology. I adopted that term from Fritz Freyhan who had been working independently from us. We didn't believe that these drugs were curative; they were not. We believed that they were powerful pharmacological agents, and the best way to use them was to look at what I called their characteristic pharmacological profile, and then apply that profile to control symptoms that were linked with the patient's disturbance. For example, if the patient was agitated, chlorpromazine and reserpine were very good drugs, because they knocked down the energy that caused the aggression. If a patient needed a stimulating drug, then Ritalin (methylphenidate), amphetamine, ephedrine, etc., were used under very careful supervision. All this took place between 1953 and 1956. We also introduced combined treatment, using drugs together with psychotherapy, but we didn't publish on this until 1960. I believe our paper was the first on combined drug treatment and psychotherapy.

GA: That is now a big issue thirty years later. You were one of the early people that indicated the importance of the combined integrative approach.

GS: Yes, we did. Now, the Second World Congress of Psychiatry was in Zurich, in 1957. The first one was in Paris. Here I have to give you just another little bit of Canadian history. The congress in Zurich was the first one I attended and it was the first one that the entire North American group involved in psychopharmacology contributed to. Remember, Deniker started with Delay to work on chlorpromazine in 1952 and Lehmann's publication on chlorpromazine appeared, I think, in 1954.

GA: 1954, yes.

GS: My first paper in psychopharmacology was published in 1955, although in 1954 we had already presented some of our findings. At the time we didn't think anything of the concentration of talent in psychopharmacology we had at McGill in those years, but later of course it became evident. We had the good fortune to have a group of very able people together, such as Charlie Shagass, Heinz Lehmann, myself, Ogle, and many, many others. Well, Ewen Cameron was talking about organizing a World Psychiatric Association (WPA) congress in Montreal. This was brought to the attention of the Canadian Psychiatric Association Board of Directors. Someone who was competing with Cameron didn't want to let him be the formal Canadian delegate to that was negotiating for this congress, and they proposed me, a young punk, to replace my professor. Well I, of course, protested violently. What happened was that Professor Cameron was confirmed as the delegate, but I was made the alternative delegate. Professor Cameron looked at me and said, "Young man, you are very lucky, so come, keep quiet and observe and learn!" I said, "Yes sir," and I did, in fact, observe and learn. It was an entrée for me to the European group.

When we went to Zurich in 1957, Nate Kline had a symposium and we were all participating in it. We met there many of our European colleagues. Some of them I already knew. I got to know Pierre Deniker very, very well, and we have remained friends until this day. I became very friendly also with Professor Delay, whom I admired. He was a remarkable man. When Professor Delay was the president of the congress of the Collegium Internationale Neuro-Psychopharmacologicum (CINP) in Washington, many years later, in 1964, I was his official guide and interpreter. Delay worked out a classification of psychotropic drugs and presented it at the Zurich meeting of the WPA and in the next year, in 1958, in Rome. Two other people had proposed alternative classifications: one was Heinz Lehmann from Montreal and the other was Nathan Kline from New York. The three classifications were remarkably similar. They used terms like neuroleptics, tranquilizers and things of that nature. Delay was a cultivated man, an aristocrat, a great scholar, and a real gentleman. He could speak English, but didn't believe he could. So he said, "Gerry, would you act as our interpreter with Nate Kline, who doesn't speak French?" There is a photograph from Rome and it's really funny. Here is Delay and here is Kline and they are talking to each other; and here I am in the mid-dle. I didn't have to say a word. Delay spoke very good English. Kline got along with him beautifully. There were many humorous things of this kind.

GA: What is amazing is how many chance encounters have shaped what was to happen subsequently.

GS: That's how they happen!

GA: I have always been impressed that you are one of the very few people who could recognize the importance of systematic observations and the context in which the treatment took place. We are still not paying too much attention to this in clinical trials, yet by now everyone recognizes it.

GS: In psychiatry, unfortunately, there are two traditions. There was the early tradition of the humane treatment of patients, which worked very well for the Conollys and the Tukes in the early years of the nineteenth century before the industrial revolution created massive overcrowded urban slums in the cities with no social services. Now when this occurred, the available hospitals that were treating patients became swamped. A good therapeutic milieu got eliminated; it was not possible any longer to individualize the care of the patients. You had one nurse for one hundred to two thousand patients, and one doctor for several hundred or even several thousand patients. So obviously they concentrated their resources in the admission services or on the agitated wards, and the rest of the patients who were chronic were given much less intensive care. This led, in an unintended way, to a Procrustean bed approach, where the patient was fitted into the programs that existed, and not what the patient needed. This development still plagues us in psychiatry to this day. When the Montreal General Hospital, the Queen Mary Veterans' Hospital and the Jewish General Hospital in Montreal started with psychiatric units, they were able to give intensive care to patients. They could follow meticulously the progress of patients. Today, there are social forces working against us: the rationing of care and the promotion of managed care to cut costs. Today we are experiencing a very rough ride, but at the time I did my research that wasn't the case. Even in the mental hospitals we were getting more funding because it was recognized that patients were ready to interact with the staff and therefore you needed more staff.

My team and I published the first Canadian teaching paper on drug-induced extrapyramidal reactions. We studied a lot of drugs that we didn't refer to because we were just another group in the American clinical trials. We studied imipramine when it was a research drug, and Nardil (phenelzine), Stelazine (trifluoperazine) and Trilafon (perphenazine). We did a whole bunch of drugs, some of which turned out not to be terribly important, but some were. We studied and published – and this is rare in terms of discussions that have gone on at this meeting – the negative results, because we felt that it was important. One antipsychotic was touted as a drug that would knock out hallucinations, delusions, and ideas of reference, and we said that this didn't sound right. So we just took the drug and gave it to patients with these three criteria to show that there was no such thing clinically, and we published the results. And there were many of these things. We started the antipsychotic school of psychopharmacology, which emerged from the state hospitals where the drug was given to treat the whole disease. The target symptom approach that we pioneered was the use of the pharmacological profile of the drug and clinical dosage to control symptoms which we felt were of significance to the patient's disturbance.

Now, Delay – if I can go back a little bit in history – was an amazing person; he was a genius in many ways. You know his biography of Gide had him admitted to the Académie Française as a writer. He had tremendous subtle political knowledge in understanding people, but he was an aristocrat and for ordinary things he was helpless. But if you talked to him about organizing this or that, or about the political consequences of X or Y, he was right there, he knew exactly what was what.

My interest in ego defenses took me into many other areas of psychiatry, so that I published not just in psychopharmacology but in many areas. And over the years it has led to my being president of a whole series of organizations, some of which have nothing to do with psychopharmacology. One of the things that emerged was an international psychiatric research society that I set up in 1958 at McGill with a meeting on what we call non-drug factors, non-direct drug factors in psychopharmacology, although we dealt with drug factors too. We ended up following the old dining societies, like the Royal Society and others in the nineteenth century where people around the dinner table discussed several topics, selected by a committee of experts, and presented by the speakers. We set up small committees, no more than fifty people in each, and people could join whichever committee they wanted to, and there was maximum discussion. We tape recorded everything and our book, *Non-specific Factors in Drug Therapy*, based on these records, was published later. The people attending the meeting loved the idea that they had so much time for discussion.

Although I hadn't intended organizing a society, they voted to meet again. They picked the topic. The second meeting was at Harvard with Milton Greenblatt running it. We didn't have a name, of course, so someone said, "Well it's the group that does not have a name, so we became known as 'The Group Without a Name'." Some very funny things happened. Hy (Herman) Denber tried to run a meeting in a nice warm place in Miami and he went to the hotel to make arrangements and said we wanted to reserve the hotel for a meeting and they said, "Yes sir." And then the guy asked, "Who is the president?" He said, "We don't have a president." Then they asked, "Who is the treasurer?" "Well, we don't have a treasurer." "Well, what's the name?" "Well, we haven't got a name." And at that point they threw him out. So after that we were called The Group Without a Name, and later on we were called the International Psychiatric Research Association.

GA: Actually you innovated something that came into the commercial sector and became known proverbially. You should have taken credit for the name. I have had the pleasure on a few occasions to participate in meetings of the Group, and I have found them very, very informative, and very conducive to extensive discussion. You have been very active in the psychodynamic and psychoanalytic area, and have also contributed extensively to developing psychopharmacology not only in Canada, but internationally. That was all happening in the 1960s when biological psychiatry was just taking off. You have kept a steady course, and I think in retrospect you are probably one of the very few that has maintained interest in both sides which is what everyone now expects.

GS: Well, I do a lot of teaching on the union of mind and brain; that the brain forms symbols and the symbols inform the mind, the psyche, and that some symbols are treated by the brain as flesh, for example the eye and the knee symbols, while other symbols are treated by the brain as imaginary playthings. I remember my first day in psychiatry at Butler Hospital when they announced the movie they would show to patients. This was not long after World War II and it happened that the movie announced was a war movie. And I said to the clinical director, George Alexander, who was a brilliant diagnostician, psychiatrist and analyst, "what happens when a schizophrenic patient sees a bomb go off and screams?" He said, "Nothing," and I didn't believe him. But of course he was right because the patient knew he was sitting in his armchair and that he was quite safe. So the brain treats many symbols as unimportant. But many symbols that deal for example with the eye and knee are treated like living flesh and the psyche becomes not a servant to the brain because the brain responds to the psyche's need as flesh. If you look at it, you still have a lot of mindless psychiatry going on, which is a disaster in my opinion.

GA: I have not always been a great admirer of the term biological psychiatry. It really may have contributed to the creation of the conflict between the two, biological and psychological, approaches to psychiatry. I think it was an unfortunate term. Yet, as you have already pointed out, they really have to come together.

GS: Yes, they should!

GA: They should. What would be your advice? I think you are right; there are still a lot of things going on which are probably not the right things to do in treating issues within the biological or psychological domains. What is your advice to the new generations?

GS: Well, my advice was unpopular in this area. I hope that this doesn't sound like arrogance, but I think my advice on this issue was correct. First of all, the early use of the term biological psychiatry antedated the developments in neuropsychopharmacology. At the time the treatments were physical: there was insulin coma, there was electric shock and there was nitrous oxide therapy. There were leucotomies and lobotomies and so on. So it was biological psychiatry, and the term was appropriate. But later we had a different context. I agree with you that if you don't know the history of it, then it becomes less appropriate. I am very, very cynical about offering new definitions of diseases of the mind every four years; they don't even talk about diseases of the mind; they only talk about signs and symptoms. I think that this is unfortunate. I think proper training can change this, but unfortunately, the financial and social pressures are against the type of training that you and I would probably wish to have. So I really don't know what to do except to keep teaching. And I keep saying that the patients will teach you if nobody else will, because, thank God, there are some bright young people coming up, and even if we don't teach them, some of them will learn from the patients. Now, that's a painful way to reinvent the wheel.

GA: You have published extensively, and I am wondering what do you think is your most important paper? It's hard to pick one paper. Usually it's a body of work, but if you had to choose one paper which one do you think has made the greatest impact?

GS: Well, it's not in one paper. The papers published from 1955 to 1961 dealing with the target symptom approach, with the psychodynamic action of drugs, with the importance of character and character defenses and how they interact with drugs, with the importance of symbols, the ego and superego conflicts and how they interact with drug effects and are influenced in terms of drug effects. I think that these are the important areas I dealt with in those papers, but I don't think one is always a good judge of one's own work in this regard.

GA: It is true; it is absolutely true; it is hard picking one favorite child among all of your children. You have been involved with and contributed to many things over the years. You were the chairman of a large academic department, a contributor to many journals and editorials, an organizer of professional bodies nationally and internationally. There were so many activities you were involved with that I don't know how you have managed to keep balance between all those activities.

GS: I am not sure that my wife would agree that I have always managed to keep balance. It's the old joke, you know, but there is truth to it. I think that I am an outgoing person, and with Cameron having introduced me to the psychiatric scene I have played a considerable role in that. I have contributed, you know, to the Sixth World Congress in Honolulu, and also quite heavily to the Montreal Congress, earlier, and to several other congresses since. If one knows people all over the world, it's an interesting life, very busy and hectic at times.

GA: So, what you are really saying is the importance of personal contacts, national and international.

GS: Yes, because I could go to a meeting with my colleagues, and sit down and tell them what I was doing and they would tell me what they were doing, and we would all exchange ideas and that's the best and easiest way to communicate.

GA: This session is for the history of psychiatry. Are there any other important historical events that you have enriched us with?

GS: Well, Ted Rothman played probably an unusually large role in the founding of the ACNP. Ted was a good psychiatrist and a good researcher, but I don't think that compared to some, he was brilliant. I mean no offense to him when I say that. I liked the formation of the American College of Neuropsychopharmacology. But earlier, before this group started we had informal research directors meetings, which was one of the developments that people don't remember because the government's involvement knocked it out very quickly. When the neuroleptic drugs came in, Henry Brill was appointed to introduce drugs into the New York State system, which was the largest state hospital system on the continent at the time. As a result, every large state hospital center was a training center with a director of psychiatric research. Sidney Merlis was one, and Nate Kline, was another, although in a different way. And we who were not in that system were in the beginning sometimes at odds with them. They were very threatened by my insistence on personal attention: I had one nurse for two patients and one doctor for every five patients. They not only envied us, they just couldn't do the kind of thing that we were doing. And we didn't have to cope with some of the problems they coped with, but we used to meet informally. The research directors would get some money from universities or drug companies and then we would meet. So, ten of us, twelve of us, fourteen of us, eighteen of us would meet every year and would sit around and talk. That led to a sort of an organization. But it was Ted Rothman more than anybody else who, several years later, got together the basic centers, the pharmaceutical industry, important professors who were not necessarily psychopharmacologists, and researchers. At the Maudsley, Sir Aubrey Lewis was very important, and at McGill Ewen Cameron. And so were some other people, such as for example Paul Hoch, who was not a professor, he was in a New York State research facility; and many, many others. That is how all these got started, and that is how progress takes place.

GA: Well, looking back into the early years of development in neuropsychopharmacology, we have gone a long way since then, yet many of the old issues are still with us!

GS: All of the old issues are still with us! All our drugs still have a 60 to 70 percent response rate and if you are lucky they will give 80 percent results on the symptoms. We still have the hardcore of placebo effects and the hardcore of non-responders. We still don't have a specifically curative drug for any of the diseases. Our drugs are safer, and have fewer side effects, especially the new ones. But, if the truth be told, they are not therapeutically more effective than the older drugs, and they don't give a higher rate of cure if you take the natural course of the illness into consideration. We have come a tremendous way and we have made tremendous progress, but we have a hell of a long way to go. I would say that we are ignorant of more things than we are knowledgeable about, and that's not a criticism of our tremendous progress. For example, what is the biochemistry of the gleam in my eye and what is the biochemistry in my smile, and the biochemistry in my frown, who knows? I think that genetics and molecular biology may help us there, to find out some of the biochemistry of thought and feeling, but there is a long way to go. But that is the nature of science. I think that we will have to have patience.

GA: Well, it sounds as though you are optimistic, and that may be part of what carried you throughout all the years from the very early days when you probably stood alone.

GS: In my own vision I have literally stood alone, but once my papers were published I very quickly did have allies all over the place. But in the beginning it was a little tough.

GA: Are you happy with how things turned out for you?

GS: Some of the things that happened, at the time they happened I thought were bad but they turned out to be very good.

GA: Yes, that is true! It is, for me, really a great pleasure to just listen to some of your early experiences. You are also one of the major Canadian figures that really contributed to psychopharmacology, so it is fascinating to hear from you first-hand about these issues. I think when you talked about these early years you were really projecting a sense of optimism about the future. What message would you leave for the younger generation now? What do you think we need to do?

GS: Well, we have to realize that we are treating people, and you have to know what a person is. If you don't know what a person is, it is very hard to work out the pharmacological or any other therapies. In other words, the difference between man and the lower animal is a very important distinction. And the distinction is in the brain and the psyche. The psyche interacts with the brain, and the brain response to the psyche is that it is living flesh. If there is an injury to the psyche, it is responded to as an injury to part of the body. And if they don't know and start with that, it is very hard to go to the pure drug effects. We tend to be getting a bit away from that because of the pressure of money, and the pressure of time, and managed care, and the pressure of a lot of things. Unfortunately doctors are not as important in controlling medicine as they used to be, and I think that is lethal. Well, that is showing my age a bit, but it shows as well my optimism when I make that kind of comment.

GA: Your work over the years, about the psychodynamic aspect of drug response, has had a tremendous impact and I think is now becoming very popular. I mean you stood alone at the beginning talking about subjective domains or subjective experiences in the lives of patients. There was one influential person who did follow your work from the beginning; the late Philip May. He was very intrigued and interested in the early work you had done about the psychodynamic aspects of drug response. We are indebted to you. Thank you very much.

GS: Thank you. You have helped me enormously in the interview.

GA: Thank you.

STEPHEN I. SZÁRA

Interviewed by Leo E. Hollister
Washington, District of Columbia, April 16, 1997

LH: Today is April 16, 1997, and we're in Washington, doing interviews on the project of the History of Early Years of Psychopharmacology sponsored by the American College of Neuropsychopharmacology. Our guest this morning is Dr. Stephen Szára.* Welcome, Stephen.

SS: Thank you.

LH: It's been a long time. That's the trouble when you retire, you get lost. Tell us, Steve, I think you have an interesting history of being educated and raised in Hungary, and then making a career in the United States. How did this come about?

SS: Well, to start at the beginning, I got my first training in chemistry. I did my DSc work in chemistry, physics and mathematics in Budapest. Then while I was doing my thesis work in organic chemistry, across the hall – across the garden, really – of the campus of the University of Budapest, there was the Institute of Biochemistry of the Medical School, which was headed by Albert Szent-Györgyi, I don't know if you remember his name.

LH: Oh, yes, of course. He was one the biggest scientists of that time.

SS: I think he got the Nobel Prize in 1937 for his work on Vitamin C and oxidative metabolism in the muscle.

LH: Muscle metabolism, yes.

SS: I was quite interested in biochemistry at that time, and while I was still working on my organic chemistry thesis, I actually took some biochemistry courses. We were allowed to cross over to another Institute. And I was really interested in it, but I wasn't involved in biochemistry until, I think, 1950. Let's go back for a moment. This was during the war, World War II, and at the end of the war, I started to take courses in medicine. I didn't really want to become a physician, a practicing physician. I wanted to do research from the beginning. So I thought, I am going to take a few courses in biochemistry, and maybe pharmacology, and maybe anatomy. And then I started to get really involved in my studies and I decided that I might as well just go through the whole thing, so that's how I got into medicine.

LH: With no intention of being a medical practitioner?

SS: No, no intention. I was primarily interested in biochemical research, and after my thesis work I got a position in the Department of Microbiology

---

* Stephen Szára was born in Budapest, Hungary in 1923, and received his PhD in chemistry at the University of Budapest in 1950, followed by a medical degree in 1951. In 1956 he left Hungary, ending up at NIMH in 1958; he joined the Center for Studies of Narcotic and Drug Abuse in 1971, which became the National Institute on Drug Abuse in 1974. He retired in 1990.

and Immunology of the Medical School. There were problems at the time that had to do with political issues, and eventually the Communist Party took control over many of the organizations at the universities, and that particular Institute was kind of disbanded; the professor disappeared, some people went to jail and I was transferred to the Department of Biochemistry. That was back in 1950; I was still in medical school, in my last year. I got my medical degree in 1951. It was in 1950 when I shifted over to the biochemistry department as assistant professor.

LH: In medical school, did you have separate institutes of different disciplines or was it all combined?

SS: No, there was a separate institute for each separate discipline.

LH: Biochemistry and all?

SS: In that particular campus that I was in, pre-medical subjects were taught in the departments of biochemistry and physiology, and the medical students came to study chemistry, physics, etc.

LH: Now, did you do any clinical work at all?

SS: Well, I did some later on. When I was in my last year in medical school, I did one year of internship, and during the internship, I met a young fellow who was working in a mental hospital in the outskirts of Budapest. He came to me one day, and said that the hospital was very much interested in doing research in the biochemistry of mental illness, and they were interested in organizing a laboratory in the hospital. He asked me whether I would be interested in starting there.

LH: Until that time you had no training in psychiatry?

SS: No, I had no training in psychiatry. I just had my year of internship.

LH: So you considered yourself a biochemist?

SS: Yes. I went to see the Director of the mental hospital, and asked her, "What should we do in the biochemistry of mental illness." You know," I told her, "mental illness is somewhere up in your brain there." And we didn't know much about the chemistry of the brain at that time. But, as it turned out, there was a publication a year before that by Hoffer, Osmond and Smythies. I don't know whether you remember it. They had two papers, I think in the *Journal of Mental Science,* in which they were proposing a biochemical hypothesis, the adrenochrome hypothesis, of schizophrenia.

LH: Hoffer, Osmond and Smythies were popular in those days.

SS: Very popular. Later on I got involved in the issue of whether adrenochrome is present in the blood.

LH: I assume by that time, in Budapest, you were able to get hands on the world literature?

SS: Yes, we had subscriptions to a lot of the prominent English and American journals.

LH: At that time, were you able to read English?

SS: Yes, I could read English, but I couldn't speak it. As a matter of fact, I studied internal medicine from an English textbook. So in 1953 I decided to accept the job in the psychiatric hospital and to start some research related to the biochemistry of schizophrenia. I got involved with the work, and became interested in LSD. We knew about LSD since Stoll, in 1947, published the first paper on the experience of Hofmann with the substance. The story had been picked up in relationship to the indole hypothesis of schizophrenia. I was thinking to do some research in that area and decided to try to get some LSD. So I wrote a letter to Sandoz, the company that made LSD, and I got back a letter essentially saying: "we are unable to send you any LSD." Well, I understood what the reasons were. This was during the peak of the Cold War and there were some allegations of brainwashing with hallucinogens, so they were reluctant to send any LSD behind the Iron Curtain. In my desperation, I was asking myself, "oh, what can I do for which I don't need LSD?" As it happened, while keeping up with the literature, I saw in 1955 in the *Journal of the American Chemical Society* an article published by Fish, Johnson and Horning about the chemical content of cohoba, the snuff used by the native Indians in South America for religious purposes. Chemical analysis had identified four compounds in it: dimethyltryptamine, bufotenine, dimethyltryptamine-N-oxide, and bufotenine-N-oxide. Bufotenine had been claimed to be psychoactive; Fabing had done some work with it, but nobody knew much about dimethyltryptamine (DMT).

LH: Who wrote that article?

SS: Fish, Johnson and Horning.

LH: I thought it might have been Dick Botnish from Harvard.

SS: Are you referring to Dick Schultes?

LH: Dick Schultes.

SS: But going back to Fish, Johnson and Horning, they identified bufotenine and said that it was probably the active ingredient. However, the Fabing report wasn't very convincing. Others who tested bufotenine reported on flushing of the face and a lot of other primarily vegetative effects with the substance. So I was not sure whether bufotenine was really the active ingredient. There was nothing about DMT in the literature, so. I decided to go back to my old institute where I did my thesis work and ask them whether they could synthesize some DMT because I would like to test it and find out what it does. This was at the end of 1955, beginning of 1956, and to make a long story short, with the help of my old friend, Miomir Mészáros, I synthesized a few grams of DMT. When I tested it in animals, first on rats, then on mice and ultimately on cats, it turned out to be active biologically and pharmacologically. From these data I guessed what would be approximately the active dose for DMT in humans. I thought it would be interesting to see whether it had hallucinogenic effects. DMT has some effects in animals, but who knows whether they're hallucinating? You can't ask them!

I decided to take DMT myself first. I started with a very small amount, like the amount Hofmann took of LSD; I used a quarter of a milligram. So, I started very carefully with a quarter of a milligram. I waited for a few hours and since it had no effect on me, I took half a milligram, then 1 milligram without any effect. And so, I went up to, I think, 100 milligrams orally. It had no effect at all. At this point I became discouraged. The substance seemed to be active in animals, but it didn't do anything to me. I knew what to expect from a hallucinogen because half a year before taking DMT, I was inspired by Huxley's book, *The Doors of Perception* and I took mescaline. But I did not get that from the oral doses of DMT. Someone in the hospital made a suggestion that maybe I should try to inject it.

LH: Yes, it was given to the animals by injection.

SS: I was hoping that maybe I could avoid getting the injection, but apparently I couldn't avoid it, so I went down to the pharmacist in the hospital and asked him to make a preparation of DMT that could be given by injection. After the preparation was ready, I started injecting it into myself, intramuscularly. Starting with a small dose, a quarter of a milligram per kg, it was inactive, I felt no noticeable effect. After increasing the dose to half a milligram per kg, I thought I saw something that started to look like visual, perceptual distortions. At the next test I injected three quarter milligram per kg, and as I weighed about 75 kg at that time, it was a total of about 55 milligrams. Two minutes after the injection I was up in seventh heaven. It was amazing. It came very fast; I could hardly keep my eyes open; everything started to move around; the faces had become distorted, in just the same way as with mescaline or LSD.

LH: So, that was your first real hallucinogenic experience.

SS: Yes, my first hallucinogenic experience with DMT. Yet half an hour later, everything was gone. Everything. I also tested DMT on a colleague of mine who was assisting me in the hospital when he told me that he would like to try it. Then, the word got around. At the time, there was no drug control, the kind we have today. It was just pure science. So the word got around and several other people volunteered. We eventually collected 36 or 37 experiences from 30 volunteers. Everyone got about 1 milligram per kg. Although this was not a scientifically designed dose-response study, it did establish in a large population that DMT was unequivocally hallucinogenic in people when given in the dose of 1 milligram per kg. This research was done in 1956. By the end of the summer, we decided that we would write it up and send it in for publication, because DMT seemed to be a very interesting new type of hallucinogen. Its effect doesn't lasts for 12 hours as does mescaline, or 6 to 8 hours as LSD. It was obviously a different kind of hallucinogen, and I thought it would be interesting to do more work with it. I thought that it was appropriate to write up our findings as a preliminary report and get it published. So I sent the report to *Experientia*, a Swiss journal. They accepted it and the paper was published the same year, I think it was in November.

But in November 1956, things were disorganized in Hungary. There was a revolution in October, and the Russian troops came in and suppressed the revolution. They decided to bring back the old Communist rule. At that point in time I realized that I didn't have a future there. I wasn't a member of the Communist Party. As a matter of fact, I found a secret report on me, when, during the revolution, the Communist Party archive was opened up. According to the report my main crime was that I was western-oriented; I was reading western literature and sent my paper on DMT for publication to a western journal. As a matter of fact, I had sent a paper before this to *Biochimica Biophysica Acta* in 1951 or 1952. So, I was western-oriented, that was my major crime in the eyes of the Communist Party.

LH: So there was, essentially, a political crusade against you?

SS: It was. I was Chief of the Laboratory in the psychiatric hospital and didn't have any chance for advancement. I had a small laboratory with 4 or 5 people working with me. During the short period of time I was working in the hospital I got involved with some clinical work and not only with human volunteers, but also with patients. Dr. Böszörményi, whom I was working with, had suggested that we should try DMT in some of our alcoholic patients and in some schizophrenic patients. We began testing the drug and we found out that it was also active in those populations. It did not have as pronounced an effect as in normals, but it was a noticeable effect as measured by the questionnaires we used.

LH: You were still using DMT?

SS: Yes, dimethyltryptamine. I also synthesized some 13 different derivatives of it. I had the diethyl, dipropyl, dibutyl and several other homologues. The dibutyl was inactive, while the dimethyl, diethyl and dipropyl were active in animals. In humans, we had only tested the dimethyl and the diethyl derivatives at that point. Then I left Hungary, I escaped illegally. I had to. There were two hundred thousand people who voted with their feet and left Hungary after the revolution, mostly through Austria. Once in Austria, I went to Vienna to see Dr. Hoff. Do you remember Dr. Hoff?

LH: Oh, he was head of pharmacology.

SS: No, he was head of psychiatry.

LH: Oh, Hoff, oh yes.

SS: H-o-f-f.

LH: Yes. He was professor of psychiatry in Vienna; I knew him only by name.

SS: I also met H. O. Arnold and G. Hofmann who were in Hoff's Institute. You may remember their names. They were publishing some interesting stuff at the time. They had done some work on LSD as well. So I decided that I'd get in touch with them. As a matter of fact, they were very kind to me. When I told them I was a refugee, they said, "there is a room here which we use for psychotherapy, and at night if you want to you can sleep in there, but by 7:00 o'clock in the morning, you'll have to clear out." But they were nice. They gave me a little shelter over my head. And while pulling out a little bottle from my pocket, I said, "I have a little dimethyl-tryptamine here with me, you know, if you are interested."

LH: You were a pusher.

SS: Then I asked them, "Could you give me some LSD to try, I would be very curious to see how it would compare with my experience with mescaline, dimethyltryptamine and diethyltryptamine." They said, "We have a proto-col here. You have to go through it and you can get tested." So I got LSD while I was there as a refugee, and it was a very interesting experience.

LH: Was it similar to dimethyltryptamine, but longer-lived?

SS: It was similar, but longer-lived. I took the LSD early in the morning, like 9:00 o'clock and at 4:00 o'clock in the afternoon, they said, by now it should be all over and you may go home. I decided to walk to a large hall where the evening meal was served for refugees in Vienna at that time and sat down for dinner. By then, it was 7:00 or 8:00 o'clock in the evening. There was a huge mural painted on the wall and as I looked at it I said, those darn things, those figures are moving.

LH: That's a late onset.

SS: Yeah, for a while they moved, and then they quieted down and everything was back to normal. The effects of LSD are longer lasting than the effects of DMT, and they come back in waves.

LH: How much had you taken?

SS: One hundred micrograms. That's a relatively small dose.

LH: That's a rather modest dose.

SS: So that was my experience with LSD. Then I decided to stay with my sister, who lived in Berlin, which at that time was still surrounded by East German and Russian troops. So the only way for me to get there, as a refugee, was to fly over the Eastern Zone to Berlin. Once I was there, I got in touch with the people at the local Free University of Berlin. It happened that I met Hanns Hippius, who was working there at that time. They had a lab at the University and they said "you are welcome to come here and do some work if you are interested." And I started to learn German. We had German in school back in Hungary. For eight years, we learned German. So the German came back pretty fast and, as a matter of fact, in a few months I gave a seminar in German about the kind of effects I had experienced with hallucinogens.

LH: I take it that you were able to speak and understand German by then?

SS: Yes. I was there for almost a year. I didn't realize that if you are a refugee, once you resettle from the first country, which was Austria, in a second country, in my case Germany, I was not considered a refugee any more. However, I wanted to come to the United States; that was my final goal. I knew that this is the place where much of the action is in the particular area I was interested in. But I had no chance or very little chance to come here, because I was already settled in a second country. But I was still interested and started correspondence with people whom I knew from the scientific literature and I did eventually get three offers: one from Bob Heath down in New Orleans, who had been looking for a psychiatrist. The second, I forget the name of the scientist who offered me a job, was in Philadelphia. And the third was from Joel Elkes at the NIMH, who was organizing a laboratory at St. Elizabeths Hospital. As I was thinking over which offer should I take, I saw a film in Berlin, which at that time was a new film with Marlon Brando. It was *A Streetcar Named Desire*, based on a Tennessee Williams play. I don't know if you're familiar with it, but the movie takes place in New Orleans. And my impression of New Orleans was so bad that I didn't want to live there. Marlon Brando was playing a bum, and everything was dirty, hot and sweaty there. I said, "I do not want to go to New Orleans; Pennsylvania would be nice, but the NIMH is more prestigious." I decided I'd take the job with Joel Elkes. So that's how I got to Washington.

LH: And, you picked a place, too, where there were many more disciplines involved. Bob Heath was kind of a loner. He worked his own path and had very innovative ideas, but no one else around would interchange with him; whereas, at St. Elizabeths, I guess Joel Elkes had a more interdisciplinary team.

SS: I was very lucky that I came here. The laboratories, however, were not ready yet. They were converting the fifth and the ground floor in the William A. White building into laboratories and offices, and the laboratories were not ready. Joel Elkes said "Listen, Stephen, there's some very interesting work going on in Building 10, at NIH, in Julie Axelrod's lab. I talked to him and you can probably stay there, and work with Julie until these labs are ready." So I went there and Julie was nice and very accommodating. He said, "Stephen, if you are interested in applying biochemistry to pharmacology and psychiatry, this is a good place to work on that." A lot of people worked there, among many others, Danny Freedman.

LH: Now, we're talking about late 1950s?

SS: Actually, it was late 1957. In 1957 I did go into Axelrod's lab and, as a matter of fact, I stayed there for about two years, because I liked it. He's a very, very innovative guy in terms of developing new methodologies. When I told him that I was interested in the metabolism of dimethyltryptamine, he immediately told me that I could study the metabolism of DMT very easily, and suggested some methodologies I might want to use. He also told me the way to detect metabolites in the blood and in the urine, so I could work out the details. I understood from him that I could probably collaborate with some people on the second floor of the NIMH; that there was a normal volunteer group there on whom they were testing new drugs, and some hypotheses, and that they also had a large chronic schizophrenic population. I teamed up with people there and studied the rate of metabolism of diethyltryptamine (DET) in normal volunteers and schizophrenic patients. We had some very interesting results that we presented at the Third World Congress of Psychiatry in Canada in 1961.

While I was in Julie's laboratory, Hoffer published a paper claiming that he detected adrenochrome in the blood of schizophrenic patients and he made a big claim that adrenochrome was the schizotoxin which produces schizophrenia. Seymour Kety got involved in the discussion, and he said "Listen, this is a very interesting and a very important finding. If it is true, it may be a breakthrough in psychiatry." But Julie said that there was some deficiency in Hoffer's methodology and there was no proof about the presence of adrenochrome at all in the laboratory tests. There were no controls, so who knew what he was measuring? So, Julie said that we should check it out.

I don't know exactly how Julie managed it, but he eventually got two milligrams of adrenochrome and told me how to develop the methodology using that two. Then I got busy and developed a spectrophotofluorometric methodology with proper controls. To prove that it was a sensitive and specific methodology I showed that we could recover as little as 0.02 microgram of adrenochrome added to plasma and measure it. And I said, "Let us try some blood from schizophrenics and see if there's indeed something to Hoffer's claims that there is adrenochrome in their blood." We tested about six or seven schizophrenic patients at the Clinical Center; we collaborated with Irv Kopin who helped us to draw some blood, and then we tested the blood samples. They were all completely negative.

I don't know exactly how but we got feedback from Hoffer, saying that only those schizophrenics who are acutely hallucinating have adrenochrome in their blood. As it happened, all the patients at the NIMH were chronic patients who were barely hallucinating any more. Dr. Kopin found out that across the street at the Naval Hospital they had a few acutely hallucinating schizophrenic patients, so we drove over and drew blood from them. We drove back to NIH and ran the samples through the test and they were also all negative.

We were quite disappointed and thought, this is probably going to go nowhere, and were ready to drop the whole project, when our lab director, Seymour Kety said to me, "You know, Stephen, this is a very important finding, even though it is negative; it is important to make a statement and publish a short note that there is no evidence that adrenochrome is present in the blood of schizophrenics." He said, "It can prevent people going up a blind alley in a wrong direction." So we published the paper in 1958 in the *American Journal of Psychiatry*. It was a one-page paper, and Hoffer reacted to it strongly. He was outraged. He wrote a letter to the editor of the *American Journal of Psychiatry* and we answered it defending our data. Subsequently, in the late 1950's in the pages of *Psychosomatic Medicine*, our paper and Hoffer's reaction spawned an open debate between John D. Benjamin and Abram Hoffer. Benjamin pointed out that the way "Szára and Axelrod approached the problem of adrenochrome in the blood was the way to do research in this area," using careful controls and proper methodologies. It was a big debate but eventually it quieted down.

LH: Well, I think one of Hoffer's contentions was that it was a very fragile molecule and could be easily reduced.

SS: It forms spontaneously when an epinephrine solution is exposed to light for an extended period of time.

LH: By oxidation.

SS: It is an oxidation product. Julie Axelrod, at that time, was involved with mapping all the catecholamine metabolism pathways, identifying all the metabolites, and he said that there was no room for metabolism to any other substance, at least in the amounts that Hoffer was claiming. Julie said that he could account for about 98 percent of the metabolites for epinephrine, so there was no room for adrenochrome. Anyway, the paper was published and that was probably the end of the adrenochrome hypothesis.

LH: Well, Abe Hoffer was an interesting person, wasn't he? He'd get an idea, a wild one, and thought it was real. But one of the interesting things about Abe's career is that his most important discovery had nothing to do with psychopharmacology. It was that nicotinic acid reduces cholesterol levels.

SS: I knew that he was using nicotinic acid.

LH: He was using nicotinic acid in those schizophrenics, and in the process they were doing a lot of chemical measuring; and it turned out that cholesterol would go down and that was the birth of nicotinic acid as a treatment for hypercholesterolemia, which is still being used.

SS: That's interesting.

LH: It's a very effective agent, so that's a paradox in his career. Now, you were doing all this work while you were at St. Elizabeths, you had a nice building there where they had laboratories on the first and top floor and the wards in between. Did you run across Tony Hordern at that time, the Australian?

SS: No, I don't think so.

LH: Well, he was a clinician, so you might not have, but didn't you write a book with Weil-Malherbe?

SS: Weil-Malherbe, yes. That was at the end of my stay at St. Elizabeths in the late 1960s that he asked me to collaborate with him. He was very much into the catecholamine business and he asked me if I want to join him in a book, which was entitled *The Biochemistry of Functional and Experimental Psychoses*. He reviewed the functional side of it, focusing on the biochemical aspects of psychoses.

LH: It was a review of almost all the biochemical aspects.

SS: It was a very nice book. I wrote a chapter on the experimental psychoses, produced by drugs such as LSD and DMT and reviewed that literature. Now, you might think if you write a review book like this it becomes just another publication in the literature and then people forget it. We also forgot about it until the end of the 1980s. In the meantime some of the ideas discussed in that book apparently inspired David Wong. I don't know if you know him from Eli Lilly. He is one of the pharmacologists who had developed Prozac (fluoxetine). He apparently did give credit in his publications for the inspiration that he got from our book for the development of Prozac, but we didn't know about it until the middle of November 1990, when Dr. Wong was giving a lecture at the NIH about developing new drugs. At the beginning he had the cover of a book on the screen for several minutes while explaining how important that book had been in inspiring him to work on new selective serotonin reuptake inhibitors such as Prozac. I didn't know about this at that time; I wasn't there, but people from the institute would come back and tell me that "your name was on the cover of the book, and you were credited for the inspiration in the development of Prozac."

LH: Did they have any idea of the importance of serotonin?

SS: The importance of serotonin is an interesting question, because most of the medical literature in psychiatry at that time was focusing on the catecholamines while serotonin was kind of pushed into the background but the review by Hans Weil-Malherbe was covering both sides. Hans tried to create a very balanced review of the involvement of both serotonin and catecholamines, and he made the point that transmitters probably don't act just alone, but are interacting with each other and serotonin may be just as important as cathecholamines. He also reviewed some of the early biochemical findings in depression and in schizophrenia. So he gave a balanced picture, and Wong apparently picked up on this because of the very interesting statement in Hans Weil-Malherbe's chapter that the metabolism of tryptamine was changed in depression.

LH: I think the reason you probably didn't follow the line of emphasing only catecholamines was because in Europe there was much more interest in serotonin; both of you were transplanted and that gave you a broader perspective than if the book had been written by a purely American author.

SS: I think you are right about the European emphasis on serotonin. It was Garattini who was interested in serotonin. He invited me to present my paper on dimethyltryptamine in 1957 at an international meeting in Milan. I don't know if you were there. That was a symposium organized by Silvio Garattini on psychotropic drugs. It was published in a monograph. It was the success of the Milan meeting that led to the founding of the CINP, the Collegium Internationale Neuro-Psychopharmacologicum.

LH: This was about in...?

SS: In May 1957. Garattini invited me to present my dimethyltryptamine work and I chose to talk about my self-experiments with the four hallucinogens: mescaline, LSD, DMT, and DET. I made as concise a comparison as possible on the basis of my personal experiences. And I think it was at that meeting that I met somebody from Joel Elkes' lab who interviewed me, and based on that interaction, Joel Elkes hired me without actually seeing me.

LH: Somewhere along the line you learned English.

SS: When I was in Berlin, I had a girlfriend, a German girlfriend, who could speak English, and we went over my paper that was written in English, so that I could learn how to pronounce the words. I gave my paper in Milan in English, but I learned to speak English only after I came here. Obviously, you don't learn a language that late – I was thirty-something – without keeping your accent.

LH: I always remember Dan Efron's famous statement, "The international language of science is broken English."

SS: That's very true.

LH: How long did you stay at that laboratory?

SS: About ten years.

LH: So, that would be 1958 to 1968.

SS: About 1969.

LH: Did you continue during that time your work on hallucinogens?

SS: Mostly hallucinogens. We did some very interesting clinical work as well. I don't know if you want to hear about that, but we tried to test the effect of DET on alcoholic patients. There was a claim in the literature that LSD and the so-called psychedelic drugs could be very useful in treating alcoholics.

LH: Again, Abe Hoffer and a couple of other Canadians.

SS: A number of claims had been made, so we decided to see what our drug could do. We set up a team that consisted of a psychotherapist whose his name was Vourlekis, and another fellow who came to work with me, whom you knew very well, because he has also worked with you, Lou Faillace. We decided to do a double-blind study on alcoholics, using what we called an active placebo. The substance we used was a derivative of DET, namely 6-fluoro-diethyltryptamine, in which we substituted the 6th position of the indole ring with fluorine. It turned out to be a substance which wasn't hallucinogenic any more, but still produced some autonomic effects so the patients felt they received something. We had maybe a dozen patients who had been chronic alcoholics for about four to ten years, and the psychotherapist, Vourlekis was involved with the patients until the effects of the drug wore off. He also conducted most of the tests and followed up the patients. We thought we did see some improvements, but they were unfortunately only temporary, lasting for about six months. We did a follow up two years later, and those patients who received DET did not differ significantly from any other alcoholic patients in their drinking habits.

LH: It's surprising that you mentioned Lou Faillace. I'd never heard of him until I did some work with STP (2, 5-dimethoxy-4-methylamphetamine), the amphetamine homologue. Sol Snyder was working on it as well at the same time. I visited Sol in Baltimore, and said, "Well, there's no use publishing our papers separately, at least for the preliminary report; why don't we combine them?" So, the paper came out, Snyder, Faillace and Hollister. I didn't know who this Faillace guy was. I guess he was a fellow at that time, doing the clinical work. And as luck would have it, in 1986, when I decided to leave California and come to Houston, Faillace became my boss. He was the Chairman of the Department in Texas when I joined. So I guess the moral of the story is, treat all of the young people gently. You never know when they'll wind up as your boss.

SS: I met him again recently. NIDA organized a meeting on hallucinogens and Lou was invited and I saw him at the meeting. That's when I last saw him.

LH: Well, I became interested in LSD in alcoholics through a group led by a guy who was essentially an engineer, named Hubbard – not Ron. They were going around the country charging people $600.00 a pop for one session with LSD with the idea that one session would cure you. So Jack Shelton and I did a study; and Joe Levine and Arnold Ludwig did a study; and perhaps it was your group, I don't know, it was a third group; all independently. None of us knew that the others were doing it. We all came to ultimately the same conclusion; that although there might have been a transitory effect, it was not long lasting, and I think that sort of finished the idea off. But it's amazing that story with hallucinogens, how it captured the imagination, and it's coming back now, isn't it?

SS: Yes, I read in the newspaper, LSD is very easily available, and people take it without a second thought; they are there for the experience. It's unfortunate, but I hope these drugs eventually prove to be useful. They are very powerful and they do produce something in our brain that affects our mind and this interaction between the brain and mind is a fascinating phenomenon. I have a preoccupation about it, because I think that their major and most important effect is probably losing the ego boundaries. After you take LSD you feel that you are one with the whole world, with the whole universe. When your ego boundary disappears you feel one with your fellow beings, so there's a very interesting social facilitating effect there, which is probably there all the time, but we are not aware of it. The hallucinogens give us a key for getting into that particular part of our brain/mind relationship that establishes a boundary of how far our ego is extended. When you drive an automobile, your ego includes the automobile and you, driving together.

LH: Another intriguing thing about LSD was that it would produce these profound mental effects in relatively small doses. 2 micrograms per kilogram was more than enough for a pretty good experience and, when you think of it, there aren't too many substances that have that potent a physiological effect. Vitamin B_{12} is one of those substances; 1 microgram per day makes a difference between having a normal blood count and having pernicious anemia. Another example is botulinum toxin; but there aren't too many compounds that are as potent. I think that LSD had a big attraction because it was feasible to consider that something equally potent or even more so, could be produced endogenously and make people schizophrenic. However, the endogenous psychotogen idea fell into disrepute and hasn't been followed up very much. A new interesting story I learned much later in life from Ernst Rothlin, the Sandoz pharmacologist;

he was visiting me and said, after Hofmann had his inadvertent experience with LSD, he decided he ought to take it again to prove it was the substance that produced the effects. He discussed with Rothlin what the dose should be. Hofmann wanted to take about 200 micrograms and Rothlin, being a cautious pharmacologist, said, oh, I think I'd only take 30 or 50. Well, Hofmann ignored Rothlin's advice and, of course, he had a whopping reaction.

SS: I hear that Hofmann took 250 micrograms.

LH: If he'd taken the dose Rothlin recommended he might have missed LSD's psychomimetic effect.

SS: Talking about LSD, a few years ago, in 1993, there was a meeting in Lugano organized by Sandoz to celebrate the 50th anniversary of the discovery of LSD and Hofmann, I think he was 86 at that time, was still very alert and very up to date with work involving LSD and the ergot alkaloids. He showed us a film about how he discovered LSD and what his experience was. It was very interesting to hear it from him on a first hand basis.

LH: Did you ever study psilocybin?

SS: No, I never got around to studying psilocybin.

LH: But you did some studies with mescaline?

SS: The only study that I had done with mescaline was taking it and experiencing it.

LH: Because they're all really a part of the same group, clinically, and virtually indistinguishable; although, the dose is different by orders of magnitude. The only person I know who is doing some work currently with hallucinogens, and we're sending him grant support, is a fellow named Rick Strassman in New Mexico or Arizona.

SS: Well, he was in New Mexico up to, I think, a year ago, and he moved to either Seattle or some other place. But at that time I was in touch with him. He had called me up a number of times, because he's the only one who is following the DMT story in a very systematic fashion. He got around the bureaucratic red tape that involves the use of these drugs, and eventually he established a good research group.

LH: So, after you finished at St. Elizabeths in 1968, what did you do then?

SS: Well, at that time, I was kind of pushed out of the laboratory. I don't want to name names, but it was a difficult situation.

LH: Had Joel left by that time?

SS: Joel had left by that time, and other people also had to go. It was a difficult time, and I had to decide what to do next. A position opened up at the Extramural Branch of NIMH. They had a Drug Abuse Center; the exact name was Center for Studies of Narcotics and Drug Abuse. Bob Peterson was involved in recruiting new people, and he thought that I could be useful to organize some new work there, so I decided to accept it, and I made the switch at that time. It was a forced switch, but I don't think that I have regretted it because I got involved with some very interesting stuff. It was not only new subjects and new drugs. I had an opportunity to meet with a variety of scientists working in that area. I became first Chief of the Clinical Studies Section, and, then in 1974, when the Center was enlarged to become the new National Institute on Drug Abuse, I became Chief of the Biomedical Branch. In the Clinical Studies section, which I first had, the main question, the main thrust, was to do some controlled clinical studies with THC (tetrahydrocannabinol) and marijuana. That was the first project I was involved in, and I remember reading in one of your books, which you had written at the time, that marijuana is probably one of the only drugs in which more experimentation had been done in humans first, rather than animals, or something like that. So, that was probably part of the impetus, among others, to do some more clinical studies and more controlled studies, because all the experimentation you referred to involved people taking drugs on their own, without knowing how much they were taking, without any controls. The main point was you ought to do some controlled clinical trials and that was my first job. In the first year when I got involved with organizing the program, I was actually sending out RFPs, Requests for Proposals. We had contract money and we decided to do a number of studies. We got a group going at UCLA, Sid Cohen was the first principal investigator on that, and then we had the San Francisco group with Reese Jones, and we also organized overseas studies in which we decided to study the health effects of marijuana in long-term users in Jamaica, Costa Rica and also in Greece. So we had a number of studies.

LH: Epidemiological studies in Jamaica and Greece.

SS: Yes, epidemiological studies including the study of medical histories and health effects, if any, as a result of chronic use. We also supported a number of other grantees studying marijuana and THC, and eventually we organized a meeting, I think it was in 1975, held in Savannah, Georgia, where we invited all the people who were involved in these studies, including you. You may not have been able to make it, but you sent in a paper, and we included that in the proceedings, as you were one of the first who studied THC. So, it was important to have documentation of what was known at that time about THC. This was also necessary, because, in my capacity at NIDA, I was responsible for sending over to the FDA reports about basic laboratory studies on THC for the Master File that FDA has to keep for any drug that is being tested for potential therapeutic use. Eventually THC has been approved, in a capsule form, to treat nausea in cancer patients on chemotherapy, so that was the only medically relevant and important result of this particular study. We also had a grantee at UCLA, Donald Tashkin, who has done some very good work about the effects of marijuana and tobacco separately and together on the lungs of chronic smokers.

LH: I think we can generalize and say, any time you take smoke in your lungs it's bad for you.

SS: Yeah, that's it. Actually it is that simple, and it's costing us millions of dollars to document it and this is the result. So that was my role in the THC studies at NIDA that I had to follow very closely. It was very important to visit all of the sites occasionally.

LH: Well, the therapeutic use of THC or marijuana is becoming a very politically sensitive issue now in states that conduct plebiscites to approve its use without any scientific basis. It's rather remarkable that in spite of all the studies on the therapeutic uses, nobody has tried to assess smoked marijuana vs. orally administered THC.

SS: Maybe they have done that in our study at UCLA in which Frank was involved.

LH: Who did it?

SS: Ira Frank. Ira Frank became the Project Director of the UCLA project.

LH: Years ago Ira incidentally found that THC lowered intraocular pressure.

SS: That was part of a study that compared smoked marijuana with smoked placebo and oral THC.

LH: I think glaucoma is a dead issue as far as the therapeutic use of THC is concerned.

SS: Sounds like it is.

LH: Most people who have glaucoma are old, and I can't see old people wanting to be stoned all day while controlling their eye pressure.

SS: Yes, as a matter of fact, it is a very unpleasant side effect for those people.

LH: Traditionally, glaucoma has been treated with local instillation, and there are now a great variety of different drugs to treat it. Besides, I think THC is not much different from alcohol in terms of the reduction of intraocular pressure, but again, who wants to be drunk all day, so I consider that a dead issue. The only three therapeutic issues I think that need to be resolved are smoked marijuana vs. oral THC in nausea and vomiting for people on cancer chemotherapy; smoked marijuana vs. oral in terms of appetite stimulation and weight preservation in people who have the wasting syndrome of AIDS. And possibly more studies, because there aren't very many, on its effect on spasticity in neurological diseases like multiple sclerosis or other diseases where you have muscle spasms. But all the other indications, I think have died out by now, or are totally unrealistic. But there could be a lot more done in that one area.

SS: The only hitch is the FDA's resistance to having a drug that cannot be well standardized. To standardize a smoke is almost impossible and the FDA is very reluctant to even consider a smoked drug to be used in any context, so that's the end.

Okay, let's just go to some other area. I understand you want to have some discussion about all the drugs that I have been involved in. At NIDA, in the early 1970s the opiates came into focus, mostly as a result of Bill Martin's initiative that there are probably more than one type of opiate receptor we have to consider. But at that time there was no known isolated opiate receptor, not even a direct demonstration that opiates are binding onto specific receptors. In 1971, we organized a meeting at the Center for Studies of Narcotics and Drug Abuse, with I think, 50 or so people attending. I don't know if you were present at that meeting, because it was related primarily to opiates. We had rounds of discussion for three days, on the question of where the Institute should put its money, in terms of opiate research. How should we proceed? Some of the conclusions were that obviously the molecular aspects of the receptors would have to be worked out in a more detailed fashion and some money should be put in that area. And this is what happened. We did establish, I think it was in 1971, eight Drug Abuse Research Centers. Some of them were almost exclusively oriented to research on opiates, like Avram Goldstein's group and a few others. Sol Snyder's group, in the beginning, was not into opiates. They were into amphetamines, primarily, and into catecholamines.

LH: I was talking yesterday to Candace Pert.

SS: I saw her recently and I was reminded that she was working with Sol as a student at that time.

LH: She said after she'd been working on the problem for a couple of months and hadn't gotten any results, Sol got impatient and said, "Well, let's go on to something else."

SS: And once they identified the opiate receptor with a reasonable certainty, using specific binding of radioactive labeled naloxone with very high specific activity, they managed to measure more reliably the localization and density of specific binding sites in the brain; that, apparently, eluded Avram Goldstein who had started this strategy earlier.

LH: Well, you know, there were so many people in the story of the opiate receptor and the endogenous ligands that it's hard to say who deserves the most credit, but I really think that Avram Goldstein was very fundamental in it, because he had started the research on the opiate receptor as early as 1971. He gave a paper at the IUPHAR meeting, in which the problem he had was distinguishing non-specific from specific binding, but that was because he didn't have ligands with high enough specific activity. And, then, a year or two later, he described something called a pituitary opioid-like material, which eventually turned out to be dynorphin, so he was right in the forefront, both in the receptor and the ligand area. But, almost simultaneously with Candace's work, along came Terenius and Eric Simon. And, of course, Kosterlitz and Hughes came in 1975 with the endogenous ligand. He must have been involved in the beginnings with LAAM, levo-α-acetylmethadol.

SS: Yes, Avram was very instrumental in pushing LAAM for the treatment of heroin addiction.

LH: Isn't it incredible it took 18 years before it got accepted?

SS: There were a number of stumbling blocks as you are clearly aware. LAAM was not a clean drug in some sense, but everybody was willing to go along without any hesitation, until eventually it became accepted. So, in 1975 and 1976, NIDA was discussing, how we should acknowledge these people's contribution to drug abuse research and they established an award. I was asked to suggest who would be the appropriate persons to get an award and we apparently settled on six of the leaders of research groups who were involved.

LH: The Pacesetter Award.

SS: Yes, it became known as The Pacesetter Award. Avram Goldstein, Sol Snyder, Eric Simon, John Hughes, Hans Kosterlitz and Lars Terenius, were the people who eventually got this award. It is obvious that Candace Pert was very upset that she was left out of this group and we did, indeed, have some serious discussion about it, but she was still a graduate student at that time.

LH: I remember when the older Governor Brown was governor of California. He made a famous statement in which he said, "Every time I appoint a judge, I make 99 enemies and one ingrate," and I think that's sometimes the way awards work, so you can't win. Well, you've had a long career both in clinical and laboratory research, as well as administration. What do you think we should do about the war on drugs? Are we going to win it, or are we losing it, or should we change our tactics?

SS: It depends on who you ask. If you ask me as a medical scientist, I would prefer that most of the available money would go to research on treatment and prevention. That would be probably better spent than putting all this money on airplanes and spraying the fields.

LH: So you would prefer treatment vs. interdictions?

SS: I would prefer that more money be put in the treatment area.

LH: And, what's the evidence for the effectiveness of these treatments? Is it all that good, once you get past methadone?

SS: Probably not, but at least it makes some people, not everybody obviously, well enough to make a contribution to society, to take a job and be a useful citizen, even though they are on methadone or continuing methadone, but they are still more respected citizens than those who are just keeping on injecting illegal stuff.

LH: Naltrexone is an ideal drug for opiate dependence. It specifically blocks the receptor. It's orally active, fairly long lasting and you don't get high on it. Nobody ever gets addicted to it. So it's a perfect drug for treating it, but nobody wants to take it. The only people who benefit from it are the high-class opiate dependent people like physicians, nurses, lawyers, and people in general who have a lot to lose if they lose their license. But if you don't have a lot to lose and you have only a very little motivation, as most of the opiate addicts do, it doesn't work

SS: It doesn't give them a buzz that they can get from methadone.

LH: Well, that's the beauty of methadone. Once you've got them hooked, they've got to stay with it, but the other problem is that as prevention, do you think a whole bunch of advertisements directed at kids are going to change the pattern?

SS: It depends on how it is being handled, I think. Some of the advertisements may provide education, perhaps making people aware of the dangers, especially if you have a child involved, because they feel themselves as invincible and think they'll live forever, so they don't care much about the dangers. But I think if the message is carefully worded and organized, it could be helpful for some people. It may not solve their personal problems, but it could benefit some people. I don't have too much hope for anything that would be spectacular in terms of cutting back on drug abuse. In a free society there is no way to have it policed effectively.

LH: The area of hope I think is with smoking cigarettes. There has been a gradual but slow decline in the number of smokers, and of course, in part, that's due to the fact that it'll kill you and you've got a constant attrition, but aside from that, I think the social pressures that have been put on smokers have had a very positive effect in either reducing the number of smokers or reducing the amounts they smoke. But that's taken a whole generation.

SS: What's interesting, I don't know if you were aware of it, but the situation you just described is probably valid only in the United States, and it may be completely different in other parts of the world. I can only speak from personal experience about the social attitude on smoking in Europe. When you go to Europe, there's cigarette smoking everywhere, and I really can get sick; I just go to a restaurant, and practically everybody is smoking around me, and I can't even smell the food. So society in general would have to recognize the potential problems, and I don't know what kind of public education would be the best, but apparently some of those that have been effective in the United States could be tried. The social acceptance of smoking is still prevalent in Europe, and we're not even talking about China and some of the other countries, where people are still smoking heavily.

LH: I guess Japanese men have the highest rate of smoking of anybody and, yes, societal attitudes play a big role, but it works so slowly that one can't get very enthusiastic. Well, you had a very interesting career, spanning several countries and several languages. I think it's very remarkable, obviously. Now, when you left Hungary, you left by yourself and no other family?

SS: Yes, I left Hungary by myself and I got married here in the States.

LH: Do you still have family there?

SS: I have a sister who stayed back in Hungary. As a matter of fact, there were five children in our family and every one of us is ended up living in a different country. My older sister is still back in Hungary. My second sister is in Berlin, Germany. My third sister is in England. Unfortunately, she had a stroke, but she's still alive. My brother is in Switzerland, and I'm in the United States.

LH: The Száras are worldwide. Well, I think you can be proud of what you did and I hope that you will keep active and interested in the field from now on as well.

SS: I'm trying to keep up with the research literature. In my spare time, I have a little computer and I'm trying to work out a model for the brain/mind.

LH: If you had to do it over again, would you do the same career? You might have a few qualifications, but on the whole, what do you think?

SS: On the whole, I'm not dissatisfied with the way things have turned out. At first, I was fretting and very distraught I had to give up laboratory research, back in 1970, but then, going into the administrative position, it gave me a slightly different perspective and a different way of leaving at least some of my footprints on the field. It was quite different than what I would have been able to do as a scientist. Eventually, I kind of settled down and made peace with myself that I did accomplish something in my life and I think the field is now moving at almost breakneck pace, which is tremendous. The only problem is that we are now deluged in a sea of data and we need some guiding principles or new tools, to find out which would be more relevant, more appropriate and more effective in trying to bridge the gap between where the drugs act at the chemical level to give rise to a behavioral response or subjective experience. How this gap could be bridged is going to be a major problem in the near future in our field, so we really need some bright ideas of how a drug acts on a receptor as a chemical, how it is translated or transformed into think-ing, feeling, and eventually action and behavior. So this is a major gap, which still needs to be bridged. There are major advances in the area of brain imaging like the PET scan and fMRI, where we can actually look into the brain and see the areas that are lighting up as a sign of increased blood flow, presumably as a result of increased neuronal activity. These are very interesting new tools for getting a handle on what's happening in our brain when we give a drug, but there is still no connection from the chemical level to the more global, neuronal level, so these gaps have to be eventually worked out before we can begin really making a major push forward.

LH: Well, maybe molecular biology is the answer.

SS: That's probably part of the answer, but not the total answer.

LH: Thank you.

SS: Leo, it was a pleasure. Thank you very much for spending the time with me.

LH: Yeah, I don't know where time goes.

SS: We may meet some other place and bump into each other as we did in the past, in Copenhagen or in Quebec, all kinds of interesting places.

LH: Well, I'll probably go to the CPDD (College on Problems of Drug Dependence) meeting in Nashville this year. I've been cursed with poor health for the last three years and I had to miss the last two meetings, but I'll go this time, maybe.

SS: Well, I will not be attending, but I will probably go to the ACNP meeting in Hawaii.

LH: Well, if we'd known you were going to be in Hawaii next year, we'd have done this interview over there.

JOSEPH WORTIS

Interviewed by Leo E. Hollister
San Juan, Puerto Rico, December 14, 1994

LH: Joe,* I suspect you are the oldest living member of the ACNP, among other distinctions.

JW: Well, how old are you, Leo?

LH: I just turned 74.

JW: You're kidding! I'm 88.

LH: Well, by god, you're going very strong.

JW: I celebrated my 88th birthday by running 5 miles, so that I could boast about it for a year.

LH: You make me feel awful with the idea of running.

JW: I also say that at my age I have no difficulty remembering. I just have trouble forgetting.

LH: Well, what we're going to do today is to see what you can remember.

JW: Too much.

LH: You've probably got a lot to tell.

JW: I'm writing my autobiography now and I've swept up all the material I have accumulated in my house and office and, as they say in the business, I'm overwhelmed by an excess of papers and I don't know how to use them all.

LH: Well, speaking of biography, when did you get started in medicine?

JW: Well, I was born in Brooklyn and I got a kind of scholarship that allowed me to go to New York University up at University Heights. I got my Bachelor's degree there. Then in the last year of my college an English writer, named Havelock Ellis, brought out a book called *The Dance of Life*; he was a writer with universal interests.

LH: And, he was also famous for his book on sex.

JW: Sex, yes, but he was also a poet, a novelist, a literary critic, and literary historian; he was into everything. H. L. Mencken, the great iconoclast, called Havelock Ellis the most civilized man in England. And Havelock Ellis became one of my heroes. I liked the fact that he was into everything. I thought, how nice! I said I'd like to be a universal man, too. I was then majoring in English, so I suddenly switched to pre-med and decided I would be a doctor, too, never intending to practice. I was an English

---

* Joseph Wortis was born in New York City in 1906, and graduated in medicine at the University of Vienna in 1932. He trained in psychiatry at Bellevue Hospital in New York, remaining on staff until 1952. He directed the pediatric psychiatry division of Jewish Hospital in Brooklyn from the early 1950s until 1968, from 1968 he did similar work at Maimonides Hospital in Brooklyn, then from 1972 until his retirement in 1976 was chief of the Division on Mental Retardation at the State University of New York, Stony Brook campus. Wortis died in 1995.

major, so it's no accident that I ended up being an editor, because I was always interested in writing and literature.

LH: And you do it very well.

JW: Then I was admitted to Yale Medical School. They had a new Dean there. I think his name was Gildersleeve, and he was interested that prospective medical college applicants have very broad interests. And when they interviewed me, they liked the fact that I had been an English major. So I was admitted. But then a schoolteacher of mine, a high school teacher, gave me a gift that allowed me to have my first trip to Europe. I went to London, Paris and Vienna. And in Vienna I met a couple of Americans studying medicine there, who persuaded me to study medicine in Europe. I was adventurous and I followed their advice.

LH: You left Yale for Vienna?

JW: Yes. I sent a letter to Yale, saying, I was staying in Europe and that maybe I'd come back next year. And they politely responded, in effect saying to hell with you.

LH: They must have told you that.

JW: So I studied in Vienna, in Munich and in Paris. I picked up foreign languages, which proved to be a useful acquisition. And I got my medical degree in Vienna. It took me five years under the European system, but I finally made it. In those years students used to say that anybody who registers and doesn't drop dead is going to graduate. You could take examinations over and over again, so, once you were registered, you had it made.

LH: As long as you took the exams. When was it that you graduated?

JW: I graduated in 1932. When I came back to the States I became a resident in psychiatry at Bellevue Hospital. Up to then, there was no psychiatric department at Bellevue Hospital or New York University. There was just a so-called observation ward.

LH: Did you choose psychiatry because you wanted to become a universal man?

JW: Well, I felt that psychiatry was virgin territory. I had an uncle who developed schizophrenia before my eyes. I was raised in the United States by European-born parents. They did not have much formal education, but they liked intellectual pursuits. My mother was trilingual. She came from a French family, attended German schools and spoke English like an American. She was a constant reader and she encouraged us children to read when we were toddlers. So I became a constant reader. My father's side was more working class than my mother's side, but they got very active in the radical movements of those times, in Socialism and so on. So I was exposed to a lot of stimulating influences. My father was a fine musician and singer. We had a lot of musical evenings at home. We'd have Italian pianists and German singers gather at our home. That was my background. I got accustomed to foreigners and always felt very international. When I elected to go to Europe, it was not out of line with the way I was brought up. I was brought up international and I was accustomed to hearing foreign languages.

LH: In fact, it almost sounds like you're more European than American.

JW: Well, paradoxically, I was raised in a Polish and Italian immigrant neighborhood and the only language my parents spoke to each other was English. I came from one of the few English speaking homes in my neighbourhood, and since I read a lot and was articulate, my teachers at school always regarded me as very indigenous American. So on the one hand, I was exposed to international influences, whereas on the other hand, I acquired a great love for the English language and I was immersed in American literature. I had both these influences.

LH: Now, what year did you go to Bellevue?

JW: In 1932, and was one of the first two residents that was ever hired at Bellevue. The hospital had only an observation ward in my time, where people picked up by the police were left to be observed, and to see whether they should be committed to a state hospital. The doctors who worked in the observation ward were called alienists. It was considered very unattractive work. They got salaries from the city as alienists. Then, the big middle building on 32nd Street was built, an eight-story building for a psychiatric institute during the administration of Jimmy Walker. It was a big graft job; they made fortunes on contracts. If they had anything that was expensive they put it into the building. The institute was run by a Napoleonic little figure without any scientific credentials. He was a very aggressive guy, his name was Menus Gregory. When they opened the psychiatric institute he needed additional help. But since he couldn't pay for any more alienists he got two young guys to put on white uniforms, Milton Abeles, who had just finished his neurology training at Montpelier, and me. And they called us residents but they didn't pay us anything. We were the first two residents in a newly created, so called psychiatric department. And the place was filled with patients. I saw an enormous number of patients. Menus Gregory was eventually fired for being a grafter. Soon after I started at Bellevue I was awarded a Havelock Ellis and Adolph Meyer fellowship that allowed me to go back to Europe for a year where I studied at Queens Square Hospital.

LH: Neurology?

JW: Yes. And then, I went to Vienna to study neuroanatomy. It was then that I had this exposure to Freud that was to become the basis of my book on

Freud. I kept a diary and published it 20 years afterwards because by that time it was no longer very personal to me.

LH: You were analyzed by Freud?

JW: Yes.

LH: I thought that was a humorous title for your book.

JW: No, that was the diary of my analysis with Freud, a daily account. I kept notes. Every day I entered notes on little index cards that I carried with me. And that's the record of what he said and what I said. It is based entirely on index cards.

LH: Well, you started off with training in neurology and psychoanalysis?

JW: Yes. Some of the interesting persons then on the staff at Bellevue were Paul Schilder and his wife Lauretta Bender. I was assigned to Lauretta Bender's ward, and I remember the first thing she asked me to do was to draw blood specimens for Wassermann tests on every new patient. And most of the tests came back positive. Apparently, in my ignorance, instead of sterilizing I cleaned each syringe in alcohol after I used it, and as a result, the same red cells were utilized in the tests. So that was my first experience with Lauretta Bender.

LH: I hope nobody got syphilis.

JW: Paul Schilder used to take me around when he saw patients. He was kind of brilliant, but not a very systematic scientist, who tried to combine psychoanalytic insights with his knowledge of neurology. Schilder was a rather peculiar looking guy with a very high-pitched voice, but he used to delight audiences because his lectures were so excellent. While I would trail after him he would dictate notes to me. I picked up a lot of information at Bellevue, but I also brought information back from Vienna, like the news on insulin shock treatment, which I observed when I was there.

LH: You met Sakel?

JW: I translated Sakel's monograph. I introduced the treatment in this country. It hit the newspapers, and, here I was in my 20s, thrust into prominence as the herald of this new first successful treatment of schizophrenia. And Karl Bowman, who was then chief of a psychiatric hospital, set me up with an insulin ward. People were flocking from all over the country to learn this wonderful new treatment of schizophrenia. And it was, indeed, a wonderful treatment.

LH: So, that was how you got into biological psychiatry?

JW: That's right, and then Farrar, the editor of the *American Journal of Psychiatry*, asked me to write a chapter on insulin shock treatment in his *Annual Review of Psychiatric Progress,* but I didn't want to be an advocate of one particular treatment, so I suggested that he change the title to "Physiological Treatment." He agreed and for 20 years, I wrote an annual review on physiological treatments. About that time psychopharmacology started. My reviews were probably among the most comprehensive reviews that appeared on psychopharmacology, because I knew foreign languages. I also developed the new technique of microfilming that fascinated me so much that I had a portable microfilming machine set up at the New York Academy of Medicine. I would check everything in the *Index Medicus* that appeared on a weekly basis that interested me. And I had my whole family sitting around the table, and my kids and my wife would slit out everything related to physiological therapies and mount them on index cards. Then my secretary would go to the Academy of Medicine and she would photograph on microfilm every item I was interested in. So I could sit in front of my machine, turn the crank and review the world's literature in all languages. As a result, I probably had the most comprehensive reviews of these new approaches to treatment. I did that for 20 years. In fact, I just threw out, these past few weeks, the thousands and thousands of index cards left over from that period that I kept because I had hoped that, sometime, I would write a book on physiological methods of treatment in psychiatry.

Now, to my amazement, Leo, when George Simpson, my friend, gave his presidential address here a couple of years ago on Treatment of Schizophrenia, he completely omitted any reference to insulin shock treatment that was one of the great historical developments in psychiatry. It was the first successful physiological treatment modality. We had of course Wagner-Jauregg's treatment of general paralysis with fever therapy. But compared to schizophrenia, general paralysis was a relatively rare disease. And George Simpson omitted any reference to its treatment with insulin shock. When I criticized him later for his omission, he said there were no good controlled studies. But he was wrong! There were some very good controlled studies. It was not a universally accepted treatment but it was a remarkably good treatment that actually induced remissions.

LH: I guess the reason it never caught on too well was that it was fairly labor intensive.

JW: That's right, and because of the introduction of pharmacological treatments, particularly chlorpromazine.

LH: Tell us about that.

JW: At the time chlorpromazine was introduced I sat on a therapeutic committee of the APA with Heinz Lehmann, who is European born. And he asked me whether I had heard about this new French treatment with Largactil, that's what they called chlorpromazine in France. And I said no. So he said, "look it up, it's very interesting." A guy, a surgeon named

Laborit, was developing it. So, I looked up the French literature and included Largactil (chlorpromazine) in my *Annual Review*. So, believe it or not, the first reference in the English language to chlorpromazine was in my *Annual Review*. And pretty soon after I published this, Smith, Kline & French got after me; Len Cook visited with me at my hospital to persuade me to use it. I was running a child psychiatric service, so I couldn't use it. But they were recommending chlorpromazine for treatment of nausea in pregnancy and so on. It was actually, I would say, a very effective sedative and it had wide applicability in a number of conditions.

LH: It was one of the first effective antiemetics.

JW: Yes, that's right. I didn't have a big patient population. I had no inpatient service. So I turned the literature over to our chief pediatric resident, a guy named Jerry Schulman, who later became a psychiatrist, a rather well established psychiatrist in Chicago. He looked over the literature and he said, "I don't think much of it," and he wouldn't allow me to use it. But the first English language reference to Largactil was in my *Annual Review*, and then for years I was covering a literature on psychopharmacology.

LH: Was that in about 1953?

JW: From about 1935 to about 1955 I was writing an annual review on physiological treatments. When Braceland took over the editorship, he changed the format of the annual reviews and it was discontinued. So my interest shifted to another area. I had several separate careers in psychiatry. In the years of the *Annual Review* people would look at me and think I was Mr. Physiological Treatment. And, when I was in the field of mental retardation for many years, they would think I was Mr. Mental Retardation. Then, I published a book on Soviet Psychiatry that got me into trouble. It came out in the McCarthy period and I was called before a Congressional Committee, and they thought I was Mr. Soviet Psychiatry. And then, I held a fellowship for sex research and people would think I was Mr. Sex Research. So, I had all these separate careers.

LH: A complete man.

JW: Well, I like to do always a little bit of the out of the way and unexpected. It's more fun.

LH: Did you ever get around to studying chlorpromazine?

JW: Yes, I did some very interesting research with chlorpromazine. I was interested in brain metabolism and had a Warburg respirometer. So, I minced rat brains, added chlorpromazine to the vials, and found that chlorpromazine had a selective action on different parts of the brain. If I remember correctly, and this was many decades ago, it depressed metabolism of the lower structures and enhanced metabolism of the cortical structures. So there you could demonstrate, by metabolic study, its selective action.

Also, I found, and I published this stuff but nobody paid any attention to it, that chlorpromazine has a biphasic action. In other words, if I sacrificed the animal at different time intervals after I administered chlorpromazine to it, I found that, at one time, in one phase, it would enhance respiratory activity, whereas in a few days, at another phase, it would depress it. I presented my findings at a meeting in Chicago and published it in the *American Journal of Psychiatry* but the work was never noticed, let alone replicated. But I did fool around with these kinds of studies.

LH: These were the kinds of biochemical studies in the beginning.

JW: Yes. I was in private practice at that time, and in order to pursue this research, I had to have a Park Avenue practice. People used to come in and lie on my couch and throw money at me. I didn't even have to listen to them. But I set up a Warburg respirometer in the laboratory in my office and the rat man used to come around to deliver rats. I had a great big paper scissor, which I still possess, and used to cut their heads off with it. It was very cruel. I would split the skull and mince the brain. And I would do my work using the Warburg respirometer in my private office.

LH: While the patients were still on the couch?

JW: Yeah. I didn't even have to listen to them.

LH: Well, were you treating any of the patients with chlorpromazine?

JW: I wasn't very actively involved in using it in treatment. Well, I ran the insulin treatment ward, and then I had something to do with the introduction of convulsive treatment. At first, we used Metrazol (pentylenetetrazol), which in Europe was called Cardiazol. I was one of the very first to introduce convulsive treatment. So, I was in charge of both insulin shock and convulsive treatment. Chlorpromazine came some years later and I had my assignment, my ward where I pursued the things that I was doing.

LH: Now, were Metrazol convulsions preferable to electrically induced ones?

JW: Janice Stephens has reviewed Meduna's work currently. Meduna's idea was Pavlovian although he didn't realize it. He observed, clinically, an incompatibility between epilepsy and schizophrena. Now, Pavlov, who in the last ten years of his life turned his attention to human psychiatric problems, had reached the conclusion that psychotic states were states of internal inhibition. That was great insight, because the thinking in dreams is actually schizophrenic thinking. In his systematic observations, he observed negativism and other catatonic phenomena at a certain stage when dogs were going into sleep. Although Meduna was not aware of it, he used the Pavlovian paradigm of inhibition versus stimulation when he produced with his powerful stimulant convulsions to relieve psychosis. Now, Janice Stephens has just written an editorial, which I'm about to publish, saying that the most effective treatments of schizophre-nia are the analeptics.

LH: Well, most of these drugs will produce seizures.

JW: I called her on the phone and asked, "Are you reviving Pavlov's theories?"

LH: She probably didn't even know it.

JW: Well, she said her library was burned up when her house was burned down, but she was very much interested in and remembered Pavlov's work. So, here we are! We've gone full circle so many years after Pavlov's death. His name is never mentioned any longer but he has been a great influence in psychiatry. His work needs to be revived.

LH: I think he was the first Nobel Laureate in the field of physiological psy-chology, wasn't he?

JW: Yes, but he would have great difficulty getting his papers published now-adays. Of course, he didn't have controls and he didn't use statistical methods. He was just a good observer.

LH: Well, I did as many controlled studies as anybody in the world, I guess, but I've always said they cannot replace observations in research.

JW: There is nothing wrong with observations.

LH: Research begins with a good observation.

JW: Darwin's work was all based on observation.

LH: Well, I think the reason that ECT is not used so much any more is that it's frightfully expensive by the time you have an anesthesiologist, and, you have to have a recovery room and all that.

JW: I gave the treatment for decades and I never used an anesthesiologist. You don't need an anesthesiologist.

LH: I know you don't, but they made it the standard to use one.

JW: ECT produces instant anesthesia.

LH: I know.

JW: In fact, it has been used as an anesthetic agent. You know who used it? Walter Freeman. He anesthesized his patients by giving an electroshock, and then stuck in his ice pick, rotating it through the orbit and producing lobotomies.

LH: That's right. But, as you know, they've raised the standards so high that it's almost impossible to do research.

JW: That's not raising standards. That's just what I call hyperscience. What we're doing, we're overdoing something and making it incorrect.

LH: For ECT I'm sure that's a deterrent, because in our hospital we figure, we don't want to do it despite the fact that we had a wonderful ECT machine. By the time you hire all these people, the cost of each treatment is about five hundred bucks.

JW: It's absurd. I used to give the treatment in my private office for 50 cents.

LH: I know.

JW: The patient would come in depressed and walk out normal.

LH: Well, it would be nice if we could get some chemical that would induce seizures so that we would get away from the electrical current.

JW: Well, Indoklon (flurothyl) was used as a convulsive agent. Now, Metrazol was used in Europe as a substitute for camphor. Camphor was used as a cardiac stimulant, but because it was administered in oil base it produced infections. They then developed the water-soluble substitute, which they called Cardiazol. And, by the time that was done, they hit upon the idea of using this as a convulsive agent. When it came to this country, it was called Metrazol. And when I started using convulsive treatment, it was Metrazol I used first. Then, Cerletti and Bini got the idea from the cattle industry, the butchering industry, to use an electrical current. They used to stun the cattle in the cattle pens with these prods, and, then, they'd slit their throat and slaughter them. And many of the animals would go into convulsions after being stunned with the prods. So Cerletti and Bini got the idea of inducing convulsions with an electric prod. What we are using today we owe to the cattle industry. That's how electric shock treatment was developed. And Kalinowsky and Impastato brought the news about electroconvulsive treatment from Italy, particularly Kalinowsky.

LH: I was going to ask you about him. How does he fit in the time frame we're talking about?

JW: He preceded me by, maybe, a few months in utilizing this treatment, but I was not far behind and, so I became Mr. Shock Treatment. I was pushing insulin shock. Everything was called shock. Well, insulin shock obviously is a misnomer, because there's nothing shocking about insulin shock. The term insulin shock came from the internists, who were afraid of diabetic patients getting an overdose of insulin and going into what they called "shock," and so that term was used. It was actually hypoglycemic coma. It was more analogous to sleep treatment. Now, I would say to you, Leo, one of the biggest challenges in psychiatry is to find out how insulin shock treatment works.

LH: Or ECT, for that matter.

JW: Or ECT, because if we discover the mechanism of how it works, we're going to have an insight into the nature of psychosis. But nobody is working on that.

LH: When you were studying in New York, were they using sleep therapy?

JW: Yes.

LH : Did you ever use it?

JW: Paul Hogan took it up and used it at Ward's Island. He used protracted sleep treatment. It's very effective and it's cheap.

LH: I guess its very labor intensive, isn't it?

JW: Well, its chief danger was the susceptibility to pneumonia, but then, with the development of antibiotics, that danger was reduced. It was also very Pavlovian. Pavlov had great confidence in the therapeutic effect of what he called "protective inhibition." Many of the animals, in whom he produced what he called neuroses – we would call them behavioral derangements – recovered if they were exposed to protracted sleep. He had the idea that there was such a thing as exhaustion of the nervous system and that this could be relieved by protracted sleep.

LH: Goes all the way back to Weir Mitchell.

JW: Yes, Weir Mitchell was also on the trail of a good idea. There were so many valuable things in psychiatry but people don't know of them.

LH: Well, that's what we're doing right now, preserving them.

JW: The history of psychiatry is full of fascinating ideas and pathways that we need to retrace.

LH: So, you got into biological psychiatry pretty early on in your career.

JW: Well, I don't know what you're interested in pursuing. I suppose your focus is on psychopharmacology. But I got into the field of sex research first because I had that Havelock Ellis Fellowship. It has a curious history, which I described in my book on Freud. But let me review the story very briefly. There was a famous and distinguished Harvard professor, Kingsley Porter. He was something of a prodigy and he produced a classic work on medieval architecture when he was still in his twenties. He was a person of great personal wealth, but he was homosexual. In those days, it was impossible for homosexuals to come out of the closet, and he was a very unhappy man. He was married and loved by his wife, who was devoted to him, and he confessed to her that he could not control what he thought was his inborn sexual drive. She was very sympathetic. He knew Havelock Ellis, and Havelock Ellis who was very advanced in his thinking, introduced him to a young man whose name was Allen Campbell. They became lovers and lived together for a short time in Cambridge. When Allen Campbell gave up this relationship, Kingsley Porter became very despondent. He was studying medieval architecture, and all the Gaelic crosses in Ireland at the time. He owned a castle, Gleanveagh Castle, that he used as a summer home, and he also had a little cottage on an island off the coast of Ireland, where he would spend quietly the weekends, away from this big castle. And one morning, he threw himself from the cliffs. His body was never recovered. His bereaved wife asked Havelock Ellis how she could use some of her money to do something for the cause of homosexuality. She felt they were entitled to their own lives, to pursue their own destiny, because they couldn't help being what they were.

LH: Sounds like an enormously modern view, doesn't it?

JW: And Havelock Ellis told her that the best thing is to invest in a young man. Being the kind of person Havelock Ellis was he had befriended me. We were corresponding. And I got this Fellowship to study sex research. Since I was at the beginning of my training in psychiatry, I would accept the Fellowship provided it saw me through my training period. Adolf Meyer was drawn in as another sponsor or monitor. So I accepted this Fellowship under the joint guidance of Havelock Ellis and Adolf Meyer, and I had a long close relationship with both of them. At any rate, it was under the terms of this Fellowship that I went back to Vienna and went through an analytic training period with Freud. When I returned to the United States, I began to publish in the field of homosexuality. One of my first stops when I was returning from Europe was in London, where I called Adrian, the great physiologist. He was very nice to me. I was a young guy in my twenties. I walked into his laboratory. He talked to me and he said, "Young man, the trouble with research in the field of 'sex' is that people think sex behavior is unconditioned. Well, it is really conditioned behavior." And that gave me the clue to realize when I studied case histories and met patients that, almost invariably, I could find the conditioning influences which created the homosexual pattern. Not only that, but I realized that heterosexual behavior was a learned behavior. Birds can build a nest and sing their songs through a series of chain reflexes, but human beings can't speak English that way. They have to learn it. Human beings can't build a house unless they learn it. And the higher, more complex forms of human behavior, and that includes sexual behavior, are learned behaviors.

LH: So we aren't doing what comes naturally.

JW: It seems natural, because we're conditioned so early. Well, the point of view I developed was at variance with the wishes and hopes of this widow, who regarded homosexuality as a congenital condition that needed to be treated with respect and forbearance. And, here I was, saying it is learned behavior. How do we raise our children? Do we let them practice incest? No, that's taboo. Do we let them masturbate? No, that's taboo. The whole so-called normal pattern of sex derives from a system of inhibitions, taboos and enticements. And that's how we become normal.

LH: So, being good means not having opportunity.

JW: After I pursued my interest and published on sexual behavior I got into mental retardation and I developed my own views there as well. Now, we have the big hullabaloo over the bell curves. Well, I learned that Binet and Simon, who were first to measure IQs, never thought that they were measuring innate intelligence. They were tied in with the French educational system and they merely wanted to learn what levels students were at, so they could be approached on the level where they stood. They didn't think that where they were at was a measure of their inborn intelligence. They said explicitly in their first monograph that the IQ of people could reflect that they came from Algiers and didn't know the French language, that they had a hearing disability and couldn't learn properly, that they had an inter-current illness and lost time from school. They were quite clear that there are all kinds of reasons why people fall behind. They complained that Terman in this country was using these tests as a measure of inborn intelligence.

LH: So, it was the influence of the Stanford group that turned the IQ into a measure of inborn intelligence.

JW: Yes. It is the American style to measure everything and to think it is the measure that is everything without analyzing it. And now we have this book, which was a best seller, with the Bell Curve, imputing that the blacks and the minorities have inferior intelligence because they test low on the IQ scale. The trouble is their poverty and educational neglect. And this has become a serious problem in social policy.

LH: Besides, I'm sure there is a tremendous overlap between two bell curves.

JW: No mental test ever devised, actually follows the Bell Shaped Curve. Even the best of tests have a bell and, then, they have a drop and, then, they have a bump. The bump, I call the bump of pathology, where you find the encephalitis, the brain injury, obstetrical injuries and so on. As a result, all these tests are skewed to the right, because there's pathology and there's no balancing hyper-health, so that IQ's need to be interpreted.

LH: Of course, in those days, when you were working with mental retardation, it was still a pretty unknown field.

JW: It was opening up as a scientific field, because the tendency was to regard mental retardation as a kind of stupidity that people were born with. We now know there are a hundred or more conditions that produce mental retardation. I mean, your own son is an example. The reason I'm so friendly with your son is that he's my material. That's what I spent my life with. I like these people.

LH: Well, he's a shining star. Unfortunately, he's handicapped.

JW: He's limited, yes, but he's human and he's appealing.

LH: The trouble is, you can never be sure of the etiologies.

JW: The etiologies we have, probably in most cases are subtle and they induce impairments. They are either genetic or toxic or birth injuries, but we seldom can make a good etiologic diagnosis. There are a number of specific etiologies but they are relatively rare.

LH: I would say probably 85 or 90 percent of the cases are still sort of idiopathic.

JW: I applied some of the Pavlovian paradigms, unsuccessfully, to see if I could tease out some basic pathophysiology that would explain mental retardation in different cases, but it was very difficult to do and I don't think we were too successful.

LH: All right, now, we've got you through several careers. How did you get to be an editor?

JW: Well, that too is an interesting story. I did brain metabolism studies with Harold Himwich for years, using the technique of jugular puncture. He was then professor of physiology at Albany. He had something to do with the earliest demonstrations that the brain only metabolizes glucose. Well, when he heard of the insulin shock treatment, he came rushing down from Albany to see if he could do brain metabolic studies on my patients, because if indeed you lowered the blood sugar, then you had arrested brain metabolic activity.

LH: So, he was puncturing the jugular vein and draining from it?

JW: That's right, and we measured the respiratory quotient and the oxygen uptake. He was one of those scientists who did everything himself. I remember the first day he plunged the syringe into the jugular and drew the barrel back and I was wondering whether it's going to be blue or red. To our great relief it was bright red, which means the blood leaving the brain had its oxygen in it. It hadn't been taken out. Brain metabolism was reduced almost to zero. That was the crucial test. And then, we pursued that in all kinds of variants. Well, Harold Himwich was one of the first members of the Society of Biological Psychiatry. I joined the Society a few years after it started, just a little bit before he did. At that point, there were maybe 20 members and we would sit around an annual dinner and tell dirty stories.

LH: That was the only biological society in psychiatry.

JW: Now, the original members were almost all neurologists, interestingly.

LH: Harold was an MD, though, wasn't he?

JW: Yes, he was an MD. Well, Harold was not one of the charter members. There were, I think, about 10 charter members, [Johannes] Neilsen, [George N.] Thompson, [Percival] Bailey, Sam Bernard Wortis my cousin, and some others. They were all neurologists. Neilsen had the idea that they had to look to neurology to explain mental illness. And, actually, the logo that's used is a neurological logo, based on a sketch that [James] Papez, the neurologist, did from the basic structures of the cortex. That's the logo.

LH: When did the Society first start publishing the journal?

JW: Well, it started publishing an annual program with abstracts of the presentations first. Then, as the Society got bigger, Henry Stratton of Grune and

Stratton suggested that it be published as a volume. Jules Masserman had very close ties with Henry Stratton. Masserman is now dead, so I can now speak ill of him, because he's dead. The Latin motto is say nothing but good of the dead, but I follow the opposite motto. Once they're dead, you can insult them. Masserman was a great careerist and he was bringing out an annual volume on psychoanalysis published by the newly formed neo-Freudian group, the American Academy of Psychoanalysis. And he got the bright idea that he would persuade Henry Stratton to publish a volume on *Biological Psychiatry*. Then he brought out the first volume. And Howard Fabing, who was then president of the Society, did not like Masserman and what he was up to. He didn't like the idea of Masserman straddling two companion publications, one on psychoanalysis, which most of our members were not too sympathetic with. He had just read my Freud book and was enthusiastic about it, and to my surprise, proposed that I take over the editorship. So, for 10 years, I edited this annual volume. During this time we changed publishers, from Grune and Stratton to Plenum, because Stratton was behaving like a kingmaker and we didn't like that. Plenum Press gave us more attractive conditions, and so Plenum Press brought out this annual volume, which I edited for 10 years. And, then, at one point, they suggested that we should convert it to a journal. Now, some of the old time members, like George Thompson and Bob Heath, didn't like the idea of a journal. They opposed it, because they thought it would run away and be too independent. But a number of the wiser members thought we could obviate that danger by making the officers of the society ex-officio members of the editorial committee and conversely making the editor ex-officio a member of the executive committee so that there would be some monitoring and control. And so, I became editor of this new journal and edited it for years until it became so successful that I couldn't keep up with it.

LH: Ending your editorship about 2 or 3 years ago?

JW: Yes.

LH: Well, it was a long period of editorship and it became a preeminent journal under your auspices.

JW: Well, my wife had died soon after I took on the editorship, and I also reached so-called retirement age at 65, almost 30 years ago, and though I continued my connection at my university, I was not on salary. So I happened, by virtue of these circumstances, to have a lot of free time. There was very little money coming in. People think that it's very charming of me to have handled my correspondence with handwriting. I couldn't afford a secretary.

LH: You were the only journal editor I ever knew…

JW: Well, there was no money for a secretary. I used to do my duplication on a little Minnesota Mining heat processed duplicating machine. I'd run the papers through, a special heat sensitive paper, and that's how I kept my copies. They all turned brown in time.

LH: Are there any careers we've missed?

JW: Well, I have a secret career. I'm now writing my autobiography and I found hundreds and hundreds of letters, to my surprise, between my late wife and me. We met at age 16, and she was a wonderful person. My voice cracks when I talk about her. But this is a unique record from a time when people didn't use telephones. We corresponded, so I have hundreds of letters of the correspondence between us.

LH: A lost art.

JW: Yes. The correspondence includes a very stormy period, when after years of being together, I fell in love with a German woman while we were in Vienna, and my wife decided to leave me and return to the United States, putting 3,000 miles between us. I had to pursue my medical studies but we continued corresponding. So our marriage began to limp after awhile, because I was stuck with my medical studies and was kind of peeved that she ran off without discussing it with me, because mine was a transient infatuation, and quite uncharacteristic of me, the only time I ever did this. Meanwhile, she got involved with a couple of other guys, and when I returned to this country, she was about to marry one of them. I rescued her, to my good fortune, at the last minute. And we had 40 years of a wonderful relationship all told in my correspondence and it makes a great love story, a great soap opera.

LH: Sounds to me like your whole life was a soap opera with many different episodes and a very charming one. Well, it was a pleasure talking to you, Joe.

JW: You didn't ask all of your questions.

LH: Well, hell, we don't go by questions. We go by what people want to talk about.

JW: All right.

LH: But, you gave us a lot of insights.

JW: Well, as I usually say when I finish a talk, I find myself in general agreement with all of the things I said.

LH: Well, I'm sure everybody is too. We're so interested in what we call the pre-history of modern psychopharmacology, and your insights into those areas.

JW: I'm glad to be regarded as part of the pre-history.

LH: Pre-historical Joe Wortis.

JW: And as I've often told, I step up to the people here. The meetings are always stratified; the higher hierarchy always speaks to people on their level and, so on. Everything is stratified here, socially. So I would always get a laugh by stepping up to somebody and saying, ah, what can you do to advance my career? Now, I say, which of you departmental chairman is in the collecting of antiques?

LH: Well, as long you keep running five miles on your birthday, I think you'll be around for awhile.

JW: I can boast about it this year, but I don't know about next year. We'll see. Thank you, Leo. One year at a time.

LH: That's the way to do it.

JW: Okay, did I give you a good time?

INDEX

Note: The page numbers for each interviewee's entry appear in boldface type.

6-hydroxydopamine, 183–85

Abbott Laboratories, 123, 124

Abeles, Milton, 313

Acetylcholine, ix, xxxii–xxxiii, 162–64, 214–15, 218, 219, 240

Adams, Roger, 163

Adrenaline/Epinephrine, ix, xxvii, xxxli, 135, 192, 236, 297

Adrenochrome hypothesis of schizophrenia, xxvii, xxx, lxii, 98, 290, 296–97

Adrian, Edgar Douglas (Lord), 214, 223, 321

Adverse effects, xxvii, xxxi, l, 6, 9, 14, 27, 45, 70, 183, 188, 208, 210, 217, 248, 270, 287, 304

Affective disorders, xxxiii, 82, 85, 89, 217, 268

Aghajanian, George, 30

Agranoff, Bernard, 162

AIDS (Acquired immunodeficiency syndrome), 155, 257, 304

Akil, Huda, 162

Alcohol/Alcoholism, 23, 32, 49, 75, 245, 252, 271, 293, 304

    LSD treatment, xxxi, 70–71, 300–1

Alexander, Franz, xxx, 266

Alexander, George, 284

Altschule, Mark, 11, 13

Alzheimer, Alois, 37

Alzheimer's disease/dementia, xlix, 22, 25, 27, 28, 37, 136–37, 186, 128, 175

American College of Neuropsychopharmacology (ACNP), xi, xliv, lxi, 16, 26, 75, 76, 100, 130, 141, 212, 261, 272

    founders/founding, xlviii, li, liii, lvi, 14, 56, 72, 88–89, 96, 286

    members, 30, 41, 52, 61, 160, 162, 179, 208, 252, 311

    neuroscience vs. clinical focus, 60, 210

American Journal of Psychiatry, lxii, 7, 73, 243, 297, 314, 317

American Psychiatric Association (APA), lx, 6, 11, 13–14, 43, 201, 252–55, 260–62, 315

Amitriptyline (Elavil), xxxi, xlviii, 22, 200

Amobarbital (Amytal), xxxiii, xlv, 214, 215, 241

Anesthesia/anesthetic agents, xxxvi, lvi, 120, 161, 164, 179, 213, 278, 318

    chlorpromazine as, xxvii, 243

Animal studies/models, xxxii–xxxiii, lix, 21–25, 35, 106–11, 128–30, 133–34, 136–37, 141, 151–52, 157, 164–67, 169, 171, 177, 179–80, 186, 192, 197, 215–16, 220, 222, 240, 247, 265, 271, 288, 291–93, 303, 317, 319, 320

Anti-anxiety agents. *See* Anxiolytics

Anticholinergic agents, xxxiii, 22, 24–25, 179, 188, 215

    antipsychotics, 12, 47, 49

Anticholinesterases, 213–16, 218, 240

Antidepressant agents, xxviii, xxxiii, 7, 9, 50–51, 72, 85, 89, 110–11, 171, 182–83, 187, 188, 203, 208, 248, 257, 283. *See also* Monoamine oxidase inhibitors (MAOI), Tricyclics

Antiemetic agents, 45, 132, 157, 316

Antihistamines, 146, 188, 242

    phenothiazines as, 12, 127, 216

Anti-Parkinson agents, lvi, 165

Antipsychotic agents, l, li, liii, 7, 12–13, 29, 41, 44–46, 49, 84–85, 89, 110, 1231, 140, 184, 283

    atypicals, l, 49, 132, 282

    chlorpromzine, xlvi, 129

    tests for, lv, 132–35

Anxiety, xxv, xxvi, lxi, 9, 134, 138, 183, 209, 269, 271
  chemically-induced, 23
  measurement, 169, 267–68, 274, 279
Anxiolytics, lv, 23, 46, 48, 84, 110, 133–35, 140, 142, 182, 267–68
Apomorphine, xxv, xxxi, lvii, 157, 181
Arieti, Silvano, 249
Attention Deficit Hyperactivity Disorder (ADHD), 76, 171
Awad, A. George, as interviewer, 277–88
Axelrod, Julius, lxii, 58, 198, 200, 220, 295–97
Ayd, Frank J., Jr., xxxi, xlviii–xix, **5–18**, 72, 78, 84
  as interviewer, 39–61
Azima, Hasan, xxx, 278

Bailey, Percival, 323
Baldessarini, Ross J., 222, 223
Ban, Thomas A., lii, lvii, lxi, 38, 85
  as interviewer, 19–34. 115–20, 191–203, 226–64, 277–88
Barbiturates, xxv, xxx, xxxii, xlv, xlvi, lvii, lix, 5, 33, 66, 125, 248
Barnes, Alan, 222
Barron, James, 200
Barton, Walter, 253
Baxter, Bruce, lvii, 181
Beecher, Harry, 17, 179, 170, 174
Behavioral pharmacology, x, xxxii, xlvii, liv–lvi, 110–12, 124, 143, 150, 154, 178
Behaviorism/behaviorist school, xxxii, lv, lvi–lvii, 108, 187
Benadryl. See Diphenhydramine
Bender, Lauretta, lx, 241–43, 314
Bender, Paul, 220
Benjamin, John D., 297
Benzedrine (amphetamine sulfate), xxvi, xlvi
Benzodiazepines, li, lxi, 48–50, 53, 109, 135, 182, 266–68
Berger, Frank, xxvii, xlviii, 123, 162, 163, 215

Biological psychiatry, lii, lx, 11, 14–15, 18, 26, 51, 97, 285, 314, 320
  Kraepelin as founder, 37
  and psychoanalysis, lvii, lxiii, 38, 203, 206–7, 284
Bipolar disorder, xxxiii, 21, 26–27, 31. See also Mania; Manic-depressive disorder
Bishop, James, 268
Blalock, Alfred, 222, 234
Bleckwenn, William, xlv
Bleuler, Eugen, 183
Bleuler, Manfred, 250
Bloom, Floyd E., 198, 220–21, 223
Bloomenfield, Michael, 257
Bodian, David, 198
Bond, Douglas, 277
Bonnycastle, Desmond, 122–24
Boren, John, 109
Böszörményi, P., 293
Bovet, Daniel, 146
Bowman, Karl, 240, 314
Braceland, Francis J., 195, 316
Bradley, Philip, xxxiii, 215–16, 224
Brady, Joseph V., xxxiii, xlvii, liv, lvii, **105–14**, 130, 142, 153, 177, 178
Brain imaging, 184, 187, 271, 273, 309
Branch, Robert, 32
Braun, Werner von, 108
Brazier, Mary, 128
Bridger, Wagner, xxxii
Brill, Henry, xlvii, 7, 13, 93, 96, 286
Brodie, Bernard B. (Steve), xxviii, lvii, 15, 58, 178–79, 182, 185, 197–98, 217, 220
Brody, Eugene B., 68, 69
Bulova, J. G. M., 237
Bunney, Benjamin S. (Steve), as interviewer, xlvi, lvii, 205–10
Bunney, William E., Jr. (Biff), 198
  as interviewer, lxi, 81–90, 265–75
Butler, Robert, 197

Cade, John, xxvi, 19–20

Caldwell, Donald, 163

Cameron, D. Ewen, 135, 277, 281, 286, 287

Campbell, Allen, 320

Cannon, Walter, xxvi

Cardin, Phillip, 197

Carlson, Anton J., 193

Carlsson, Arvid, 30, 52, 57
    as interviewer, lvi, 177–88

Carpenter, William T., Jr., 73, 75

Carr, Charles Jelleffe, xxli, xlv, liv–v, **115–20**

Carr, Sallie, 118–19

Carroll, Bernard J., 32–33

Carter, Jimmy, 202

Carter's Little Liver Pills. *See* Wallace
    Laboratories

Catania, Charles

Catatonia, xxvi, xxxii, xlv, lix, 184, 214–16,
    317

Catecholamine(s), x, lvii, 30, 134, 179–85,
    198, 297–99, 305

Center for Studies of Narcotics and Drug
    Abuse, lxii, 302, 306. *See also*
    National Institute on Drug Abuse
    (NIDA)

Center for the Study of Drug Development,
    lvii, 172

Central nervous system (CNS), xxxiii, lix, 22,
    123, 188, 214
    drugs/drug effects, xxvi, liv, 24, 28, 99,
    106, 126–27, 137, 146, 177, 179,
    210
    neurotransmitters, ix, 219, 223

Cerletti, Ugo, 319

Child psychiatry, 148, 240–41, 250, 255, 316
    psychoanalysis, 194, 266
    psychopharmacology, xxvi, xxxi, lx, 171,
    242–43, 248, 261, 263

Childhood schizophrenia, 241, 245

Chlordiazepoxide (Librium), xxxi, 47–48, 53,
    133–34, 140, 267

Chlorpromazine (CPZ) (Thorazine; Largactil),
    xxxix, xxxi, l, lvii, lxii, 89, 129
    acquisition by Smith, Kline & French,
    124–25, 127, 131–32, 154
    discovery and early use, ix, xxviii, xlvi–xl-
    vii, 6, 8–9, 11–12, 35–37, 41, 56, 68,
    83–87, 92, 157, 278, 280–81, 315–17
    pediatric use, lx, 242–47, 266
    studies/trials, lii, lv, lix, 26, 29, 42–47,
    68, 70, 114, 133, 134, 177–79, 184,
    216–17, 279

Cholden, Louis, 67, 70

Cholinergic system/mechanisms, 28, 31, 136,
    162–63, 215

Cholinesterase, 218, 240
    inhibitors, xxxiii, 22, 24–25, 152

CIBA (Swiss pharmaceutical company), xxvii,
    6–7, 41, 43, 224

Clark, John Kapp, 127, 130

Classification, psychiatric, xxv, lx, 17. *See
    also* Diagnosis, psychiatric; *DSM*;
    Nosology
    psychotropic drugs, 281

Clausen, John, 197, 198

Clinical Neuropharmacology Research
    Center. *See* St. Elizabeths Hospital
    (Washington, DC)

Clinical trials, xxxi, xxxii, xlvii, li, lii, lvii, 19,
    53, 83, 85, 173, 207, 244, 267, 282,
    303. *See also* Controlled trials/
    studies

Clinton, James, 58

Cohen, Mabel, 193–96, 201

Cohen, Robert A., xxix, lvii, **191–203**, 218,
    219

Cohen, Sidney, 303

Cole, Charles, 146

Cole, Jonathan O., liv, 14, 23, 24, 33, 41, 42,
    57, 58, 67, 96, 116–17, 146, 162,
    197, 251

Coleman, Jules, xlvi, 206–7

Collegium Internationale Neuro-
     Psychopharmacologicum, xi, xiii,
     xxix, 14, 51, 52, 256, 281, 299
Compton, Arthur Holly, 265
Conditional/conditioned reflex (CR), xxxii, liv, 125
Conditoned avoidance, xxxii, lv, 125–27, 129,
     131–35
Conditioned emotional response (CER), xxxii,
     liv, 106
Conflict test, 133, 134, 182
Congress (U.S.), lvii, 79, 316
     psychopharmacology funding, 14–15, 57,
     60, 173, 199
Conolly, John, 282
Content analysis of speech, xxx, lxi, 267–69,
     271, 274
Controlled trials/studies, xxxi, xxxii, l–li, lvi–
     lvii, lix, lxii, 20, 26, 41, 42, 47, 50,
     53, 72, 169, 171–74, 185, 206, 207,
     216–17, 243, 303, 315, 318
Convulsive treatment, xxxix, 317, 319.
     See also Electroconvulsive ther-
     apy (ECT); Insulin coma therapy;
     Pentylenetetrazol
Cook, Leonard, xxxii, xlvi, lv, **121–43**, 154,
     316
Cooke, Robert, 222
Cori, Carl, 265
Cori, Gerty (Radnitz), 265
Costa, Erminio (Mimo), 58
Courvoisier, Simone, 126
Coyle, Joseph, 222
Crane, George, xxviii, 71
Cyclazocine, xxxi, lxi, 247–48

Dale, Henry Hallett, 149, 214
Dancey, Travis, 277, 279
Davidson, Arnold, 142
Davis, Brian, 23
Dawson, Wolfgang Siegried, 23
Day, Richard, 244

De Beer, E. J., 146
Defenses, ego/psychic, xxx, lxii, 279–80, 283
Delay, Jean, xxvii, 83, 84, 127, 278, 281–83
Dementia, xxxii, 22, 28, 136, 257. See also
     Alzheimer's disease/dementia
     praecox, xxv. See also Schizophrenia
Deniker, Pierre-Georges, xxviii, 16, 83, 84,
     127, 278, 281
Depression, xxviii, xxx, xlv, xlvi, l, lvi, 9, 10, 30,
     33, 50, 56, 76, 81–82, 85, 90, 169,
     188, 206, 248, 257, 263, 271, 299
     and reserpine, xxvii, 70
Detre, Thomas, xxxi, xlvi, xlix, l, lvii, 31, 32,
     205–10
Dews, Peter B., xxxii, lv–lvi, 125, 142, **145–56**,
     178
Diagnosis, psychiatric, xxvii, lii, 37, 59, 82, 85,
     235, 256, 267, 274, 279, 322
Diagnostic and Statistical Manual, American
     Psychiatric Association (DSM)
     DSM-I (1952), 59
     DSM-II (1968), 253–54
     DSM-III (1980), 59, 256
     DSM-IV (1994), 256
Diazepam (Valium), 48–49, 267
Diethyltyptamine (DET) lxii, 294, 296, 299, 300
Dimethyltryptamine (DMT), xxx, lxii, 291–94,
     296, 298–99, 302
Diphenylhydantoin. See Phenytoin
Diphenhydramine (Benadryl), xxxi, lx, 242–44
Ditran (N-ethyl-2-
     pyrrolidylmethylphencyclopentyl gly-
     colate hydrochloride and N-ethyl-3
     piperidyl phenylcyclopentyl glycolate
     hydrochloride), xxxiii, 22, 24
Dodge, Donald, 195
Domino, Edward F., xxx, lvi, **157–68**
Dopamine, ix, lvii, 29–30, 57–58, 77, 134–35,
     180–81, 184–86, 188, 216
     agonists, xxxii–xxxiii, 165
Dreyfus, Jack, liii, 99–100

Drug abuse/addiction, xxxi, liv lvi,, lxi, 99,
    107, 110–12, 163, 245–49, 251–52,
    261, 271, 306–7
    Centers/programs, lxii, 140, 271, 302–3,
    305
Drug companies. See Pharmaceutical
    industry
Drug development, 52, 59, 172, 174, 176,
    178, 187. See also Center for the
    Study of Drug Development
Drug discovery, liv–lv, 137–40
Drug discrimination/screening, liv, 57, 106,
    107, 110, 111, 136, 182
Drug efficacy. See Efficacy, therapeutic
Dryer, Donna, 74
Dufresne, Todd, lxiii
DuPont/DuPont-Merck, 136–37, 140, 142, 249
Dystonic reactions, 45–46, 49

Early Clinical Drug Evaluation Unit (ECDEU)
    program, xxxi, liii
Efficacy, therapeutic, xi, xxxi, xlviii, lv, 6, 20–
    21, 53, 132, 172–73
Efron, Daniel H., 299
Ehrlich, Paul, 212, 241
Einstein, Albert, 212
Eisenberg, Leon, 251
Electrical brain activity, xxxiii, lix, 215
    brain stimulation, 179, 180, 191
Electroconvulsive therapy (ECT), xlviii,
    xlix, lxiii, 5, 9–11, 18, 21, 31, 83,
    105–6, 235, 248, 249, 251, 263, 285,
    318–19
Electroencephalography (EEG), lii, 7, 24–25,
    27, 128, 159–60, 166, 240–41, 257–
    58, 266–67
Elion, Gertrude B., 146
Elkes, Charmian, lix, 214, 216
Elkes, Joel, xxxii–xxxiii, lviii–lx, 42, 69, 71, 78,
    197–98, **211–24**, 295, 299
Ellis, Havelock, lxii, lxiv, 311, 320—21

Engelhardt, David M., 91
Engelhardt, Jo Ann, as interviewer, 91–101
Epilepsy, xxv, xxvi, 35, 99, 240, 266–67, 317
Epinephrine. See Adrenaline
Erin, Charles, 40
Erlanger, Joseph 265
Etts, Susan, 95
Evans, Joseph, 40
Everett, Edward, 196, 197
Extrapyramidal reactions, l, 282

Fabing, Howard, 18, 291, 324
Faillace, Louis, 300
Farrar, Clarence B., 314
Fazekas, Joseph, 235
Feldberg, Wilhelm, 148, 149
Felix, Robert, lviii, 195–96, 198–99, 218–19
Ferenczi, Sándor, 205
Ferris, Steven, 27, 28
Ferster, Charles, 130–31, 147, 150, 153, 154
Feuerstein, Reuven, 245
Finean, Bryan, 213
Fink, Max, xlix, 24, 96, 247–49, 251, 257
Fish, Barbara, 242
Fisher, Seymour, 117, 252, 261, 291
Fixed interval schedule(s)/test, xxxii, lv, 133–
    34, 151
Flexner, Louis, 218
Fluoxetine (Prozac), 183, 298
Folch-Pi, Jordi, 281, 233
Food and Drug Administration (FDA), li, lvii,
    56, 58, 170, 172, 174, 303, 305
    drug approval/regulation, xlix, 7, 28, 83, 119
Fortino, Marileena, 94
Fox, Herbert, xxviii
Frank, Ira, 304
Frank, Jerome, 222
Frazer, Alistair, 213
Freedman, Alfred M., xxxi, lx–lxi, **225–64**
Freedman, Daniel X., xlvii, 207, 2521, 296
Freeman, Walter, 318

French, Audie, 231

French, Thomas, xxx, 266

Freud, Sigmund, xxix, lii, lxi–lxiv, 82, 90, 179, 193, 205, 213, 314, 320–21

Freyhan, Fritz, xxxvii, 12, 43, 50, 57, 78, 84, 220, 255, 280

Friedhoff, Arnold, xlix, 25, 26

Fromm-Reichmann, Frieda, xxix, lviii, 195, 201, 202

Fuxe, Kjell, 180

Gaddum, John, 148, 149

Galambos, Robert, 105

Gantt, Horsley, xxxii, 202, 222

Garattini, Silvio, 299

Geller, Irving, 109, 182

Genetic aspects of psychiatry/psychophar-macology, xi, 60, 61, 91, 94–95, 99, 101, 168, 210, 229, 262, 263, 271, 273, 274, 287, 322

Gerard, Margaret Wilson, 194

Gerard, Ralph, xlix, lvi, lvii, 14, 22–23, 42, 162, 191–94, 197–98, 201, 202

Geriatric programs/research, 27–28, 31, 161

Gershon, Eliot, 95

Gershon, Samuel, xxxiii, xlix–1, **19–34**

Gesell, Joseph, 194

Gibson, Robert, 201

Gillespie, Hamp, 48

Gillin, Christian J., lvi; as interviewer, 157–68

Gjessing, Rolv, xxv

Gleser, Goldine C., 268

Goethe, Johann Wolfgang von, 212

Gold, Harry, 42, 170

Goldman, Douglas, 6, 18, 62, 84

Goldstein, Avram, 305, 306

Goldstein, Menek, 30

Goodman, Louis, 141, 154

Goodwin, Frederick K., 198, 200

Gordon, Myron, 228–29, 231

Gorham, Donald, 55

Gorman, Mike, 15

Gottlieb, Jacques, 161m 163

Gottschalk, Louis A., xxx, lxi, **265–75**

Greenblatt, Milton, 10, 253

Gregory, Menus, 313

Grinker, Roy R., 193–94, 266, 280

Grinspoon, Lester, 252

Grof, Stanislaus, 71

Hallucinogens, ix, lxii, 13, 72, 74–75, 97–99, 291–93, 295, 299–302

Haloperidol (Haldol), xxx, 26, 54, 61, 132, 262

Halpern, Abraham, 260

Halpern, Bernard, 146

Hamburg, David, lviii, 197, 198

Hamilton, Max, 14, 220

Hardman, Harry, 163

Harris, Geoffrey, 216, 218, 221, 223

Harris, Titus, 6, 18

Harvey, A. McGehee, 222

Harvey, John A., as interviewer, 145–56

Healy, David, xiii, 38

Heath, Robert, 295, 3245

Heroin, 245, 247, 248, 261, 306

Herrnstein, Richard, 109

Hill, Bradford, 173–74

Hill, Dennis, 191

Hill, Lister, 13, 15–16, 199

Himwich, Harold, 235–37, 239–40, 242, 328

Hippius, Hanns, xxx, l, **35–38**, 250, 255, 295

Hirschberg, Carl, 245

Hitchings, George H., 59, 146

Hitler, Adolf, lii, 81, 228, 229, 233, 237

Hökfelt, Tomas 236

Hoch, Paul, 13, 57, 257

Hoff, Hans, lxii, 293–94

Hoffer, Abram, xxxi, 70, 290, 296–97

Hoffman, Jay, 198

Hoffmann-LaRoche, 134–35, 140, 142, 251. *See also* Roche Laboratories

Hofmann, Albert, xxxvi, 67, 291, 292, 302

Hollister, Leo E., xxxi, xlviii, l–li, **39–61**, 96, 300
    as interviewer, lxii, lxiii, 5–18, 63–79,
        106–14, 289–309, 311–26
Holtz, William, 142
Homosexuality, liii, 320–21
    removal from DSM, xl, 253–54
Hordern, Anthony, 14, 298
Hornykiewicz, Oleh, 57
Hoskins, Roy, 192
Hough, Lindsey, 165
Howard, Jack, 7
Hubbard, Alfred Matthew, 70, 301
Hubel, David H., 148–49
Hughes, John, 306
Hunt, Howard, 105–6. 154
Huxley, Aldous, 292
Hypertension, 20, 40, 61, 271
    and reserpine, x, xxxviii, li, 41, 43
Hypnotic agents, xxxii, lvi–lvii, 171

Imipramine, ix, xxvii–xxviii, xxx, xxxi, lii, 9, 10,
        14, 22, 30, 71, 85, 199, 248, 282
Impastato, David, 319
Informed consent, 66, 69, 83
Insulin coma therapy, xxix, lvii, 5, 55, 83, 249,
        277–78, 285, 314–15, 317, 319, 323
Iproniazid (Marsilid), ix, x, xxviii, xxi, lii, 7,
        9–10, 50
Isoniazid, x, 9–10
Itil, Turan, 24, 257

Jacobsen, Carlyle, 265
Jaffe, Milton, 58
Jarvik, Murray, 42
John, Erwin Roy, 251–52, 257
Jones, Reese, 24, 303

Kabat, Herman, 234, 235, 236
Kalinowsky, Lothar, 18, 249–50, 319
Kandel, Eric, 203
Kanner, Leo, 241

Kaplan, Harold, ix, 250
Katz, Bernard, 149
Kefauver–Harris amendments (Food and Drug
        Act), 172
Kelleher, Roger, 130–31, 142
Kennedy, John F., 246
Kennedy, Robert F., 246
Kesey, Ken, li
Kety, Seymour, lviii, lx, 196, 218–19, 221, 223,
        296, 297
Kielholz, Paul, 52, 250, 255, 256
Killam, Eva King, 159
Killam, Keith, 159
Kinross-Wright, John, 8, 13, 41
Klein, Donald F., 76
    as interviewer, 169–76
Kleitman, Nathaniel, 193
Klerman, Gerald, 24, 57, 257
Kline, Nathan Schellenberg, li, 7–9, 13, 16,
        41–44, 52, 57, 70–71, 84, 96, 279,
        281–82, 286
Kolb, Lawrence Coleman, 194, 251
Kopin, Irving, 182, 197, 198, 296–97
Kosterlitz, Hans, 306
Kraepelin, Emil, ix, l, 37–38, 82, 85
Krajeski, James, 254
Krantz, John, 115, 120
Krayer, Otto, 146–47
Kretschmer, Ernst, 37
Krumholz, Wilhelm, liii
Kuhn, Roland, xxxvii–xxxviii, lii, 85
Kupfer, David, 208, 210
Kurland, Albert A., xxxi, li, **63–79**

Lasagna, Louis C., xxxi, lvi–lvii, **169–76**
Lasker, Mary, 15, 16
Lasker Award, xxx, 7, 9, 16, 42
Lasko, Michael, 165
Lehmann, Heinz Edgar, xxx, lii–liii, 8, 12, 16,
        18, 24, 65, **81–90**, 96, 117, 278,
        281, 315

Lerer, Bernard, 31

Levine, Joseph, 301

Levine, Maurice, lxi, 33, 272

Lewis, Aubrey, 267

Lewis, Nolan, 14

Lewis, Sinclair, 227

Lithium, xxvi, xxxiii, xlix, 19–21, 26–27

Lobotomy, 285, 318

Long, William, 6

Lorr, Maurice, 55

Ludwig, Arnold, xxxvii, 301

Lysergic acid diethylamide (LSD), ix, xxvi,
    xxxi, li, lxi–lvxii, 58, 67, 70–72,
    74–75, 197, 291–93, 294, 298–99,
    300–302

Lytic cocktail, lxii, 278

Macher, Jean-Paul, 259–60

Macht, David, ix

MacLean, J. Ross, 70

McPherson, Aimee Semple, 239

Malitz, Sidney, 89

Managed care, 7, 71, 76, 287, 288

Mania, xxvi, xlix, 16, 20–21, 26, 30, 45, 84,
    279

Manic-depressive illness, ix, xxxiii, xlix, 7, 21,
    83, 201, 235, 278

Marijuana, lxii, 112, 145, 47, 163, 303–4.
    See also Tetrahydrocannibinol
    (THC)

Marshall, Wade, 192, 197

Martin, William, 158, 306

Marrazzi, Amadeo, 179

Mason, John, 106, 107

Masserman, Jules, xlvi, 324

Matsuoka, Shigeaki, 165

May, Phillip, 288

Meduna, László, 317

Mészáros, Miomir, 291

Melancholia, xxvi, xlvi, 9

Meltzer, Herbert Y., 73

Memory, xxxiii, 5, 110, 135–37, 140, 158,
    289

Mental hospitals. See Psychiatric hospitals

Mental illness. See Psychiatric illness

Mental retardation, 16, 316, 321–23

Mentors/mentoring, lvii, 18–19, 26, 28, 33,
    122–23, 161, 163, 77, 266, 272

Mephenesin, xxvii, xxxiii, xlviii, 5, 214, 215

Meprobamate (Equanil, Miltown), xxvii, xxxi,
    xlvi, lvii, 6, 11, 46–47, 50, 53, 109,
    133–34, 140, 163, 182, 242

Merck (pharmaceutical company), 123, 124–
    25, 137, 154, 157

Mescaline, xxvi, xxxii, 58, 292–93, 299, 302

Methadone, liv, 306–7

Meyer, Adolf, 194, 198, 202–3, 221, 223,
    321

Michael, Richard, 221

Milner, Peter, liv, 177

Mirsky, Arthur, 238, 272

Mitchell, Silas Weir, 320

Molecular approaches, x–xi, xxxiii, 44, 60, 85,
    990, 108–9, 151, 167–68, 171, 175,
    187, 210, 213, 219, 263, 287, 305,
    309

Molitor, Hans, 124

Money, John, 222

Monoamine(s), x–xi, xxvii

Monoamine oxidase (MAO) inhibitors, xxviii,
    lii, 7, 9–10, 30, 71, 107, 208

Morphine, ix, xxv, 17, 157, 174, 175

antagonists, xxxiii, 21–22, 32, 33

Moussaoui, Driss, 258

Nalorphine, 157–58

Naloxone, xxxi, lxi, 248–49, 306

Naltrexone, 249, 307

Narcotics, xxxi, 76, 160, 257, 266. See also
    Drug abuse/addiction; Heroin;
    Opiates

antagonists, lxi, 157–58

National Institute of Mental Health (NIMH), li, lvii, lviii–lix, 13, 58, 67–69, 71, 96, 195, 199, 200–1, 203, 271, 295–97, 302
   Early Clinical Drug Evaluation. *See* Early Clinical Drug Evaluation Unit (ECDEU) program
   funding/grants, 23, 27, 29, 164
   Intramural Research Program, xxx, 207
   Psychopharmacology Service Center. *See* Psychopharmacology Service Center (PSC)
National Institute of Drug Abuse (NIDA), lxii, 140, 142, 271, 301, 303–306
National Institutes of Health (NIH), xxxix, lvii, lxi–lxii, 58, 67, 116, 199, 210, 220, 244, 266, 267, 296–98
Nauta, Walle, 108
Negative symptoms, 29, 54–55, 73, 279
Neilsen, Johannes, 323
Neuroleptics, lxix, liii, lxiii, 7, 26, 72, 77, 274, 278, 281, 286. *See also* Antipsychotic agents; Tranquilizers, major
Neuropharmacology, x, xxxviiii, 159–62, 167–68, 181, 214
Neuroscience, xlvii, lviii, 60, 77, 89, 209, 223
Neuroses, xlm, lii, 82, 320
Neurotransmitters, ix–xi, xxxlii, xlvi, xlvii, 29, 57, 58, 178–79, 210, 218
Nickerson, Mark, 160
Nicotine, 136, 162, 163–66
Nicotinic acid, xxv, 91, 298
Nishizono, Masahisa, 254
Nobel Prize/Laureates, 8, 58–59, 200, 265, 299, 318
Noradrenaline/Norepinephrine, ix, x, xxvi–xxviii, 29–30, 180–82, 184–85, 215, 219
Nosology, lx, xxviii, liii, 88. *See also* Classification, psychiatric; Diagnosis, psychiatric

Ogle, William, 279–81
Olds, James, liv, 177–78
Opiates/opioids, 140, 186, 247–48, 305–307
   receptor, 58, 305
Osmond, Humphry Fortescue, xxxvi–xxxvii, xxxi, 70–71, 290
Ostow, Mortimer, xxx, 279
Overall, John E., 51, 54, 55
Overholser, Winfred, 198

Pahnke, Walter N., 71
Paraldehyde, ix, 241
Parke-Davis Company, 99, 161
Parkinson's disease/Parkinsonian symptoms, 49, 57, 164, 242
Pavlov, Ivan Petrovich, xxxii, 222, 317–18, 320
Paykel, Eugene, ix
Pentylenetetrazol (Cardiazol, Metrazol), xxix, 83, 317, 319
Pentobarbital, lvi, 66, 179
Perphenazine (Trilafon), xxx, 14, 282
Perris, Carlo, 21
Pert, Candace B., 305, 306
Peterson, Robert, 302
Pharmaceutical industry, ix, xi, xxxviii, xlvi, xlvii, liv, iv, 97, 109, 120, 122–24, 137–39, 141, 143. 165–66, 170, 172, 176, 181, 267
Pharmacokinetics, 15, 53, 268, 272
Pharmacology, xxxii, lvi, 15, 32, 154, 157, 159, 161, 164, 169, 170–72
Phencyclidine (PCP; Sernyl), xxx, xlix, 22, 161, 164
Phenelzine (Nardil), xxx, 10, 282
Phenobarbital, 44, 45, 148
Phenothiazines, l, liii, 12, 45, 46, 50, 109, 127, 149, 184, 278
Phenomenology, xxxvi, 28–29, 85
Phenytoin (Diphenylhydantoin, Dilantin), xxvi, xxxi, liii, 99–100
   active, 44, 300

Pichot, Pierre, 250, 255–56, 258
Pinner, Max, 231, 232, 236, 239
Placebo(s), lvii, 10, 26, 28, 42, 46, 170, 174,
    216–17, 267, 304
  active, 44, 300
  in controlled trials, xxii, lvi, 47, 169, 243,
    267
Pletscher, Alfred, xxviii
Pomara, Nunzio, 31
Porter, Kingsley, 320
Porter, William, 107
Positive reinforcement, 162, 177
Positron emission tomography (PET) scan-
    ning, 32, 165–66, 271, 309
Psychiatric hospitals, xi, xxxi, xlviii, 36, 40–41,
    59–60, 64, 66, 81–92, 87, 93, 153,
    214–17, 221, 247, 282, 290, 291,
    293, 314
Psychiatric illness, x, xi, xxv, xlv, 6, 106, 155,
    263, 274, 323
  biochemical aspects, xxxvii, lx, 239, 290
  genetic aspects, 94–95
Psychoanalysis, xxix–xxx, xxxi, xlv–xlvi, xlix,
    lvii, lx, 64–65, 92, 93, 194–95, 205,
    250, 272, 314, 324
  dispute over homosexuality, 254
  dominance, 13, 36, 38, 50, 59, 87, 206,
    2566–67
  and psychopharmacology/biological
    psychiatry, lii, lix, lxi–lxiii, 37, 99, 165,
    200, 222, 251, 275, 284
Psychopathology, xxv–xxvi, xxxi, xxxiii
Psychopharmacology Service Center (PSC),
    xxxi, xlv, lii, liv, 14, 24, 33, 50–51, 57,
    116, 200
Psychoses, xi, xxv, xlv, lii, lvi, 82, 156, 184, 319
  AIDS-related, 155
  drug-induced/experimental, xxv, 22, 24,
    298
  organic, 84, 87, 162
  treatments, xxvii, l, 51, 83, 89, 278, 317

Psychotherapy, xxvi,m xxviii, xlvi, li, lii, 11, 15,
    36, 86, 90, 100, 207, 208, 266, 267
  combined/integrated treatment, 37, 257,
    280
Psychotropic drugs, ix–xi, xxviii, xxx–xxxii,
    36–37, 49, 96, 116, 200, 206–8, 257,
    262, 263, 281, 299
Punishment effects/paradigm, 133, 182–83,
    260

Quastel, Juda Hirsch, 214
Quitkin, Frederic, 10

Rafaelsen, Ole, 52
Raffel, Sidney, 46
Rating scales, xxxi, li, 54–55, 73
Ray, Oakley, xii, 179, 180
Redlich, Fritz, lvii, 198, 206–7, 251
Reed, Walter, 227
Regional neurochemistry, lix, 218–19, 224
Reinforcement, xxxii, lv, 131, 142, 151, 152,
    177, 179–81, 184–87, 271
Reserpine, ix–x, xxvii-xxviii, xxxi–xxxii, lio,
    6–9, 11, 40, 43, 46, 55, 70, 84, 106,
    109, 111, 177, 206, 242, 279–80
Reward effects/theory, xxxii, lvii, 131, 134,
    152, 117–86
Rhône-Poulenc, xxvi, 6, 65, 83, 125–27, 131,
    154, 157, 278
Richards, Richard K., 41, 42, 123–24
Richmond, Julius, 244
Richter, Curt, 222
Richter, Derek, 223
Richter, Dietmar, 214, 218
Rinkel, Max, 277
Rioch, Daniel, 106, 201, 265, 266, 268
Risperidone (Risperdal), 7, 46, 61
Robins, Lee, 111
Roche Laboratories, xxviii, 47, 48, 50, 142,
    256
Roosevelt, Franklin Delano, 228, 232

Roth, Lloyd, 154

Roth, Martin, 250

Rothlin, Ernst, 301–2

Rothman, Theodore, xlviii, 51, 52, 286, 287

Rotrosen, John, 30

Sabin, Al, 40

St. Elizabeths Hospital (Washington, DC), lix, lxii, 78, 198, 218–221, 223, 295, 298, 302

Sakel, Manfred, lxiii, 314

Salmoiraghi, Nino, 220, 223

Salter, William, 121, 122

Sams, Josephine, 196

Sandoz, xxvi, l, lxi, 291, 301, 302

Sargant, William, 10

Sarwer-Foner, Gerald J.,xxx, lxii–lxiii, **277–88**

Saunders, Lawrence, xxviii, 7 Savage, Charles, li, 67, 70, 71, 72, 197

Schedules/scheduling, xxxli, liv–lvi, 131, 142, 148, 150–53

Schilder, Paul, 241, 314

Schizoaffective disorder, xlix, 26

Schizophrenia, ix, xxviii, xlvi, lii, lxiii, 16, 17, 57, 59, 82, 85, 87, 94–96, 100, 201, 235, 277, 299, 312, 315
    causation hypotheses, xvii, xxvi, lvii, lxii, 224, 296
    in children. See Childhood schizophrenia
    chronic, 5–6, 296
    research/studies, xlix, 22, 23, 26–30, 130, 133, 155, 183–84, 189, 279, 290–91
    treatments, xvii, xxxi, 60, 73, 129, 134, 269, 314, 318

Schmitt, Francis, 213

Schou, Mogens, 27

Schulman, Jerry, 316

Schultes, Richard Evans, 98, 291

Schuster, Robert, 130, 142

Scopolamine, xxv, 177

Secobarbital (Seconal), 238

Sedative agents/effects, xxv, xxxii, xlv, xlvi, 6, 12, 46, 127, 135, 163, 316

Seizures, 12,, 48, 240, 266, 318, 319; See also Epilepsy

Selective serotonin reuptake inhibitors (SSRI), 183, 188

Selling, Lowell, xxxvii

Sepinwall, Jerry, 142

Serotonin (5-hydroxytriptamine), ix–x, xxvii, xviii, xxxlii, 30, 49, 135, 180–83, 186, 219, 271, 298–99

Sexual behavior/research,. lxiii, 183, 221, 222, 320–21. See also Homosexuality

Shagass, Charles, 281

Shakow, David, 197–98

Shannon, James, 199, 200, 219–20

Shaw, George Bernard, 212

Shelton, Jack, 74, 301

Sherrington, Charles Scott, 214, 223

Shopsin, Baron, 26, 30

Side effects. See Adverse effects

Sidman, Murray, 106, 109

Siegel, Mary, 93

Signals (behavioral studies), xxxli, lix, 107, 108, 126; (CNS transmission), xxxiii, 186

Simon, Eric, 305, 306

Simon, Théodore, 321

Simpson, George, 50, 315

Skinner, Burrhus Frederic (B.F.), 131, 147, 150

Sleep agents/studies, xxv, lvi, 120, 126, 163, 193, 215

Smith, Colin, 70

Smith, Kline & French (SK&F), xliv–xlvi, xlvii, lv, 6, 8–9, 11–12, 45, 66, 69, 123–27, 132–42, 154, 157, 243, 316

Smythies, John, xxxvi, xxxvii, 290

Snyder, Solomon, 58, 108, 222, 300–1, 305, 306

Sokoloff, Louis, xvii, 197

Spectrophotofluorometry, ix–x, xlvii, 296

Squibb, xlviii, 5, 242

Stanley, Michael, 31
Stanton, Alfred, 201
Steck, Hans, xxvii
Stein, Larry, xxxiii, xlvi, lvii–lviii, 109, **177–88**
    as interviewer, 121–43
Stephens, Janice, 317
Stoll, Arthur, 291
Strassman, Rick, 74, 302
Stratton, Henry, 323–24
Stress, xxvi, 64, 86
Striker, Edward, 209
Substance P, ix, 65
Succinic acid, 21, 22, 32
Succinylcholine, 5, 219
Suicide, lxiii, 33, 238–39
Sullivan, Harry Stack, 202
Supeer, Edwards, 192
Symptoms, psychiatric, xxv, xxxiii, xlv, liii, lxiii,
        9, 28, 75, 26, 155, 188, 235, 279–80,
        285, 287
    negative. See Negative symptoms
    psychotic/schizophrenia, 83, 84, 183,
        206
    target, 37, 84, 280, 283, 285
Szára, Stephen, xxx, lviii, lxi–lxii, 220,
        289–309
Szent-Györgyi, Albert, 289

Tamminga, Carol, 73, 76
Tardive dyskinesia, 46, 50, 71
Tarjan, George, 253
Tashkin, Donald, 304
Terenius, Lars, 306
Terman, Lewis, 322
Tetrahydroaminoacridane (THA), xxxiii, 21–22,
        24–25, 28
Tetrahydrocannabinol (THC), 163, 303–4
Thioridazine (Mellaril), 49, 57, 269, 270
Thompson, George N., 323, 324
Thompson, Travis, 153
Tone, Andrea, as interviewer, 35–38

Toxicology, xxxi, liv, 14, 110, 118–20, 170
Tricyclic antidepressants, xlvii, 10, 23, 50
Tranquilizers, xlvi, 163
    major, 106, 107, 134, 171, 269.
        See also Antipsychotic agents;
        Neuroleptics
    minor, 107, 134, 163. See also Anxiolytics
Tranylcypromine, 9, 10
Trautner, Edward, xxxiii, xlix, 19–20
Tricyclic antidepressants, xlviii, 1, 10–11, 23
Trifluoperazine (Stelazine), xxx, xxxi, 11, 12,
        45, 85, 96, 131, 292
Tuberculosis, xxxviii, 9, 46, 71, 92, 169, 236
Tuerk, Isador, 68
Tuke family, 282
Turner, William J., xxxi, liii, **91–101**

Ullett, George, 24
Unger, Sanford M., 71
US Public Health Service (USPHS), xl, lxiii, 9,
        169, 266
Unna, Klaus, 157, 160, 161, 162

Vane, John, 148–49
Vartanian, Felix, 254
Verhav, Thomas, 109
Veterans Administration (VA) hospital system,
        li, lii, lvi, 5, 12, 40, 42, 56, 59–60, 64,
        91–92, 179, 181
    cooperative studies program, li, 49–51, 53
Voelkel, Arno, xlvi

Waelsch, Heinrich, 218, 223
Wagner-Jauregg, Julius, 315
Walker, James, 315
Walker, Stuart, 174
Wallace Laboratories, xxxvii, 123
Walter Reed Army Hospital/Research
        Institute, lvii, liv, lvii, 106, 105, 108–9,
        113, 117, 179, 201, 166, 167
Watson, Samuel, 162

Weil-Malherbe, Hans, 220, 298, 299

Weissman, Myrna M., 58

West, Louis Jolyon (Jolly), 253

Wheatley, David, 14

Whipple, George Hoyt, 231

Whitehorn, John C., 221, 265

Wiesel, Torsten, 148–49

Wikler, Abraham, x, 131, 247, 248

Wilk, Sherwin, 30

Will, Otto, 201

Wilson, Charles, 212

Winkelman, William, 8, 86, 278

Winter, Charles, 212

Withdrawal reactions/symptoms, xxxi, 47, 48, 52, 247

Witt, Peter, 147

Wittenborn, Richard, 52

Wong, David, 298–99

World Health Organization (WHO), 197, 252, 254, 256, 259, 263

Wortis, Helen, 245

Wortis, Joseph, xxix, lxiii–lxiv, **311–26**

Wortis, Samuel B., 25, 240

Wright, Almroth, 212

Wright, David Graham, 277

Wyeth Laboratories, lvii, 12, 181–82

Wynn, Victor, 20

Wynne, Lyman C., 198

Yensen, Richard, 74

Yohimbine, 22–23

Yolles, Stanley, 95

Yuwiler, Arthur, xlix

Zilboorg, Gregory, lxii, 277

Zimelidine, 188

www.ingramcontent.com/pod-product-compliance
Lightning Source LLC
Chambersburg PA
CBHW081103170526
45165CB00008B/2312